Geriatrics

Rehabilitation Medicine Quick Reference

Ralph M. Buschbacher, MD
Series Editor

Professor, Department of Physical Medicine and Rehabilitation
Indiana University School of Medicine
Indianapolis, Indiana

■ Spine
Andre N. Panagos

■ Spinal Cord Injury
Thomas N. Bryce

■ Traumatic Brain Injury
David X. Cifu and Deborah Caruso

■ Pediatrics
Maureen R. Nelson

■ Musculoskeletal, Sports, and Occupational Medicine
William Micheo

■ Geriatrics
Kevin M. Means and Patrick M. Kortebein

Forthcoming Volumes in the Series

Neuromuscular/EMG

Prosthetics

Stroke

Geriatrics

Rehabilitation Medicine Quick Reference

Kevin M. Means MD

Professor and Chair
Department of Physical Medicine and Rehabilitation
University of Arkansas for Medical Sciences
Little Rock, Arkansas

Patrick M. Kortebein MD

Assistant Professor
Department of Physical Medicine and Rehabilitation
University of Arkansas for Medical Sciences
Little Rock, Arkansas

demosMEDICAL
New York

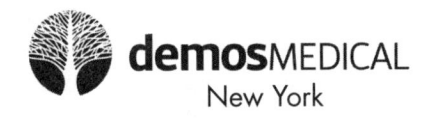

Visit our website at www.demosmedpub.com

ISBN: 9781936287093
e-book ISBN: 9781617050305

Acquisitions Editor: Beth Barry
Compositor: Newgen Imaging

© 2013 Demos Medical Publishing, LLC. All rights reserved. This book is protected by copyright. No part of it may be reproduced, stored in a retrieval system, or transmitted in any form or by any means, electronic, mechanical, photocopying, recording, or otherwise, without the prior written permission of the publisher.

Medicine is an ever-changing science. Research and clinical experience are continually expanding our knowledge, in particular our understanding of proper treatment and drug therapy. The authors, editors, and publisher have made every effort to ensure that all information in this book is in accordance with the state of knowledge at the time of production of the book. Nevertheless, the authors, editors, and publisher are not responsible for errors or omissions or for any consequences from application of the information in this book and make no warranty, express or implied, with respect to the contents of the publication. Every reader should examine carefully the package inserts accompanying each drug and should carefully check whether the dosage schedules mentioned therein or the contraindications stated by the manufacturer differ from the statements made in this book. Such examination is particularly important with drugs that are either rarely used or have been newly released on the market.

Library of Congress Cataloging-in-Publication Data

Geriatrics / [edited by] Kevin M. Means, Patrick M. Kortebein.
　　p. ; cm.—(Rehabilitation medicine quick reference)
Includes bibliographical references and index.
ISBN 978-1-936287-09-3—ISBN 978-1-61705-030-5 (e-book ISBN)
I. Means, Kevin M. II. Kortebein, Patrick M. III. Series: Rehabilitation medicine quick reference.
[DNLM: 1. Geriatrics—Handbooks. 2. Aging—physiology—Handbooks. WT 39]

618.97—dc23

2012016482

Special discounts on bulk quantities of Demos Medical Publishing books are available to corporations, professional associations, pharmaceutical companies, health care organizations, and other qualifying groups. For details, please contact:
Special Sales Department
Demos Medical Publishing, LLC
11 West 42nd Street, 15th Floor
New York, NY 10036
Phone: 800-532-8663 or 212-683-0072
Fax: 212-941-7842
E-mail: rsantana@demosmedpub.com

Printed in the United States of America by Bang.
12 13 14 15 / 5 4 3 2 1

Contents

Series Foreword ix
Preface xi
Acknowledgments. xi
Contributors xiii

I Assessment and Aging

1. Aging: Theories and Epidemiology 2
2. Age-Related Changes: Bone 4
3. Age-Related Changes: Cardiovascular 6
4. Age-Related Changes: Central Nervous System and Cognitive 8
5. Age-Related Changes: Gastrointestinal. 10
6. Age-Related Changes: Hearing and Vestibular 12
7. Age-Related Changes: Muscular. 14
8. Age-Related Changes: Posture and Balance .15
9. Age-Related Changes: Pulmonary. 17
10. Age-Related Changes: Renal. 19
11. Age-Related Changes: Sensory. 21
12. Age-Related Changes: Skin. 23
13. Age-Related Changes: Visual 25
14. Decision Making. 26
15. History 28
16. Examination: Cognitive 30
17. Examination: Musculoskeletal 33
18. Examination: Neurologic 35
19. Electrodiagnosis: Nerve Conduction Studies 38
20. Electrodiagnosis: The Needle Exam—Electromyography 40
21. Evaluation of Balance and Mobility 42
22. Evaluation of Depression 52
23. Evaluation of Function 55
24. Evaluation of Osteoporosis: Detection of Significant Bone Loss 56

II Organ System Diseases and Disorders

25. Anemia 58
26. Blood Disorders. 60
27. Cancer 63

28. Cardiovascular: Amputation....66
29. Cardiovascular: Peripheral Arterial Disease....69
30. Cardiovascular: Syncope and Orthostatic Hypotension....72
31. Cardiovascular: Thromboembolic Disease....74
32. Depression....76
33. Diabetes Mellitus....80
34. Diabetes: The Diabetic Foot....84
35. Functional Decline: Deconditioning....87
36. Functional Decline: Frailty....89
37. Functional Decline: Sarcopenia....91
38. Gastrointestinal: Constipation....93
39. Gastrointestinal: Fecal Incontinence....96
40. Musculoskeletal: Arthritis of the Ankle and Hind Foot....101
41. Musculoskeletal: Arthritis of the Thumb, Fingers, and Wrist....104
42. Musculoskeletal: Dupuytren's Contractures and Trigger Finger....106
43. Musculoskeletal: Hip Fracture....108
44. Musculoskeletal: Joint Replacement....111
45. Musculoskeletal: Low Back Pain....114
46. Musculoskeletal: Neck Pain....117
47. Musculoskeletal: Osteoarthritis....120
48. Musculoskeletal: Osteoporosis and Vertebral Fractures....124
49. Musculoskeletal: Posterior Tibial Tendon Dysfunction....127
50. Musculoskeletal: Shoulder....129
51. Musculoskeletal: Spinal Stenosis....132
52. Neurologic: Alzheimer's Disease and Other Neurodegenerative Disorders....135
53. Neurologic: Amyotrophic Lateral Sclerosis and Other Neuromuscular Disorders....138
54. Neurologic: Balance Disorders....141
55. Neurologic: Carpal Tunnel Syndrome....143
56. Neurologic: Charcot Foot....145
57. Neurologic: Delirium....148
58. Neurologic: Dizziness and Vertigo....151
59. Neurologic: Dysphagia....157
60. Neurologic: Falls....159
61. Neurologic: Gait Disorders....162
62. Neurologic: Homonymous Hemianopsia....165
63. Neurologic: Parkinson's Disease....167
64. Neurologic: Parkinson's Disease—Postural Instability, Freezing, and Falls....171

65. Neurologic: Spinal Cord Injury 173
66. Neurologic: Stroke 176
67. Neurologic: Traumatic Brain Injury 179
68. Rheumatologic: Fibromyalgia 182
69. Rheumatologic: Giant Cell Arteritis 185
70. Rheumatologic: Polymyalgia Rheumatica 187
71. Skin: Pressure Sores 189
72. Skin: The Problem Wound 192
73. Special Senses: Hearing 196
74. Special Senses: Vision—Cataracts 199
75. Special Senses: Vision—General 201
76. Special Senses: Vision—Glaucoma 204
77. Special Senses: Vision—Macular Degeneration 206
78. Urinary Incontinence 208

III Special Topics

79. Aging With a Developmental Disability 212
80. Aging With a Spinal Cord Injury 215
81. Alternative Medicine 218
82. Driving Evaluation 221
83. Ethics 224
84. Exercise 226
85. Home and Environmental Modifications 228
86. Medicolegal Concerns 231
87. Pain Management 233
88. Pharmacology: General 235
89. Pharmacology: Management of Polypharmacy 238
90. Prescription Writing: Drugs and Therapy 241
91. Rehabilitation Settings: Evaluation for Postacute Rehabilitation 243
92. Rehabilitation Settings: Home Health Care 245
93. Rehabilitation Settings: Inpatient Rehabilitation, Acute 248
94. Rehabilitation Settings: Long-Term Acute Care
    Hospital and Adult Day Care 251
95. Rehabilitation Settings: Subacute Rehabilitation 253
96. Rehabilitation Settings: Palliative Care 255
97. End-of-Life Care 257

Index 259

Series Foreword

The Rehabilitation Medicine Quick Reference (RMQR) series is dedicated to the busy clinician. While we all strive to keep up with the latest medical knowledge, there are many times when things come up in our daily practices that we need to look up. Even more importantly…look up quickly.

Those aren't the times to do a complete literature search, or to read a detailed chapter, or review an article. We just need to get a quick grasp of a topic that we may not see routinely or just to refresh our memory. Sometimes a subject comes up that is outside our usual scope of practice, but that may still impact our care. It is for such moments that this series has been created.

Whether you need to quickly look up what a Tarlov cyst is, or you need to read about a neurorehabilitation complication or treatment, RMQR has you covered.

RMQR is designed to include the most common problems found in a busy practice and also a lot of the less common ones as well.

I was extremely lucky to have been able to assemble an absolutely fantastic group of editors. They in turn have harnessed an excellent set of authors. So what we have in this series is, I hope and believe, a tremendous reference set to be used often in daily clinical practice. As series editor, I have of course been privy to these books before actual publication. I can tell you that I have already started to rely on them in my clinic—often. They have helped me become more efficient in practice.

Each chapter is organized into succinct facts, presented in a bullet point style. The chapters are set up in the same way throughout all of the volumes in the series, so once you get used to the format, it is incredibly easy to look things up.

And while the focus of the RMQR series is, of course, rehabilitation medicine, the clinical applications are much broader.

I hope that each reader grows to appreciate the RMQR series as much as I have. I congratulate a fine group of editors and authors on creating readable and useful texts.

Ralph M. Buschbacher, MD

Preface

Persons at or over 85 years of age represent the fastest growing segment of U.S. society. As our population ages and becomes increasingly susceptible to a myriad of acute and chronic disabling and potentially disabling conditions, there will be an increased opportunity to seek care from physiatrists and other rehabilitation professionals. Accordingly, in the near future, few of us in the rehabilitation field will be able to ignore meeting the increasing health care needs of the aging population.

The goal of this book is threefold: to provide sound, practical, useful, and readily available information about the "normal aging" process as manifested in several body systems of interest to rehabilitation professionals and assessment methods to measure these manifestations; to provide essential information about common aging-associated diseases and disorders affecting relevant organ systems, including central and peripheral neurologic systems, the musculoskeletal and rheumatologic systems, among others; and finally, to provide information about a broad range of special geriatric rehabilitation topics, from aging with a disability, exercise and pain management in the elderly person to polypharmacy, and rehabilitation in several different health care settings.

Armed with this information, we anticipate that the physician and other providers will be better able to care for and provide education and prevention for older patients to keep them healthier, happier, and more functionally independent.

Kevin M. Means, MD
Patrick M. Kortebein, MD

Acknowledgments

This book was a true collaboration. We appreciate Dr. Ralph Buschbacher, the editor of this series, for his assistance with reviewing and editing many of the chapters. We wish to sincerely thank all of the many contributing authors. They represent our colleagues in the Department of Physical Medicine and Rehabilitation as well as other Departments within the University of Arkansas for Medical Sciences College of Medicine, and other rehabilitation, aging, and other specialists across the U.S. We would also like to thank our respective wives, Barbara Means and Betsy Kortebein, and families for their support during the many hours of planning and writing of this book. We owe special thanks to Jennifer Crow for her tireless and excellent assistance coordinating and communicating with the authors.

Contributors

Carlo E. Adams, MD
Staff Physician
Physical Medicine & Rehabilitation Service
Central Arkansas Veterans Healthcare System
North Little Rock, Arkansas

Monica Agarwal, MD
Assistant Professor of Medicine
Division of Endocrinology, Department of Internal Medicine
University of Arkansas for Medical Sciences
Staff Physician, Central Arkansas Veterans Healthcare System
Little Rock, Arkansas

Audra Arant, APN
Department of Dermatology
University of Arkansas for Medical Sciences
Little Rock, Arkansas

Cheryl A. Armstrong, MD
Professor and Chair
Department of Dermatology, College of Medicine
University of Arkansas for Medical Sciences
Dermatology Section Chief
Central Arkansas Veterans Healthcare System
Little Rock, Arkansas

Konstantinos Arnaoutakis, MD
Assistant Professor of Medicine – Division of Hematology/Oncology
Associate Program Director, Hematology/Oncology Fellowship
Winthrop P. Rockefeller Cancer Institute
University of Arkansas for Medical Sciences
Little Rock, Arkansas

Samuel R. Atcherson, PhD
Assistant Professor, Audiology
Director, Auditory Electrophysiology and (Re)habilitation Laboratory
Department of Audiology and Speech Pathology
University of Arkansas at Little Rock
University of Arkansas for Medical Sciences
Little Rock, Arkansas

Ozun Bayindir, MD
Department of Physical Medicine and Rehabilitation
Indiana University School of Medicine
Indianapolis, Indiana

Nabil K. Bissada, MD
Professor
Oklahoma City VA Medical Center
Oklahoma City, Oklahoma

Martin B. Brodsky, PhD
Assistant Professor
Department of Physical Medicine & Rehabilitation
Johns Hopkins University
Baltimore, Maryland

Derek S. Buck, MD, DC
Resident Physician
Department of Physical Medicine and Rehabilitation
University of Arkansas for Medical Sciences
Little Rock, Arkansas

Lois Buschbacher, MD
Department of Physical Medicine and Rehabilitation
Indiana University School of Medicine
Indianapolis, Indiana

Ralph M. Buschbacher, MD
Professor
Department of Physical Medicine and Rehabilitation
Indiana University School of Medicine
Indianapolis, Indiana

Tanya Cabrita, MD
Resident Physician
Department of Rehabilitation Medicine
Emory University School of Medicine
Atlanta, Georgia

Joseph Canvin, MD
Memorial Hospital of Martinsville & Henry County
Martinsville, Virginia

Joseph G. Chacko, MD
Associate Professor of Ophthalmology and Neurology
Director of Neuro-Ophthalmology
Jones Eye Institute, UAMS
Little Rock, Arkansas

Gary P. Chimes, MD, PhD
Sports & Spine Rehabilitation
Fellowship Director, Musculoskeletal Sports & Spine Fellowship
PM&R Director, UPMC Monroeville
Assistant Professor
Department of Physical Medicine and Rehabilitation
University of Pittsburgh
Monroeville, Pennsylvania

Kimberly A. Curseen, MD
Assistant Professor of Geriatric Medicine
Director of Geriatric Palliative Care Program Clinical Services
University of Arkansas for Medicine Sciences
Baptist Hospice Medical Director; Baptist Healthcare System
Department of Geriatrics
University of Arkansas for Medical Sciences
Little Rock, Arkansas

Romona LeDay Davis, MD
Assistant Professor of Ophthalmology
Jones Eye Institute
University of Arkansas for Medical Sciences
Little Rock, Arkansas

Jamil R. Dibu, MD
Neurology Resident
University of Arkansas for Medical Sciences
Little Rock, Arkansas

Willliam L. Doss, MD, MBA
Assistant Professor
Department of Physical Medicine and Rehabilitation
University of Arkansas for Medical Sciences
Little Rock, Arkansas

Gail L. Gamble, MD
Physical Rehabilitation Medicine
Northwestern Memorial Hospital
Chicago, Illinois

Kimberly K. Garner, MD, JD, MPH, FAAFP
Geriatrician/Researcher, Geriatric Research Education and Clinical Center
Department of Veteran Affairs
Assistant Professor, Department of Geriatrics
University of Arkansas for Medical Sciences
Little Rock, Arkansas

Andrew Geller, MD
Resident Physician
Department of Rehabilitation Medicine
Emory University School of Medicine
Atlanta, Georgia

Hugh H. Gregory, MD, JD
Medical Director, Inpatient Rehabilitation
Wellspan Health
York, Pennsylvania

Rani Lynn Haley, MD
Assistant Professor
Department of Physical Medicine and Rehabilitation
University of Arkansas for Medical Sciences
Little Rock, Arkansas

Stephanie Hansen, DO
Nevada Hospitalist Group
Las Vegas, Nevada

Sarah E. Harrington, MD
Assistant Professor of Medicine
UAMS Department of Internal Medicine
Division of Hematology/Oncology
Department of Geriatrics
Little Rock, Arkansas

Jamie Harrison, MD
Resident Physician
Department of Physical Medicine and Rehabilitation
University of Arkansas for Medical Sciences
Little Rock, Arkansas

Danielle L. Hinton, MD
Medical Director
Baptist Skilled Rehabilitation Unit Germantown
Baptist Memorial Medical Group – Physiatry
Germantown, Tennessee

Shahla M. Hosseini, MD, PhD
Resident Physician
Department of Physical Medicine and Rehabilitation
University of Pittsburgh Medical Center
Pittsburgh, Pennsylvania

Elizabeth Huntoon, MD
Department of Physical Medicine and Rehabilitation
Mayo Clinic
Rochester, Minnesota

Lisa C. Hutchison, PharmD, MPH, BCPS
Professor
College of Pharmacy
Department of Pharmacy Practice
University of Arkansas for Medical Sciences
Little Rock, Arkansas

Vivek S. Jagadale, MD
Assistant Professor Orthopaedics
CAIMS Medical College
Satara, Maharashtra

Larry G. Johnson, MD
Professor of Internal Medicine
Director, Division of Pulmonary and Critical Care Medicine
University of Arkansas for Medical Sciences
Little Rock, Arkansas

Vitaly Kantorovich, MD
Assistant Professor of Medicine
Division of Endocrinology, Department of Medicine
University of Arkansas for Medical Sciences
Medical Director, UAMS Weight Control Program
Staff Physician, Central Arkansas Veterans Healthcare System
Little Rock, Arkansas

Florian S. Keplinger, MD
Baptist Health Rehabilitation Institute
Little Rock, Arkansas

Salah G. Keyrouz, MD
Assistant Professor, Neurology and Neurosurgery
Medical Director, Neurology and Neurosurgery Intensive Care Unit
Washington University School of Medicine
St. Louis, Missouri

Thomas S. Kiser, MD
Associate Professor
Department of Physical Medicine & Rehabilitation
Medical Director of the Arkansas Spinal Cord Commission
University of Arkansas for Medical Sciences
Little Rock, Arkansas

Ravinder R. Kurella, MD
Oklahoma Center for Orthopaedic & Multi-Specialty Surgeries
Oklahoma City, Oklahoma

Ted A. Lennard, MD
Springfield Neurological & Spine Institute
Cox Health Care Systems
Springfield, Missouri
Department of Physical Medicine and Rehabilitation
University of Arkansas for Medical Sciences
Little Rock, Arkansas

LaTanya Lofton, MD
Assistant Professor
Carolinas Rehabilitation
Director of Spinal Cord Injury Rehabilitation
Charlotte, North Carolina

Ayman Mahdy, MD
Assistant Professor of Urology
Director of Voiding Dysfunction and Female Urology
University of Cincinnati College of Medicine
Cincinnati, Ohio

Issam Makhoul, MD
Departments of Hematology & Medical Oncology and Internal Medicine
Winthrop P. Rockefeller Cancer Institute
University of Arkansas for Medical Sciences
Little Rock, Arkansas

A. Bilal Malik, MD
Assistant Professor of Medicine
Program Director, Nephrology Fellowship Program
Division of Nephrology
University of Arkansas for Medical Sciences &
The Central Arkansas Veterans' Healthcare System
Little Rock, Arkansas

Sara Rebecca Martin, MD
Fellow, Pulmonary Disease and Critical Care Medicine
University of Arkansas for Medical Sciences
Little Rock, Arkansas
Private Practice
Mountain Home, Arkansas

Terry H. McCoy, AuD
Advanced Practice Audiologist
Central Arkansas Veterans Healthcare System
Adjunct Faculty, Department of Audiology and Speech Pathology
University of Arkansas at Little Rock
University of Arkansas for Medical Sciences
Little Rock, Arkansas

Robert A. Ortmann, MD
Senior Medical Advisor
Diagnostic and Experimental Medicine
Lilly Research Laboratories
Indianapolis, Indiana

Jeffrey B. Palmer, MD
Lawrence Cardinal Shehan Professor and Director
Department of Physical Medicine and Rehabilitation
Professor of Otolaryngology/Head and Neck Surgery and Functional Anatomy/Evolution
Johns Hopkins University School of Medicine
Physiatrist-in-Chief
The Johns Hopkins Hospital
Chairman, Department of Physical Medicine and Rehabilitation
Good Samaritan Hospital of Maryland
Baltimore, Maryland

Christopher Parks, MD
Resident Physician
Department of Orthopaedic Surgery
University of Arkansas for Medical Sciences
Little Rock, Arkansas

K. Rao Poduri, MD
Chair and Associate Professor
Department of Physical Medicine and Rehabilitation
University of Rochester Medical Center
Rochester, New York

Danielle K. Powell, MD
Assistant Professor
Department of Physical Medicine and Rehabilitation
University of Alabama at Birmingham
Birmingham, Alabama

Nathan Prahlow, MD
Department of Physical Medicine and Rehabilitation
Indiana University School of Medicine
Indianapolis, Indiana

Deepthi S. Saxena, MD
Medical Director, Acute Inpatient Rehabilitation
Desert Springs Hospital Medical Center
Las Vegas, Nevada
Director of Affiliated Medical Rehabilitation
Avant-Garde Medicine
Las Vegas & Henderson, Nevada

Aparna Wagle Shukla, MD
Assistant Professor
Center for Movement Disorders and Neurorestoration
University of Florida
Gainesville, Florida

Debra L. Simmons, MD, MS, FACE, FACP
Professor of Medicine
Division of Endocrinology, Department of Medicine
Director, UAMS Arkansas Diabetes Program
University of Arkansas for Medical Sciences
Staff Physician, Central Arkansas Veterans Healthcare System
Chief, CAVHS DM/ENDO Firm
Little Rock, Arkansas

Mehrsheed Sinaki, MD, MS
Professor of Physical Medicine and Rehabilitation
Mayo Clinic College of Medicine
Rochester, Minnesota

Melissa Sinkiewicz, DO
Resident Physician
Department of Physical Medicine and Rehabilitation
Emory University School of Medicine
Atlanta, Georgia

Gayle R. Spill, MD
Associate Professor
Department of Physical Medicine and Rehabilitation
Feinberg School of Medicine of Northwestern University
Cancer Rehabilitation Program
Rehabilitation Institute of Chicago
Chicago, Illinois

Vikki Stefans, MD
Associate Professor
University of Arkansas for Medical Sciences College of Medicine
Departments of Pediatrics and PM&R
Arkansas Children's Hospital
Little Rock, Arkansas

Dale C. Strasser, MD
Associate Professor
Department of Rehabilitation Medicine
Emory University School of Medicine
Atlanta, Georgia

Jonathan M. Stuart, DO
Resident Physician
Department of Physical Medicine and Rehabilitation
University of Arkansas for Medical Sciences
Little Rock, Arkansas

Jonathan Swenson, MD
Resident Physician
Department of Physical Medicine and Rehabilitation
University of Arkansas for Medical Sciences
Little Rock, Arkansas

Reginald D. Talley, MD
Resident Physician
Department of Physical Medicine and Rehabilitation
University of Arkansas for Medical Sciences
Little Rock, Arkansas

Jordan Lee Tate, MD, MPH
Resident Physician
Department of Rehabilitation Medicine
Emory University School of Medicine
Atlanta, Georgia

Andre Taylor, MD, MBA
President
Dependable Home Care, Inc.
Brooklyn, New York

Junell Taylor, RN, MA
Nursing Administrator/Director
Dependable Home Care, Inc.
Brooklyn, New York

Ruth L. Thomas, MD
Professor, Department of Orthopaedics
University of Arkansas for Medical Sciences
Little Rock, Arkansas

Heikki Uustal, MD
Medical Director, Prosthetic/Orthotic Team
Department of Rehabilitation Medicine
JFK-Johnson Rehabilitation Institute
Edison, New Jersey

Sami Uwaydat, MD
Assistant Professor
Jones Eye Institute
Little Rock, Arkansas

Jennifer May M. Villacorta, MD, PTRP
Resident Physician
Department of Physical Medicine and Rehabilitation
University of Arkansas for Medical Sciences
Little Rock, Arkansas

Brad P. Wilson, DO
Resident Physician
Department of Physical Medicine and Rehabilitation
University of Arkansas for Medical Sciences
Little Rock, Arkansas

Theresa O. Wyrick, MD
Assistant Professor
Section Chief, Hand and Upper Extremity Surgery
Department of Orthopaedics Surgery
University of Arkansas for Medical Sciences
Arkansas Children's Hospital
Little Rock, Arkansas

Shadi R. Yaghi, MD
Resident Physician
Department of Neurology
University of Arkansas for Medical Sciences
Little Rock, Arkansas

Tamara Zagustin, MD
Pediatric Physiatrist at Children's Healthcare of Atlanta
Assistant Professor
Department of Rehabilitation Medicine
Emory University School of Medicine
Children's Rehabilitation Associates
Atlanta, Georgia

Richard D. Zorowitz, MD
Associate Professor
Department of Physical Medicine and Rehabilitation
The Johns Hopkins University School of Medicine
Chairman
Department of Physical Medicine and Rehabilitation
Johns Hopkins Bayview Medical Center
Baltimore, Maryland

Geriatrics

I

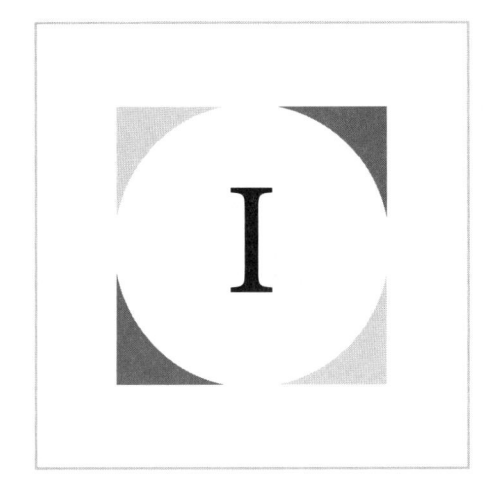

Assessment and Aging

Aging: Theories and Epidemiology

Deepthi S. Saxena MD

Description
- Aging involves an inevitable loss of homeostasis or breakdown of maintenance in molecular structures and pathways, causing a decline and deterioration of functional reserves at the cellular, tissue, and organ levels.
- Molecular and cellular changes with aging can occur at two levels:
  1. Specific cells and tissue in organs.
  2. Multiple organs, which affect the functional capacity.
- Aging itself is not synonymous with pathology. However, it paves the way for disease, without leading to overt disease in the absence of pathogenic stimuli.
- The prevalence of many diseases increases with aging, but how these diseases are related to the primary aging processes remains to be defined.
- Since aging is universal, an understanding of its epidemiology and the theories of aging helps to elucidate factors that contribute to geriatric syndromes.

Epidemiology
- Currently, 12% of the U.S. population, that is 35 million people, are 65 years and older.
- It is estimated that by 2030, this population will double to 70 million.
- Life expectancy has increased to 75 and 80 years in men and women, respectively, from 48 and 51 years in 1900.
- People above 75 years in age comprise the majority of users of health services.

Theories of Aging
- Evolutionary: why we age, and
- Physiologic: how we age.

Evolutionary

Mutation accumulation theory
- Proposes that aging is a nonadaptive trait caused by late—acting deleterious gene mutations.

Antagonistic pleiotropic theory
- Pleiotropy is the process by which a single gene produces two or more apparently unrelated effects.
- This theory states that aging is an adaptive trade-off by early—acting genes, choosing between reproductive capacity and longevity.

Disposable soma theory
- Suggests that of the four functions of growth, reproduction, maintenance, and repair, the body compromises on allocating energy to the repair function as a trade off to the others, allowing cumulative damage to the soma cells, leading to aging.

Physiologic
- The normal cellular response to stressors comprises the same three main defenses implicated in aging:
  - Apoptosis
  - Senescence
  - Repair

Apoptosis
- This is the orderly process of cellular self-destruction, which is as important to survival as cell division; as it helps by eliminating damaged cells.
- Too much apoptosis causes tissue degeneration, whereas, too little allows dysfunctional cells to accumulate.
- Apoptosis correlates inversely with aging.

Immune theory and senescence
- Cellular senescence is a physiologic suppressive response to potential cancer and oxidative stress, and to DNA damage.
- Senescence is the process by which high numbers of cell divisions (40–60) cause gradual shortening of the telomere region of chromosomes. When a critically short length is reached, DNA can no longer be replicated, leading to an arrest of cell proliferation.
- The immune theory supposes that during aging, immune cells undergo senescence and enter into a nonreplicating state. In this state, their genetic program changes to produce proinflammatory cytokines, such as interleukin (IL)-6.
- The aging immune system is characterized by a low-grade, chronic, systemic inflammatory state causing an increase in morbidity and mortality.

Epigenetic theory
- The individual's phenotype results from the interaction of its genotype with the environment.
- Epigenetic modifications, which can be heritable, are those resulting from external rather than genetic influences.
- The epigenetic theory supposes that environmental toxins change gene expression by processes such as DNA methylation to switch cells into a senescent phenotype, causing aging.

Mitochondrial free radical theory and repair
- According to this hypothesis, free radicals produced as by-products of normal metabolism cause oxidative damage in proteins, lipids, and DNA, resulting in mutations that alter functions such as adenosine triphosphate (ATP) production.
- There is dysregulation of autophagy, causing enzymes to be driven away from their normal substrates, and therefore, not allowing repair.

Protein modification theory
- Aging is caused by alteration in protein structure, which modifies chemical reactions and cellular transport.

Protein error theory
- Molecules with damaged RNA and proteins spread, causing biologic mistakes, leading to aging.

Target theory of genetic damage
- Hypothesizes that genes are susceptible to inactivation from radiation and other damages, causing aging.

Endocrine theory
- Speculates that multiple hormonal deficiencies alter homeostasis, causing aging.

Rate of living theory
- Speculates that the faster the metabolism, the faster the aging, as organisms possess a finite amount of "vital substance" to survive.

Stem cell/progenitor cell theory
- Suggests that a shift in the commitment of bone marrow stem cells, away from bone and muscle cell pathways and toward the adipocytic cell line, causes aging.

Biology of Aging and Rehabilitation
- Aging occurs across multiple systems and contributes to geriatric syndromes. In the context of these theories, it can be supposed that dysregulation of apoptosis contributes to sarcopenia and frailty, and that the inflammatory state seen in frailty could be caused by senescence.
- With an understanding of these theories, geriatric rehabilitation supports adding life to years by promoting disability-free years.

Suggested Readings
Fedarko NS. The biology of aging and frailty. *Clin Geriatr Med*. 2011;27:27–37.

Holliday R. *Aging: The Paradox of Life*. Dordrecht: Springer; 2007.

Yao X, Li H, Leng SX. Inflammation and immune system alterations in frailty. *Clin Geriatr Med*. 2011;27(1):79–87.

Age-Related Changes: Bone

Vikki Stefans MD

Description
Bone changes with aging can have a profound effect on quality of life. Reduced strength of the bones is due in part to physiologic changes but is also influenced by activity levels.

Epidemiology
- The incidence of fractures from low-impact trauma and spinal deformities related to bony insufficiency increases with age.
- These problems are more pronounced in postmenopausal females, but can also be noted in males.
- About 10 million Americans have osteoporosis; an additional 34 million have osteopenia.
- About half of all postmenopausal women will experience an insufficiency fracture during their lifetime; about a quarter of these are vertebral, and about 15% involve the femoral neck.
- There is a 15% to 25% decrease in expected survival during the year following a hip fracture. Half of these fractures lead to long-term use of an assistive device for walking, and about one fourth lead to long-term care placement.

Growth and Development
- Protein matrix is normally added to the skeleton throughout the years of growth.
  - Peak rates of bone accrual occur during adolescent growth spurts.
  - Total bone mineral content and density peak during young adulthood, around age 30.
  - After this, there is a slight and slow decline, until menopause for females and until about age 60 for males; after that bone loss substantially accelerates.
  - Insufficiency ("pathologic") fractures do not occur earlier in life in the absence of pathology that has reduced bone density or bone quality.
  - Pediatric-onset physically disabling conditions, limited weight-bearing activity, serious nutritional deficiencies, eating disorders, and chronic inflammatory diseases (e.g., rheumatologic conditions and inflammatory bowel disease) can cause early-onset bone loss and increase the risk of severe bone insufficiency and fractures in later life.

Normal Bone
- Details of bone cell functions and biochemical signaling are still being elucidated.
- The major mature cell types in bone are the osteocytes and osteoclasts.
- Osteocytes start as preosteoblasts and progress through osteoblast and preosteocyte stages, where they begin to mineralize their surrounding collagen matrix (osteoid). The mature osteocyte lives in a small lacuna with a little bone fluid immediately surrounding it; dendrites extend out into the mineralized tissue, which completely surrounds the osteoclast.
- There is a complex network of tiny (about 7 nm) canaliculi, which communicate with the bone's vascular supply and permit the exchange of small molecules, including nutrients, vitamins, hormones, and other intercell signaling substances. Their chief function may be to mediate responses to demands for mineral exchange and to create localized increases in structural stability in response to mechanical stresses.
- Osteoclasts seem to undo the work of the osteocytes, but are critical to allow the bone to serve as the reservoir for bodily calcium and phosphate; they allow the renewal and remodeling of bone to correspond to the stresses to which it is subjected during daily activities.
- Osteocytes can use osteoclast-like mechanisms to release calcium from the perilacunar areas when needed for physiologic processes, for example, lactation.

Abnormal Bone
- Most causes of low bone density are polygenic or multifactorial, but some severe cases may be due to specific polymorphisms in vitamin D and estrogen receptors, or milder abnormalities in the *COL1a* and *COL1b* genes that are associated with osteogenesis imperfecta.
- Bone cell autophagy may occur with stress or undernutrition; this prevents apoptosis (programmed cell death) by removing damaged organelles that might otherwise trigger the apoptosis. Although autophagy limits mineralization, some compounds that inhibit autophagy promote apoptosis, and therefore may not be therapeutic.

- Glucocorticoids cause autophagy at low doses (1.4 mg/kg/day) and apoptosis at higher doses (2.8 mg/kg/day). Parathyroid hormone (PTH), calcitonin, prostaglandin-3 (PGE-3), and mechanical loading can partially block these effects.
- Smoking is a known contributor to poor bone mineralization, possibly through restriction of nutrient supply via impaired circulation and/or decreased appetite and intake.
- Obesity may be osteoprotective for cortical bone, but is also associated with impaired spinal mineralization, possibly through confounders in dietary intake patterns or increases in inflammation. Tumor necrosis factors and other inflammatory cytokines can also cause osteocyte death.
- Continuous hypersecretion of PTH occurs with renal disease and with parathyroid gland hyperfunction due to tumor or hyperplasia, resulting in bone loss. An elevated PTH level is a sensitive marker for renal disease. However, intermittent administration of PTH analogs stimulates osteoblasts more than osteoclasts and is anabolic to bone overall.
- Antiresorptive therapies (e.g., bisphosphonates) inhibit osteoclast function; this has a disadvantage of decreasing remodeling capability and leading to a higher risk of atypical fractures distal to the usual femoral neck location. These fractures are uncommon and overall fracture incidence is still reduced. Drug holidays and time-limited treatment courses may ameliorate this risk.
- Hypothyroidism and its treatment unfavorably alter bone metabolism via either lack of thyroxine and possibly of thyroid stimulating hormone (TSH), which reduce bone mineralization.
- Hyperthyroidism greatly increases bone turnover and also reduces bone mineral density.
- Exposure to nonorganic molecules such as aluminum, fluoride, and lead have varying, but probably overall negative influences on bone strength, even though measured bone density may be increased. Strontium ranelate, though structurally similar to calcium and capable of increasing bone density by both stimulating and antiresorptive effects, has problematic side effects at doses sufficient to reduce fracture risks.
- Alcohol use may favorably affect hormonal influences on bone for both males and females at moderate intake levels, but abuse is associated with lower bone density (except perhaps at the hip) and higher risk of fracture overall.

Bone Physiology in Aging
- Normally, trabecular bone accounts for 70% of bone strength and load bearing, and marked thinning of trabeculae is typically noted with aging.
- Cortical bone is less metabolically active and is affected to a lesser degree.
- The etiology of age-related bone loss is multifactorial and includes
  - General age-related declines in osteoblast function and increased osteoclast activity.
  - Decreased function of kidneys, intestines, gonads, and thyroid, resulting in lower production of, and responsiveness to, biochemical signals that normally maintain ideal bone strength and density; this may be more severe with individual genetic variants of cellular receptors.
  - Lack of estrogen or oxygen causes osteocyte death by apoptosis or necrosis, leaving areas of micropetrosis which are either empty or filled-in lacunae, with surrounding areas of hypermineralized matrix. Without the living cells, these areas cannot be remodeled, resulting in brittle bone.
  - Aging also indirectly affects bone via changes in neuromuscular transmission, muscle bulk, and strength, partly due to less weight-bearing exercise.
  - Poorer protein, calorie, mineral, and vitamin D intake also contribute to net bone loss.
  - Aging is associated with a higher prevalence of chronic inflammatory conditions.

Helpful Hints
- In aging, decreased catabolism as well as production and secretion of thyroid hormone requires lowering of dosage to maintain the euthyroid state; this adjustment is commonly overlooked and leads to suboptimal mineralization.

Suggested Readings
National Osteoporosis Foundation. *NOF Clinician's Guide to Prevention and Treatment of Osteoporosis*. Washington, DC: National Osteoporosis Foundation; 2010. www.nof.org/professionals/clinical-guidelines.

U.S. Preventative Services Task Force Screening for osteoporosis: Recommendation statement [published online ahead of print January 17, 2011]. *Ann Intern Med*. 2011;154:1–40. www.annals.org/content/154/5/356.full?sid=c8552006-4b5c-4b8f-bc31-4a21f847807b.

Zhang K, Adjemian CB, Ye L, et al. E11gp38 selective expression in osteocytes: Regulation by mechanical strain and role in dendrite elongation. *Mol Cell Biol*. 2006;26(12):4539-4552.

Age-Related Changes: Cardiovascular

Deepthi S. Saxena MD ■ K. Rao Poduri MD

Description
Increasing age leads to a progressive decline in cardiovascular reserve capacity and substantive alterations in clinical presentation, response to therapy, and prognosis. These changes, occurring at different rates in each individual, are accentuated by comorbid conditions, such as hypertension and diabetes mellitus.

Pathogenesis

Blood vessels
- Increased collagen cross-linking and degenerative changes in elastin fibers cause arterial dilation and increased stiffness of large arteries.
- This increases systolic blood pressure (SBP) and impedance to left ventricular (LV) ejection, increasing afterload.
- Basement membranes thicken; increased matrix synthesis causes intimal sclerosis.
- Endothelial cells become irregular; smooth muscle cells and blood-derived macrophages infiltrate.
- Elasticity of the media decreases due to thinning of the lamina, elastin fiber fragmentation, and replacement by collagen.
- Calcification increases, and lipids accumulate intracellularly and extracellularly.

Heart
The heart increases in size and weight.
- Calcium release from contractile proteins and calcium reuptake by the sarcoplasmic reticulum are impaired, attenuating myocardial relaxation.
- Microscopic changes in the endocardium and myocardium, including lipofuscin deposits, fatty infiltration, and myocyte hypertrophy (to compensate for the increased afterload), cause ventricular stiffness.
- The combination of impaired myocardial relaxation and decreased compliance decreases LV filling in diastole. To preserve the LV end diastolic volume by increasing its contraction, the left atrium dilates and hypertrophies, predisposing to atrial fibrillation and diastolic heart failure, even if left ventricular ejection fraction (LVEF) is preserved.
- Macroscopically, the LV wall increases in thickness, but the size of the LV cavity does not change.
- The endocardium, myocardium, and heart valves thicken and calcify.
- Endothelial dysfunction contributes to the pathogenesis and progression of atherosclerosis, leading to age-related coronary artery disease (CAD) and peripheral arterial disease (PAD).

Conduction system
- Fibrosis, myocyte hypertrophy, and calcium deposition slow conduction at the sinoatrial (SA) and atrioventricular (AV) nodes.
- Degenerative changes in and around the sinus node cause a 10% loss per decade in sinus pacemaker function.
- By age 75, over 90% of SA pacemaker cells cannot initiate an electrical impulse, causing symptomatic "sick sinus syndrome," an indication for pacemaker implants.
- Calcification of the cardiac skeleton increases infranodular conduction abnormalities such as left anterior fascicular and bundle branch blocks.

Oxygen consumption
- Maximal oxygen consumption ($\dot{V}O_2$max), an objective measure of exercise and peak aerobic capacity, declines with advancing age due to decline in maximal heart rate (HR), maximal cardiac output (CO), and muscle extraction of oxygen from the blood.
- In the Baltimore Longitudinal Study on Aging, $\dot{V}O_2$max in healthy adults aged 80 and free of cardiovascular disease was similar to that in middle-aged people with New York Heart Association (NYHA) Class II congestive heart failure (CHF).
- Due to decreased nitric oxide (NO) synthase activity causing decreased availability of NO, the primary endothelium-dependent vasodilator, there is decreased coronary blood flow in response to increased myocardial oxygen demands, causing "demand ischemia."
  - Demand ischemia is precipitated by a sudden increase in myocardial oxygen demand, for

example, due to tachycardia or severe hypertension (HTN), even in the absence of CAD.
- As endothelium-independent vasodilation is unaffected by age, the vascular response to exogenous nitrates, such as nitroglycerin, is similar to that in younger individuals.

Cardiovascular responsiveness
- The heart becomes less responsive to beta-adrenergic stimulation and does not speed up as much when stimulated by exercise or stress, causing the maximal attainable sinus HR to decrease.
- Maximal HR is equal to 220 minus age. Because CO is the product of HR and stroke volume (SV), maximal CO declines with age.
- Beta 1-adrenergic-mediated peak ventricular contractility and beta 2-adrenergic-mediated peripheral vasodilation decline. Decrease in peripheral vasodilation decreases blood flow to exercising muscles leading to impaired thermoregulation.
- Poor responsiveness to carotid baroreceptors and a decreased capacity to rapidly adjust HR, blood pressure (BP), and CO in response to abrupt changes in cerebral blood flow, as occurs with postural changes, can cause orthostatic hypotension, falls, and syncope.
- This predisposition to orthostasis is aggravated by medications used to treat cardiovascular disorders.

Response to stress
- In healthier older adults, though clinically relevant effects on cardiac hemodynamics at rest are well preserved, the capacity to respond to increased metabolic demands due to exercise or illness declines.

Response to treatment
- Although the benefits of current treatments for acute coronary syndrome are similar to that in younger adults, the elderly are at an increased risk for complications.

Suggested Readings
Lakkatta EG, Levy D. Arterial and cardiac aging: major shareholders in cardiovascular disease enterprises. *Parts I, II & III: Circulation.* 2003;107(3):490–497.

Shock NW, et al. *Normal Human Aging: The Baltimore Longitudinal Study of Aging.* NIH-84-2450. Washington, DC: Superintendent of Documents, U.S. Government Printing Office; 1984.

Table 1 Summary of the Physiologic Cardiovascular Changes With Aging

Arterial stiffness	↑
Afterload	↑
Systolic blood pressure	↑
Myocardial compliance	↓
Baroreceptor responsiveness	↓
Maximal heart rate	↓
Maximal cardiac output	↓
$\dot{V}O_2$max	↓
Peripheral vasodilation	↓
Exercise response	↓

Age-Related Changes: Central Nervous System and Cognitive

Patrick M. Kortebein MD

Description
Normal "brain aging" can be described as the aging of the central nervous system (CNS) in the absence of clinically diagnosed neurodegenerative or psychiatric diseases or related pathology.

Etiology/Pathogenesis
The exact etiology of aging of the nervous system is not known and is understudied. Structural and functional changes include
- Decreased brain volume, with the frontal cortex most affected.
- Hippocampal volume decline with normal aging, though not as much as with Alzheimer disease.
- Brain volume changes are minimal up to middle age and more accelerated after age 70.
- Resting cerebral blood flow decreases with aging, as does vascular reactivity and cerebral metabolic rate.

Epidemiology
A 2010 report indicates that one of eight (13%) people aged 65 have Alzheimer disease. This is expected to increase with the aging of the U.S. population.

Risk Factors
- Protective:
  - Aerobic exercise
  - Moderate alcohol intake (1–2 drinks per day)
  - Diets high in vegetables/fish
  - Cognitive training
- Adverse/exacerbating:
  - Cardiac disease, especially cardiac bypass surgery
  - Hypertension; treatment reduces the risk, although in untreated individuals this should be done gradually to avoid hypoperfusion.
  - Chronic obstructive pulmonary disease (COPD); oxygen supplementation is modestly beneficial.
  - Diabetes; optimal management, including a focus on reducing insulin resistance, improves cognitive function.
  - Sleep apnea; severity of hypoxemia appears related; continuous positive airway pressure (CPAP) improves cognition.
  - Hypothyroidism; thyroid replacement may not return cognition to baseline.
  - Obesity; increased saturated fat levels
  - Tobacco abuse
  - Alcohol intake; none or excessive
  - Nutritional deficiencies (e.g., folate)
  - Head trauma; more severe injury has a greater effect.
  - Apolipoprotein E epsilon 4 genotype

Clinical Features
Preserved cognitive functions during aging include
- "Crystallized" abilities (i.e., experience-related information and skills)
- Verbal intelligence
- Primary attention span
- Remote/procedural/semantic memory
- Language comprehension and vocabulary
- Simple visuospatial skills

Cognitive functions that decline with aging include:
- "Fluid" nonverbal ability (e.g., flexible reasoning and problem solving)
- Speed of information-processing/reaction time
- Divided attention tasks
- Learning/recall of new information
- Spontaneous word-finding/verbal fluency
- Complex visuospatial skills (e.g., mental rotation, complex copy)

Differential Diagnosis
- Depression
- Delirium
- Dementia
- Medication includes opiates, benzodiazepines, anticonvulsants, antipsychotics, antidepressants, antiparkinsonian, antihistamines, and central nervous system stimulants.

Suggested Readings

Drag LL, Bieliauskas LA. Contemporary review 2009: Cognitive aging. *J Geriatr Psychiatry Neurol.* 2010;23:75-93.

Glorioso C, Sibille E. Between destiny and disease: Genetics and molecular pathways of human central nervous system aging. *Prog Neurobiol.* 2011;93:165-181.

Halter JB, Hazzard WR, Ouslander JG, et al. Cognitive changes associated with normal and pathological aging. In: Craft S, Cholerton B, Reger M, eds. *Hazzard's Geriatric Medicine and Gerontology.* 6th ed. New York, NY: McGraw Hill; 2009:751-766.

The American Geriatrics Society. *A Guide to Dementia Diagnosis and Treatment.* Philadelphia, PA: The American Geriatrics Society; 2011. www.dementia.americangeriatrics.org

Age-Related Changes: Gastrointestinal

Deepthi S. Saxena MD ■ Ravinder R. Kurella MD

Description
Gastrointestinal changes are not as obvious, or as visible as changes in other, more visible, body systems, but changes do occur with aging, and they can have an important impact on function. Normal physiologic changes in the gastrointestinal (GI) tract include
- Connective tissue changes, which limit the elasticity of the gut.
- Changes in the nerves and muscles due to neurodegeneration and loss of excitatory enteric neurons impair motility.

Organ-Specific Changes With Aging

Tongue
- Varicosities and decreased production of saliva predispose to oral infections, such as candida. Use of anticholinergics, antihypertensives, and antihistamines exacerbates this by decreasing salivary flow.

Esophagus
- Peristaltic amplitude of the esophagus decreases due to weakening of its smooth muscle.
- Disordered nonperistaltic spontaneous contractions can occur (without symptoms).
- Dysphagia in the elderly can be caused by subtle changes in the oropharyngeal region and upper esophageal sphincter, causing aspiration and pneumonia.
- Another common cause of dysphagia is Zenker's diverticulum, an out-pouching of the esophagus just above the upper esophageal sphincter.
- The incidence of achalasia rises with age.

Gastroesophageal junction
- There is decreased esophageal acid clearance, leading to increased esophageal contact with the acid.
- This, along with an increased incidence of hiatal hernia and decreased salivary neutralization of the acid, leads to gastroesophageal reflux disease (GERD).
- Symptoms correlate poorly with the severity of GERD due to reduced visceral sensitivity.

Stomach
- There is atrophy of the stomach mucosa and muscularis mucosa with loss of gastric glands.
- Decreased production of intrinsic factor from the parietal cells leads to decreased absorption of vitamin B_{12} and can cause deficiency of this vitamin.
- Increased incidence of *Helicobacter pylori* infection causes increased risk of peptic ulcer disease(PUD), especially with nonsteroidal anti-inflammatory drug (NSAID) use.

Small intestine
- Generally, aging does not affect the absorption of food and its passage through the small bowel.
- There is increased small bowel bacterial overgrowth, exacerbated by diverticula.
- There is decreased iron and calcium absorption.
- Chronic mesenteric ischemia due to atherosclerosis is common.

Large intestine
- There is reduced peristalsis of the large bowel with aging, mucosal atrophy, hypertrophy of the muscularis mucosa, and infiltration with connective tissue.
- Constipation, a common problem, causes increased pressure in the colon. This can lead to diverticulitis and diverticulosis.
- There is an increased incidence of diarrhea due to microscopic colitis in the elderly, especially in those taking NSAIDs.

Liver
- There is decrease in the size of the liver with a diminished capacity for regeneration in case of damage.
- Decreased clearance of drugs due to decreased metabolism leads to increased medication side effects.

Pancreas
- Duct hyperplasia, increased cyst formation, deposition of lipofuscin granules in acinar cells, and increased fatty deposition occurs.

Gall bladder
- Age increases the lithogenecity of bile. The incidence of gall stones is 35% in women and 20% in men by age 70.

Risk Factors for Weight Loss in the Elderly
- Physiologic factors associated with weight loss include an age-related decrease in taste and smell sensitivity, delayed gastric emptying, early satiety, and impairment in the regulation of food intake.
- Age raises the threshold for odor detection and lowers perceived odor intensity. The number of taste buds remains constant, but thresholds for recognition of salt and other specific tastes increase.
- A decrease in the rate of gastric emptying in the elderly causes antral distension, reduced hunger, and increased satiety.
- Early satiety occurs due to dysregulation of peripheral signals such as glucagon, leptin, ghrelin, and cholecystokinin.
- *Anorexia*—a decrease in appetite, is influenced by these multiple changes. Food intake diminishes with age due to reduced physical activity, decreased resting energy expenditure (REE), and/or loss of lean body mass.

Suggested Readings
Crane SJ, Talley NJ. Chronic gastrointestinal symptoms in the elderly. *Clin Geriatr Med.* 2007;23:721–734.

McCrea GK. Pathophysiology of constipation in the older adult. *World J Gastroenterol.* 2008;14(17):2631–2638.

Zarowitz BJ. Pharmacologic consideration of commonly used gastrointestinal drugs in the elderly. *Gastroenterol Clin North Am.* 2009;38(3):547–562.

Age-Related Changes: Hearing and Vestibular

Samuel R. Atcherson PhD ■ Terry McCoy AuD

Description
The prevalence of hearing loss and vestibular-related disequilibrium in older patients is high. Normal age-related changes are often a contributing factor associated with anatomic, physiologic, and/or functional deficits. Both the organ of hearing and vestibular apparatus reside in the temporal bone and receive innervation from cranial nerve VIII and blood supply from the vertebrobasilar arterial system, Age-related changes in hearing and in vestibular function are not well correlated with each other as they each degenerate at different rates.

Etiology/Types
- Hearing loss
  - Sensorineural hearing loss (SNHL; cochlear)
  - Conductive hearing loss (CHL; outer or middle ear)
  - Mixed hearing loss (combination of SNHL and CHL)
  - Retrocochlear/neurologic hearing loss
  - Unilateral or bilateral hearing loss
- Vestibular dysfunction
  - Labyrinthine
  - Saccule, utricle, or semicircular canals
  - Unilateral or bilateral

Epidemiology
- Hearing loss is highly associated with aging (presbycusis) after age 65 (35% of the U.S. population).
- As many as half of the U.S. elderly population have a vestibular dysfunction.
- One third of older adults between the ages of 65 and 75 report some type of disequilibrium.
- Dizziness is the most common complaint to physicians in patients over the age of 75.

Pathogenesis
- Hearing
  - Sensory (hair cell loss)
  - Neural (spiral ganglion fiber loss)
  - Strial (striavascularis dysfunction)
  - Cochlear conductive (mechanical dysfunction)
  - Mixed (additive)
  - Intermediate (biochemical changes)
  - Central (central nervous system [CNS] changes)
- Vestibular
  - Sensory (hair cell loss and/or otoconia displacement)
  - Neural (vestibular nerve fiber loss)
  - Intermediate (biochemical changes)
  - Central (CNS changes)

Natural History
- Progressive hair cell loss/neural degeneration
- Biochemical and metabolic changes
- Changes in vestibuloocular reflex, vestibulospinal reflex, and so on

Risk Factors
- Age (greater than 65 years), but presentation may begin as early as the fifth decade
- Hereditary
- Vocational or lifestyle noise exposure
- Ototoxicity due to medications

Clinical Features
- High-frequency or flat hearing loss that progressively worsens with age
- Greater difficulty understanding speech in the presence of competing/background noise
- Maladaptive communication or balance behaviors
- Anxiety and other socioemotional issues

Differential Diagnosis

Hearing
- Tinnitus
- Central auditory processing disorder (CAPD)
- Vestibular schwannoma
- Neuropathy
- Cognitive impairment

Vestibular
- Vestibular schwannoma
- CNS disorder
- Cerebellar degeneration

- Meniere's disease/endolymphatic hydrops
- Vestibular neuritis or labyrinthitis
- Vertebrobasilar insufficiency
- Orthostatic hypotension
- Benign paroxysmal positional vertigo (BPPV)
- Psychological (anxiety or panic) disorders

Helpful Hints
- Maintain face-to-face communication, avoid "Elderspeak," and minimize background noise.
- Encourage use of earplugs during noisy activities.
- Consider nonrolling chairs with arms, rails on walls, nonslip/nontrip flooring, and so on.
- Properly fitted corrective lenses are important.
- Quality of life should improve with sensory aid compliance, motivation, and consistent use of compensatory strategies.
- Vestibular disorders may have favorable prognosis through spontaneous recovery, habituation and substitution exercises, or repositioning maneuvers (BPPV).

Suggested Readings
Hnath-Chisholm T, Willott JF, Lister, JJ. The aging auditory system: Anatomic and physiologic changes and implications for rehabilitation. *Int J Audiol.* 2003;42(Suppl. 2):S3–S10.

Huang Q, Tan J. Age-related hearing loss or presbycusis. *Eur Arch Otorhinolaryngol.* 2010;267:1179–1191.

Matheson AJ, Darlington CL, Smith PF. Dizziness in the elderly and age-related degeneration of the vestibular system. *New Zeal J Psychol.* 1999;1:10–16.

Park JJ, Tang Y, Lopez I, et al. Age-related changes in the number of neurons in the human vestibular ganglion. *J Comp Neurol.* 2001;431:437–443.

Weinstein BE, ed. *Geriatric Audiology.* New York, NY: Thieme Medical Publishers; 2000.

Age-Related Changes: Muscular

Carlo E. Adams MD

Description
Various age- and disease-related physiologic changes, including a natural decline in muscle strength, occur with aging. The decrease in strength is partially due to loss of muscle mass, called sarcopenia.
- Sarcopenia is a natural nonreversible process, which can be mistaken for atrophy, a disease and inactivity-related process that may be reversible.
- Strength is generally described as the amount of force produced by maximal muscle contraction, while power is the ability to rapidly generate force (work/time).

Progression of Strength and Muscle Changes
- Maximal strength is reached during the second and third decades.
- Some studies show isometric strength significantly decreasing after age 70.
- Concentric strength is maintained longer.
- On average, strength starts to decline for sedentary people about 1% per year in the 50s and increases to a 3% decline per year in the 70s.
- Upper extremity muscle strength generally changes less than lower extremity strength.
- Women have been found to have a slower decline of upper extremity strength than men.
- On average, muscle mass will decrease by 16% and strength by 25% over time; sedentary individuals may lose as much as 40% of their muscle mass.
- Muscle mass is replaced by increased fat and connective tissue within the muscle belly during aging.
- Power decreases faster than strength with age.
- Muscle structural changes in aging include loss of all types of fibers, along with loss of type II fiber diameter.
- The overall percentage of fat-free mass (FFM) declines with age.
- Loss of muscle mass is directly related to weakness, but exactly to what degree is still unknown.
- Previously, a decline in physical activity was thought to be the main contributor to loss of strength in the elderly, but a host of other factors may be just as significant.
- Chronic disease, poor muscle blood flow, and changes in motor unit mechanisms, such as modulation of contractile elements, fiber type group, and neural and metabolic mediators, have been found to greatly affect muscle strength.

Clinical Features
- Increasing functional difficulty with common daily activities may be an initial sign of weakness.
- Weakness can also lead to increased mortality from bone fractures after falls.
- Sarcopenia does not account for all age-related loss of strength.
  - Although muscle mass is strongly linked to strength, other factors also play major roles. These include nutrition, cardiovascular status, work activities, neural factors, and the level of physical activity.

Differential Diagnosis
- Focal disuse atrophy
- Myopathy/myositis
- Peripheral vascular disease
- Poor activity tolerance from cardiopulmonary disease
- Central (i.e., stroke) or peripheral nervous system injury
- Debility following illness and/or poor nutrition
- Metabolic disorders limiting neuromuscular pathways
- Hormonal deficiency
- Poorly controlled chronic disease

Maximizing Strength and Function
- Aerobic and endurance training, rather than strength training, has traditionally been prescribed for geriatric strengthening, but slow progressive resistance training has also been found to be effective and well tolerated.
- Baseline evaluation, including cardiovascular status, strength, and balance, should be assessed prior to training.

Suggested Readings
Delmonico MJ. Longitudinal study of muscle strength, quality, and adipose tissue infiltration. *Am J Clin Nutr.* 2009;90(6):1579–1585.

Frontera W. Muscle fiber size and function in elderly humans: A longitudinal study. *J Appl Physiol.* 2008;105(2):637–642.

Goodpaster B. The loss of skeletal muscle strength, mass, and quality in older adults: The Health, Aging and Body Composition Study. *J Gerontol: Med Sci.* 2006;61A(10):1059–1064.

Age-Related Changes: Posture and Balance

Jamie Harrison MD

Description
Posture is the biomechanical alignment of each part of the body relative to gravity, and the orientation of the body as a whole to expend the least amount of energy needed to maintain an upright position with adequate balance. Healthy posture plays a key role in maintaining normal balance.

Normal balance requires proper posture and several physiological systems being in tune with each other, including the muscular system and three sensory systems: visual, vestibular, and somatosensory.

Epidemiology
- Roughly 9% of adults aged 65 or above report having difficulty with their balance.
- The common "elderly posture" of forward head flexion and increased kyphosis can restrict movement that increases the risk of falls, most commonly in the backward direction.

Pathogenesis
- With aging comes a natural loss in disc height that exaggerates age-associated postural changes.
- Osteoporosis can lead to compression fractures that can cause postural changes due to wedging of the anterior portion of the vertebrae; thereby increasing kyphosis and decreasing lumbar lordosis.
- Changes in the lumbar spine can result in alterations in pelvic tilt and knee position.
- Elderly patients have a more anterior center of gravity above the hips.

Risk Factors
Impaired posture and balance including the following:
- Physical inactivity
- Prolonged sitting
- Arthritis
- Osteoporosis
- Infection
- Fatigue
- Alcohol use
- Certain medications and polypharmacy
- Cardiac problems, including blood pressure abnormalities
- Problems with blood circulation
- Dementia

Clinical Features
- Decreased spine and pelvic flexibility
- Stooped forward posture with head and shoulders flexed forward and bent knees
- Increased kyphosis
- Decreased height
- Leaning to one side
- Increased sway and unsteadiness

Natural History
- As age increases, so does the risk of developing a condition that will lead to enhanced degeneration of neural and/or musculoskeletal systems.
- Elderly patients are often less physically active. This inactivity leads to muscular weakness. The muscles also fatigue more quickly, which puts the individual at risk for postural imbalance.

Diagnosis

Differential diagnosis
Impaired balance
- Polypharmacy
- Ear disorders—vertigo and Ménière's disease
- Orthostatic hypotension
- Vision impairment
- Substance use
- Neuromuscular disease
- Myopathy
- Neuropathy
- Dementia
- Infection
- Brain tumor

Impaired posture
- Osteoporosis
- Compression fracture

- Neuromuscular disease
- Myopathy

History
- Dizziness
- Musculoskeletal pain
- Weakness
- Fatigue
- Prior fall
- Fear of falling

Examination
Posture
- View anteriorly, laterally, and posteriorly
- Plum line may be helpful

Balance
- Assess footwear
- Ability to maintain side-by-side, semitandem (one foot in front of the other, as if taking a step), and full tandem stance (heel of one foot directly in front of toes of the other) for 10 seconds
- Ability to resist a nudge while standing
- Stability during 360° turn
- Quadriceps strength—rising from armless chair without the use of arms
- Functional reach test (Appendix 1)
- Berg Balance Scale (Appendix 2)
- Fullerton Advance Balance Scale (Appendix 3)
- Tinnetti Balance and Mobility Subscale (Appendix 4)

Testing
- Vision testing
- Audiological testing
- Cardiac and/or vascular testing
- Tilt table testing
- Imaging of the spine and/or brain
- Lab tests of electrolytes and nutrients
- Bone density testing
- Force plate balance systems, with or without filming systems, to observe volitional, anticipatory, and reactive postural control, as well as sensory organization and integration.

Treatment
- Balance and posture-enhancing exercises such as Tai Chi, standing yoga, one-leg standing, tandem standing and walking, stair climbing, turning, heel standing, and toe standing
  - The exact dose and intensity needed for balance improvement are not clear.
  - Intensity is increased by decreasing the base of support, sensory input, or changing the center of mass.
- Balance master—force platform system
- Wii therapy
- Aquatic therapy

Suggested Readings

Wood-Dauphinee S, Berg K, Bravo G, et al. The Balance Scale: responding to clinically meaningful changes. *Can J Rehabili.* 1997;10:35–50.

Hazzard William, Blass JP, Halter JB, et al. *Principles of Geriatric Medicine and Gerontology.* 5th ed. New York, NY: McGraw-Hill; 2003.

Leukoff S, Chee YK, Noguchi S. *Aging in Good Health Multidisciplinary Perspectives.* New York, NY: Springer; 2001.

Spirduso W, Francis KL, MacRae PG. *Physical Dimensions of Aging.* 2nd ed. Champaign, IL: Human Kinetics; 2005.

Woodhull-Mckneal A. Changes in posture and balance with age. *Aging Clin.* 1992;4(3):219–225.

Age-Related Changes: Pulmonary

Sara Rebecca Martin MD ■ Larry G. Johnson MD

Description

Important changes in lung structure, lung function and physiology, and immunologic responses occur as a result of the normal aging process. These changes may play an important role in lung responses to infection and to environmental and oxidant stress.

Lung Changes With Age

Lung development and growth
- The lung is immature at birth. Alveolar septal formation and microvascular development continue postnatally, generally nearing completion at age 2 to 3 years, followed by a phase of rapid lung growth.
- This phase of rapid lung growth, occurring during the first two decades of life, culminates in maximal lung function at age 20 in females and 25 in males.
- Lung function remains steady from 20 to 35 years of age, but begins to decline thereafter.
- The estimated rate of decline in lung function, measured as the forced expired volume in 1 second from a maximal inhalation (FEV1), is 25 mL/yr to 30 mL/yr starting at age 35, but can double to 60 mL/yr after age 70 (with significant person-to-person variability).

Structural changes in the elderly
- Aging effects in the pharynx lead to changes in the pharyngeal component of swallowing, resulting in slowing of transit times and reduced pharyngeal sensation, which can contribute to aspiration.
- An increase in upper airway resistance during supine sleep is often present in healthy older persons, and may initiate sleep disordered breathing.
- A stiffer chest wall and thoracic cage (less compliant) may restrict lung function.
- Kyphoscoliosis can cause a restrictive effect on pulmonary function.
- Homogeneous degeneration of the elastic fibers around the alveolar ducts starts around 50 years of age, resulting in enlargement of airspaces.
- This "senile emphysema" pattern reflects a reduction in supporting tissue, resulting in premature closure of small airways during normal breathing, which can potentially cause air trapping and hyperinflation.

Pulmonary function changes in the elderly
See Table 1.

Exercise capacity in the elderly
This parameter is highly variable, due its dependence upon individual fitness and regular physical activity.
- Maximum oxygen consumption ($\dot{V}O_2$max), a surrogate measure of fitness, peaks between 20 and 30 years of age, then declines by a rate of about 1% per year, depending upon the individual level of physical activity.
- CO_2 production is higher in older adults compared with younger individuals, suggesting a possible increase in dead space ventilation (nonperfused lung).
- Additional age-related changes, including reduced heart rate response, cardiac output, and peripheral muscle mass, may account for part of the decline in $\dot{V}O_2$max.

Table 1 Physiologic Changes of Lung Aging

Maximal expiratory flows (FEV1, FVC)	↓
FEV1/FVC ratio	↓
Diffusing lung capacity (gas exchange)	↓
Respiratory drive for hypoxia, hypercarbia, and resistive loads	↓
PO_2/SaO_2 ratio (due to V/Q mismatch)	↓
PCO_2	↔
Respiratory muscle strength and endurance	↓
Vital capacity	↓
Total lung capacity	↔
Functional residual capacity and residual volume	↑
Airway responsiveness (without change in bronchodilator response)	↑

Note. FEV1, forced expiratory volume in one second; FRC, functional residual capacity; FVC, forced vital capacity; PCO_2, partial pressure of carbon dioxide; PO_2, partial pressure of oxygen; RV, residual volume; SaO_2, arterial oxyhemoglobin saturation; V/Q, ventilation/perfusion.

Immunologic changes in the elderly
- Bronchoalveolar lavage (BAL) fluid in healthy, older subjects shows an increased proportion of neutrophils and a lower percentage of macrophages compared with younger adults.
- An age-associated increase in immunoglobulins IgA and IgM occurs in BAL fluid.
- The BAL fluid CD4+/CD8+ lymphocyte ratio increases with age, suggesting the presence of a primed T-cell response from repeated antigenic stimuli of the lower respiratory tract.
- Alveolar macrophages in the elderly exhibit an increased ability to release superoxide anion in response to stimuli.
- Persistent low-grade inflammation in the airways may cause proteolytic and oxidant-mediated injury to the lung matrix resulting in loss of alveoli and impaired gas exchange across the alveolar membrane seen with aging.
- The composition of the epithelial lining fluid (ELF), which consists of superoxide dismutase, catalase, metal-binding proteins, glutathione, and vitamins C and E that provide antioxidant defenses and minimize oxidative injury to the respiratory epithelium following toxic exposure, is altered with increasing age. This alteration increases the susceptibility of the elderly to environmental and toxin exposures.

Clinical Features
- An increased risk of aspiration occurs with age.
- Changes in lung structure and function lead to impaired cough, impaired airway clearance, and decreased ventilatory responsiveness to hypoxemia, acidosis, and resistive loads.
- Maximal exercise capacity is reduced and may be further exacerbated by reduced maximal cardiac performance and reduced muscle mass. However, maintenance of a high level of physical fitness may be protective.
- An increased risk of pneumonia and an increased severity of lung infection, lung injury, and environmental lung toxicity may occur as a result of chronic low-grade inflammation, changes in lung immune cell populations and antioxidants, and a primed antigen response.

Suggested Readings
Crausman RS. Pulmonary problems in the elderly. In: Gallo JJ, Busby-Whitehead, Rabins PV, et al., eds. *Reichel's Care of the Elderly: Clinical Aspects of Aging*. 5th ed. Philadelphia, PA: Lippincott Williams and Wilkins; 1999:156–165.

Enright, P. Aging of the respiratory system. In: Halter JB, Ouslander JG, Tinetti ME, et al., eds. *Hazzard's Geriatric Medicine and Gerontology*. 6th ed. New York, NY: McGraw-Hill Companies; 2009:983–986.

Meyer KC. Aging. *Proc Am Thorac Soc*. 2005;2:433–439.

Sharma G, Goodwin J. Effect of aging on respiratory system physiology and immunology. *Clin Intervent Aging*. 2006;1(3):253–260.

Ware JH, Dockery DW, Louis TA, et al. Longitudinal and cross-sectional estimates of pulmonary function decline in never-smoking adults. *Am J Epidemiol*. 1990;132:685–700.

Webster JR, Jr. Evaluation of the elderly patient with pulmonary disease. In: Cassel CK, et al. *Geriatric Medicine: An Evidence Based Approach*. 4th ed. New York, NY: Spring-Verlag; 2003:856–868.

Age-Related Changes: Renal

A. Bilal Malik MD

Description
Senescent histologic and physiologic changes in the aging kidney are the rule but do not universally lead to clinical disease. The prevalence of nephrosclerosis increases markedly with age from 2.7% (18–29 years) to 73% (70–77 years).

Structural Changes
- **Glomerular:** capillary tuft collapse and global sclerosis; a total of 30% to 50% loss of cortical glomeruli by the seventh decade
- **Vascular:** diffuse arteriosclerosis with preferential decrease in cortical flow per unit of mass
- **Tubulointerstitial:** tubular simplification, atrophy, and interstitial fibrosis

Physiologic Changes
- Progressive fall in glomerular filtration rate (GFR) of about 8 mL/min/1.73 m2/decade and renal blood flow by 10% per decade after age 40
- Decrease in functional reserve
- Decrease in concentrating and diluting capacity
- Defective renal acidification

Functional Consequences
- Increased susceptibility to nephrotoxic agents
- Predisposition to both fluid overload and dehydration
- Acidosis can lead to sarcopenia, wasting, frailty, and osteoporosis

Epidemiology of Chronic Kidney Disease in the Elderly
- **Definition**
  - GFR less than 60 mL/min/1.73 m2 and/or kidney damage for ≥3 months
- **Prevalence**
  - 13% of the total U.S. population
  - 6.71% of ages 40–59, compared with 46.3% in those aged above 70
- **Risk factors**
  - Older age
  - Diabetes mellitus
  - Hypertension
  - Recurrent episodes of acute kidney injury (AKI)
  - Male gender
  - Nonwhite ancestry
  - Iatrogenic insults
  - Rate of GFR decline

End-Stage Kidney Disease Burden in the Elderly
- The elderly are the fastest growing segment of the U.S. population initiating dialysis, with the median age at initiation increasing from age 56 to 64.4.
- For those aged more than 75, this accounts to an increase of 11% in incidence and 28% in adjusted prevalence rate since 2000.

Impact on Morbidity and Mortality
- One-year mortality rate for those aged above 80 initiating dialysis is 46% (compared with 23% overall)
- Major deficits in quality of life (QOL) and functionality
- High incidence of frailty

CKD and Frailty
Developing insidiously over time, frailty leads to increased incidence of morbidity, functional decline, hospitalization rates, and death.
- **Definition of frailty (≥3 of the following)**
  - Unintentional weight loss (≥10 lb in 1 year)
  - Self-reported exhaustion
  - Weakness (reduced grip strength)
  - Slow walking speed
  - Low physical activity
- **Prefrailty**
  ≤2 of the components
- **Functional decline/disability**
  - Diminishing ability to perform activities of daily living (ADLs), impaired mobility, and recurrent falls with hip and spine fractures
  - Increases in a graded fashion with kidney dysfunction
- **Scope of the problem**
  - Prevalence of frailty (6%) and disability (7%) in the elderly doubles with the onset of chronic kidney disease (CKD) to 15% and 12%, respectively.

- In end-stage kidney disease (ESKD) population, frailty developed in 78.8% of those ≥80 years compared with 44.4% in those younger than 40 years.

CKD-Related Risk Factors for Frailty

The following risk factors for frailty have a high prevalence in elderly patients with CKD:

- Inflammation
  - Higher levels of C-reactive protein (CRP), fibrinogen, interleukin (IL)-6, and so on
- Hormonal deficiencies
  - Testosterone, dehydroepiandrosterone (DHEA), growth hormone, insulin-like growth factor (IGF), and so on
- Anemia
- Depression
- Sarcopenia
- Malnutrition
  - Physiologic anorexia in elderly is aggravated by uremia.
  - Large protein losses occur during dialysis, particularly peritoneal.
  - Chronic acidemia results in protein energy malnutrition (PEM), catabolism, muscle wasting, and cachexia.
  - High prevalence of hyperhomocysteinemia, deficiency of trace elements and vitamins in elderly with CKD and ESKD.
  - Optimal survival on dialysis requires 35 to 40 kcal/kg/day of total calorie intake and protein intake of between 1.1 and 1.4 g/kg/day.

Suggested Readings

Fried LF, Lee JS, Shlipak M, et al. Chronic kidney disease and functional limitation in older people: Health, Aging and Body Composition Study. *J Am Geriatr Soc*. 2006;54:750–756.

Johansen KL, Chertow GM. Significance of frailty among dialysis patients. *J Am Soc Nephrol*. 2007;18:2960–2967.

Shlipak MG, Stehman-Breen C, Fried LF, et al. The presence of frailty in elderly persons with chronic renal insufficiency. *Am J Kidney Dis*. 2004;43:861–867.

Weinstein JR, Anderson S. The aging kidney: Physiological changes. *Adv Chronic Kidney Dis*. 2010;17(4):302–307.

Age-Related Changes: Sensory

Jamil R. Dibu MD ■ Salah G. Keyrouz MD

Description
Structural and functional decline of the somatosensory system is among the many physiologic changes that accompany the process of aging. Our senses (vision, hearing, taste, smell, touch) become less acute, with the degree of change varying from person to person.

Changes in Vision
- Progressive decrease in pupillary size
- Presbyopia (decrease in the ability to adjust to near/farsighted vision); usually noticed between the age of 40 and 50
- Decrease in visual acuity and narrowing of visual fields
- Impairment of color discrimination
- Restriction in upward gaze and insufficient convergence
- Diminished dark adaption and hypersensitivity to glare

Changes in Hearing/Vestibular System
- Presbycusis (progressive sensorineural hearing loss)
- Decrease in sensitivity to high-frequency tones.
- Decrease in tone discrimination
- Vestibular changes, leading to disequilibrium

Changes in Olfaction and Taste
- Perception of both sensations decreases with age.
- Taste sensation diminishes because of a decline in the number of, and atrophy of, taste buds.
- Sweet and salt tastes seem to be affected first.
- Chronic irritation from smoking contributes to the decrease in taste sensation.

Changes in Somatosensation
Impairment in perception of sensory stimuli in the elderly is caused by a loss of tactile acuity, with a reduction in the number and density of myelinated peripheral nerves. It is associated with a risk of falling and functional decline.
- Diminished monofilament and two-point discrimination testing
- Difficulty in processing multimodality sensory information
- Diminished vibration perception:
  - Most common change, progressing with age
  - Mainly impaired in the lower extremities
  - Ascending pattern, starting from the toes
- Proprioception-position sense
  - Affected, but to a lesser extent
  - Usually follows a distal-to-proximal pattern loss
  - Manifests as mild swaying during the Romberg test (however, position sense perception should not be grossly affected on examination)
- Pain and temperature sensation
  - Slightly diminished; increased threshold to pain and difficulty in differentiating temperature
  - Asymptomatic, unless other pathologic causes are present

Differential Diagnosis

Vision
- Decrease in visual acuity might be due to pathological etiologies (i.e., cataract and macular degeneration).
- Decline in ability to detect motion in the visual field can be due to glaucoma.
- Decline in the ability to detect color contrasts can also be due to macular degeneration and Parkinson's disease.

Hearing
- Severe hearing loss is not part of aging (check for sensorineural hearing loss causes, i.e., inner ear, auditory nerve, central nervous system pathology, or conductive hearing loss etiologies, i.e., outer ear, middle ear, or tympanic membrane pathology).

Olfaction
- Most overlooked sensory modality during neurologic examination
- Loss of smell can be associated with neurologic diseases, that is, Parkinson's disease, neurodegenerative diseases—mainly Alzheimer's disease, and frontal lobe tumors.

Helpful Hints

- Studies have shown that correction of sensory deficits (i.e., eye glasses, hearing devices) decrease the rate of mortality and improve the quality of life in the elderly.
  - Counseling to avoid driving at night
  - The perception of taste and odors is intertwined, and therefore impairment in one could lead to impairment of the other.
  - The elderly with olfactory and taste loss are at risk of: poor hygiene (unable to smell body odor), asphyxia (unable to detect environmental hazards/fumes), malnutrition (due to a decrease in interest in food intake), and worsening of their hypertension (the elderly add more salt to their food due to loss of salt taste).
  - Sensory impairment affects both quality of life and functional status of an elderly person.
  - Patients themselves, family members, and physicians often overlook somatosensory decline in the elderly.
  - Patients with sensory senescence might be misdiagnosed with dementia, although their intellectual function is relatively intact.
  - Decreased sensation with age might lead to higher risk of injuries, including pressure ulcers.
  - Among the many sensory declines, hearing loss is the most socially disabling, since hearing is essential for social interaction and safety.

Suggested Readings

Nussbaum NJ. Aging and sensory senescence. *South Med J.* 1999;92(3):267–275.

Ropper AH, Samuels MA. *Adams & Victor's Principles of Neurology.* 9th ed. New York, NY: Mc-Graw Hill; 2009.

Shaffer SW, Harrison AL. Aging of the somatosensory system: A translational perspective. *Phys Ther.* 2007;87:193–207.

Age-Related Changes: Skin

Cheryl A. Armstrong MD

Description
The functional properties of the cells that populate the skin undergo genetically determined changes with age that lead to detectable changes in skin appearance. Some skin disorders and conditions are more common in the geriatric population.

Etiology/Types
- Intrinsic aging of skin
  - Normal age-related physiological changes that are not the result of exogenous environmental agents; for example, thinning of skin, decrease in lipids, decrease in cell numbers, and decrease in collagen.
- Extrinsic aging of skin
  - Decades of exposure to ultraviolet irradiation (photoaging), cigarette smoke, and other environmental agents lead to significant skin damage.
  - Results in coarseness, wrinkling, mottled pigmentation, telangiectasia, and premalignant and malignant neoplasms
  - With age, sun-exposed skin shows changes of photoaging that are superimposed on normal age-related changes.

Epidemiology
- All individuals experience intrinsic aging of the skin.
- There are poorly understood genetic factors that cause people in some ethnic groups to exhibit intrinsic skin aging in later decades of life, so that normal skin aging is delayed.

Physiologic Changes With Aging
- Age-related changes in epidermis
  - Renewal of stratum corneum decreases
  - Epidermis becomes thinner
  - Decrease in lipid content
  - Volume of keratinocytes decreases
  - Melanocyte population decreases
  - Langerhans cell population decreases
- Age-related changes in dermis
  - Dermis becomes thinner
  - Fibroblasts decrease in number and size
  - Alteration and reduction in collagen, elastin, and ground substance, including a decrease in proteoglycans
  - Change in vascular tissue in dermis, including dilation of lymphatic channels
- Age-related changes in subcutaneous tissue
  - Reduced adipose tissue in some regions of skin, including face, shins, hands and feet, abdomen, and thighs
- Age-related changes in adnexal structures
  - Reduction in number and size of eccrine glands
  - Increase in size of sebaceous glands, but reduction in secretory output
  - Attenuation of apocrine gland function
- Age-related changes in nails
  - Nails become thinner and more brittle
  - Nail plate grows slower
  - Nails become more susceptible to fungal infections
- Age-related changes in hair
  - Reduction in density of hair follicle per unit area on the face and scalp
  - Decrease in rate of hair growth
  - Decrease in hair shaft diameter on most hair-bearing skin
  - Development of thick terminal hairs on ears, nose, and eyebrows of men and upper lip and chin in women

Clinical Features
- Skin appearance becomes loose and lax instead of plump and smooth.
- Reduced pigmentation of skin and impaired tanning response to ultraviolet light
- Alterations in cutaneous immune function
- Decrease in wound-healing capabilities
- Increased susceptibility to blister formation
- Increased risk of wound infections
- Thermoregulatory disturbances
- Vascular and lymphatic disorders

Natural History
- Normal age-related changes of the skin progresses in a genetically determined manner in each individual.

Skin Disorders With High Prevalence in the Geriatric Population
- Alopecia
- Bullous pemphigoid
- Cherry angiomas
- Herpes zoster
- Onychomycosis (fungal infection of nails)
- Seborrheic dermatitis
- Seborrheic keratoses
- Spider veins and varicose veins
- Stasis dermatitis
- Stasis ulcers
- Xerosis (dry, scaling skin without redness)

Helpful Hints
- The physiologic changes associated with normal aging of the skin correlate with the types of clinical conditions that develop in geriatric patients.
- Patients may be reassured to know that some changes they can see on their skin are a normal part of the aging process.
- The majority of basic research studies of normal age-related changes of the skin are being performed by pharmaceutical and cosmetic companies with the proprietary results not available for general review.

Suggested Readings
Fenske NA, Lober CW. Structural and functional changes of normal aging skin. *J Am Acad Dermatol.* 1986;15:571–585.

Jenkins G. Molecular mechanisms of skin ageing. *Mech Ageing Dev.* 2002;123(7):801–810.

Leyden JJ. Clinical features of ageing skin. *Br J Dermatol.* 1990;122(35):1–3.

Sunderkotter C, Kalden H, Luger TA. Aging and the skin immune system. *Arch Dermatol.* 1997;133(10):1256–1262.

Age-Related Changes: Visual

Romona LeDay Davis MD

Description
Eyesight generally declines as a normal part of aging.

Etiology/Types
- Presbyopia
  - Near vision declines at about 40 years of age.
- Dry eyes
- Pupillary changes with aging
  - Pupil becomes miotic.
  - Pupil dilates less in dim illumination.

Epidemiology
- Patients above age 40 experience difficulty with near vision.
- Over 50% of those above 50 years of age experience dry eye symptoms.
- Most 60-year-olds require three times more illumination than 20-year-olds for reading.

Pathogenesis
Presbyopia
- Lens fibers harden and become less pliable during accommodation.
- Lens power cannot increase for near tasks.

Dry eyes
- Poor tear production
  - Hormonal changes
  - Medications
- Environmental driers
  - Air-conditioners
  - Central heaters
  - Fans

Pupillary changes
- Pupillary dilation in dim illumination decreases.

Risk Factors
- Aged above 40 years (presbyopia)
- Female (dry eyes)
- Medications (dry eyes)
  - Antihistamines
  - Diuretics
  - Birth control pills
  - Isotretinoin-type drugs
- Menopause (dry eyes)
- Previous refractive surgery (dry eyes)

Clinical Features
- Slow, progressive decline in vision, especially near vision
- Vague complaints of visual decline and discomfort
- Intermittently blurred vision
- Difficulty in transitioning from light to dark areas

Natural History
Presbyopia
- Worsened near vision
- Increased dependence on "reading glasses"

Dry eyes
- Foreign body sensation
- Decline in vision
- Epiphora "watery eyes" with tears flowing onto the face

Pupillary changes
- A delay in visual recovery when going from areas of high-lighting to low-lighting; may be progressive

Differential Diagnosis
- Refractive error
- Ocular diseases
  - Cataract
  - Diabetic retinopathy
  - Glaucoma
- Sjogrens syndrome
- Rheumatoid arthritis

Suggested Readings
Dry-eye syndrome. In: Ehlers JP, et al., eds. *The Wills Eye Manual: Office and Emergency Room Diagnosis and Treatment of Eye Disease.* 5th ed. Philadelphia, PA: Wolters Kluwer Health Lippincott Williams & Wilkins; 2008:52–53.

Hammond CJ, Snieder H, Spector TD, et al. Factors affecting pupil size after dilation: The Twin Study. *Br J Ophthal.* 2000;84(10):1173–1176.

Decision Making

Kimberly Garner MD

Description
Medical decision making is the mental process of addressing the relationships between multiple diseases and conditions, medical options, guidelines, uncertain outcomes, uncertain benefits and harms, and the preferences and values of patients for these outcomes.

Special Considerations
- Current approaches to patient decision-making focus on people's use of systematic decision strategies, such as weighing the pros and cons of different options.
- However, when making health decisions, people often decide using nonsystematic strategies, such as past experiences, memories, and beliefs about health.

Key Procedural Steps
- It is essential to distinguish between problem analysis and decision making. The concepts are entirely different from one another.
- Problem analysis is done initially, and then the information gathered in that process may be used in medical decision making.
- This can be illustrated with a patient who presents with abdominal pain.

Problem analysis
Problem analysis involves the following:
- Analyzing the situation, what should be the presentation against what is actually present (i.e., normal abdominal examination vs. right lower quadrant abdominal pain)
- Problems are deviations from normal (i.e., abdominal pain).
- Problems must be precisely identified and described (i.e., description of right lower quadrant pain with associated signs and symptoms, such as anorexia and vomiting).
- Causes of problems can be deduced by analyzing the problem (differential for abdominal pain).
- The most likely cause of a problem is the one that most closely explains all findings.

Decision making
Decision making involves the following:
- Establishing objectives (confirming the cause of abdominal pain)
- Ranking of objectives
- Ordering of objectives (in the order of importance)
- Exploring potential actions to achieve the objectives (i.e., serial abdominal examinations, surgery, etc.)
- Evaluating potential actions against all the objectives
- The potential action that is able to achieve all the objectives is the tentative decision.
- The tentative decision is evaluated for possible consequences (i.e., risks of surgery).
- The decisive actions are taken (i.e., patient taken to surgery).
- Additional actions may be taken to prevent any adverse consequences from becoming problems and starting both systems (problem analysis and decision making) all over again.
- Note of caution: Even though we have used a simple problem to illustrate problem analysis and decision making, most elderly patients have multiple medical problems and do not present with typical signs and symptoms that a younger patient might. This complicates the decision making by increasing the level of uncertainty in the medical decision-making process.

Anticipated Problems
Biases can creep into our decision-making processes. Below is a list of some of the more common biases.
- Selective search—tendency to be eager to gather evidence for facts that support certain conclusions, but disregard facts that may support other conclusions.
- Premature termination—tendency to accept the earliest alternative that is feasible.
- Inertia—tendency to be disinclined to alter past thought patterns in the face of new situations or circumstances.
- Selective perception—tendency to screen-out evidence that we do not initially perceive as important.

- Wishful thinking or optimism bias—tendency to see evidence from a positive perspective that can distort perception and thinking.
- Repetition bias—tendency to believe what we have been told most often or by the greatest number of sources.
- Anchoring and adjustment—tendency to be unduly influenced by initial evidence that shapes our subsequent evidence collection.
- Group thinking—tendency to conform to the opinion held by the majority or the group.
- Source credibility bias—tendency to reject evidence if we have a preconceived notion against the person, organization, or group.
- Underestimating uncertainty and the illusion of control—tendency to underestimate future uncertainty because we tend to believe we have more control over events than we actually do.

Helpful Hints

Patients should reasonably expect that their health care provider will

- Make a good-faith effort to explain treatment options to them in a language that they can understand.
- Guide them through a process to align their understanding with the area in which the patient is an expert—their own values, preferences, and life goals.
- Use all available resources, including decision aids, to support them in reaching a decision.
- Work to persuade patients to consider their expert opinion, when one option seems optimal, but also resolve that the patient has the final say.

Suggested Readings

Braddock CH. The emerging importance and relevance of shared decision making to clinical practice. *Med Decis Making*. 2010;30:5S–7S.

Fried TR, Tinetti ME, Iannone MA. Primary care clinicians' experiences with treatment decision making for older persons with multiple conditions. *Arch Intern Med*. 2011;171(1):75–80.

Legare F, Ratte S, Stacey D, et al. Interventions for improving the adoption of shared decision making by healthcare professionals. *Cochrane Libr*. 2010;5:CD006732.

Zikmund-Fisher BJ, Couper MP, Singer E, et al. The DECISIONS Study: A nationwide survey of United States adults regarding 9 common medical decisions. *Med Decis Making*. 2010;30:20S–34S.

History

Deepthi S. Saxena MD

Description
- Geriatric history in habilitation setting is a multifaceted approach, with a goal of determining a path to optimizing disability-free years.
- History includes the following domains:
  - Physical
  - Cognitive
  - Psychological
  - Social
- Since all geriatric history is based on function, it behooves rehabilitation professionals to perform functional assessment.
- A complete geriatric history is often obtained with caregiver or family input.
- The key to obtaining an efficient history is the provider's clinical skill and communication rather than time.

Method
- Rapid screening of targeted areas
- Comprehensive history of areas of concern

Strategies for Effective Communication
Due to the increased prevalence of sensory deficits in the elderly, the environment in which the history is obtained is very important.

Facilitating factors
- Providing good lighting
- Facing the patient
- Sitting at eye level
- Addressing patient by name
- Speaking slowly
- Asking open-ended questions
- Allowing adequate time for the patient to answer.
- Using amplification devices, if needed

Limiting factors
- Backlighting (behind examiner)
- Noise and interruptions
- Raising tone and volume while talking to the patient. (Do not assume hearing deficits.)
- Low health care literacy of patient and caregivers. (Provision of appropriate educational materials helps.)
- "Talking down" to the patient; both literally, by standing over them, and figuratively, by equating disability with loss of intellect.

Rapid Screening

Instrumental activities of daily living
- Ability to use a telephone
- Shopping and groceries
- Meal preparation
- Housekeeping and laundry
- Transportation and driving
- Medication management and compliance
- Money management

Activities of daily living and mobility
- History is followed by assessment of activities of daily living (ADLs) and mobility with specific tests, such as "Timed Up and Go" test.

Nutrition (weight loss of greater than 10 lb in the last 6 months)
Poor nutrition indicates the following:
- Depression
- Dementia
- Medical illness
- ADL/IADL decline
- Financial hardship

Vision
- Ability to drive, watch TV, or read a newspaper or magazine with corrective lenses.
- Though accommodation worsens with age, the elderly may be unaware of their deficits.

Hearing
- Hearing loss may be associated with depression.
- Assess for cerumen impaction.
- A positive history of hearing loss calls for an audiology consult.

Cognition
- Minimental status exam
- Short-term recall
- The elderly often do not report memory loss, unless specifically asked.

Depression
- Self-reported or decreased pleasure and interest in activities. Subthreshold depressive symptoms in older adults are primarily somatic, with an absence of pathology; for example, fatigue and insomnia.
- Subclinical depression causes poorer outcomes in rehabilitation and an increase in disability.

Pain
- Older adults may minimize pain or do not report pain due to language or cognitive impairments. This and the provider's hesitation to administer adequate analgesics for the fear of worsening the patient's cognition lead to undertreatment of persistent pain.
- Pain-related behaviors while taking history become important clues. Resistance to giving a history, withdrawal, and inappropriate, combative, abusive, and disruptive behaviors are clues to the presence of pain.

Falls
- Fall history, especially, for those with greater than 2 falls/year, should include
  - Medication
  - Chronic medical illness
  - Vision
  - Circumstances of the occurrence
  - Alcohol
  - Substance abuse

Urinary incontinence
- History should include
  - Lower urinary tract pathology
  - Urinary tract infections
  - Cognitive issues
  - Medication
  - Mobility

Social assessment
- Background: ethnic, spiritual, and cultural
- Caregiver need and role
- Caregiver burden
- Home safety
- Financial resources and stability
- Neglect and abuse: According to a telephone survey in Boston, 3.2% of elders were victims of mistreatment at least once, since they turned 65 years.
- Current medication and allergies

Comprehensive History
- This is imperative in the rehabilitation setting, as acute and severe functional decline can be brought on by insidious illness in the elderly due to their poor reserve capacity and compensatory mechanisms to handle disease, putting them at a high risk of subsequent disability. Often, in a person with a reduced reserve capacity, a small physical deficit can cause a disproportionately large loss of function.
- A good comprehensive history will lead to the assessment of two important syndromes in the elderly:
  - *Failure to thrive (FTT):* A syndrome of global decline, associated with frailty, functional disability, and neuropsychiatric impairment.
  - *Frailty:* Weight loss, exhaustion, weakness, slow gait, and decreased physical activity.

Suggested Readings
Cigolle CT, Langa KM, Kabeto MU, et al. Geriatric conditions and disability: The Health and Retirement Study. *Ann Intern Med.* 2007;147(3):156–164.

Gill TM, Allore HG, Gahbauer EA, et al. Change in disability after hospitalization or restricted activity in older persons. *JAMA.* 2010;304(17):1919–1928.

Examination: Cognitive

Kimberly Curseen MD

Description

Evaluation of baseline cognition is very important when assessing the elderly patient's functional status and current/future care needs.

- Delirium is defined as acute onset and fluctuating mental status changes, which include deficits in attention, changes in cognition, and severe disorganization of behavior. It is a symptom of an underlying disease and requires treatment of the underlying process. Delirium is an independent risk factor for mortality. Common causes include
  - Acute/critical illness
  - Medications
  - Constipation
- Dementia is defined as a class of disorders in which patients experience significant cognitive decline in at least two areas of cognitive function (memory, thinking, language, judgment, executive function, and behavior), which is severe enough to cause a functional decline. Irreversible dementias are terminal diagnoses.

Etiology/Types

Irreversible causes

- Mild cognitive impairment (MCI): deficits in cognitive function which are abnormal but do not affect daily living.
  - Usual presentation is a mild memory deficit ("amnestic MCI").
  - May be at risk for Alzheimer dementia (AD).
- Alzheimer dementia (AD): most common dementia.
  - Gradually progresses over 8 to 10 years.
  - Memory deficit is the most prominent early feature and progresses to debilitating motor and sensory impairment. AD has characteristic neurophysiologic changes in the brain.
  - Diagnosis is usually clinical; gold standard is brain autopsy.
  - Deficits in language and visual–spatial disturbances
  - Patients may show signs of indifference, delusions, or agitation as the disease progresses.
  - Average age of onset is above 65.

- Vascular dementia: cognitive deficits associated with vascular changes in the brain caused by ischemia.
  - Progression follows a stepwise pattern; patients experience sudden loss in function followed by periods of plateaus.
  - Risk factors include: hypertension, diabetes, and high cholesterol.
- Lewy body dementia: identified by cognitive deficits, including poor visuospatial abilities out of proportion to memory deficits, visual hallucinations, fluctuating cognition, and parkinsonian signs.
  - Second-most-common dementia
  - Progresses faster than AD.
  - Age of onset is above 60.
  - Hypersensitivity to antipsychotic medications
- Frontotemporal dementia (FT): defined by cognitive deficits in executive function, language, and behavior (disinhibition and apathy).
  - Memory deficits are not a primary feature.
  - Age of onset is above 60; may have rapid progression.
  - May exhibit hyperorality and personality changes
  - Often atrophy in the frontal and temporal lobe is visible on magnetic resonance imaging (MRI).
- There are several dementias associated with chronic diseases, including Parkinson's disease, multiple sclerosis, Huntington's disease, progressive supranuclear palsy, HIV, chronic alcohol abuse, radiation exposure, and obstructive sleep apnea.

Reversible causes

- Nutritional deficiencies: vitamin B_{12} deficiency, pellagra, and malnutrition
- Infection: syphilis and Lyme disease
- Endocrine disorders: thyroid disorders, hyperparathyroidism, adrenal, and pituitary disorders
- Normal pressure hydrocephalus
- Exposure to heavy metals
- Metabolic causes: hyponatremia, uremia, hypercalcemia, and porphyria
- Pseudodementia: depression in the elderly can present with signs of cognitive decline.
- Medications: can cause mental status changes

- Antihypertensives, opioids/opiates, benzodiazepines, anticonvulsants, antibiotics: fluoroquinolones, mycins, antipsychotics, muscle relaxants, antihistamines, nonsteroidal anti-inflammatory drugs (NSAIDs), tricyclic antidepressants, and cholinergic medications

Evaluation of the Patient With Cognitive Deficits

- History and physical: verbal skills, vital signs, hearing, and visual impairments (cataract, glaucoma, macular degeneration)
- Evaluate for dementia risk factors: age, atrial fibrillation, depression, Down's syndrome, and family history
- Evaluate for pain, constipation, sleep disorders, and dehydration
- Review medication history, past medical history, and recent hospitalizations
- Assess functional status: gait, continence, activities of daily living (ADLs), and instrumental activities of daily living (IADLs)
- Evaluate for delirium: assess for acute onset of mental status change, inattention, disturbed concentration, and for fluctuating levels of consciousness
- Screen for depression
- Evaluate for health care literacy and language

Common Screening and Evaluation Tools

- Minimental status exam (MMSE)
  - Pros: commonly used; can be used to follow treatment of dementia; low scores correlate closely with severity of dementia
  - Cons: copyrighted; can be influenced by education and other mental disorders; limited use in patients who are illiterate, who have visual impairment, or who are unable to write
- Minicog assessment instruments for dementia
  - Pros: less influenced by education level; takes less than 5 minutes
  - Cons: limited use in patients who have visual impairment or who are unable to write
- Saint Louis University mental status exam (SLUMS): validated screening tools to quantify cognitive function and screen for cognitive loss (not diagnostic tools)
  - Pros: SLUMS and MMSE have similar sensitivities and specificities; SLUMS is possibly better at detecting MCI, not copyrighted, adjusted for education.
  - Cons: limited use in patients who have visual impairment or who are unable to write
- Geriatric Depression Scale (GDS): screen for depression that can be helpful for evaluating pseudodementia
  - Pros: validated; simple to administer; can be used in ill patients
  - Cons: loses validity in demented patients; it fails to identify depression in mild-to-moderate dementia.
- Clock drawing test (CDT): can screen for general memory/executive function deficits, how people process information, and vision; can also offer clues about the area of change or damage in the brain. A normal clock drawing almost always predicts normal cognitive abilities.
  - Pros: CDT is good for screening moderate and severe dementia.
  - Cons: not good for screening MCI; scoring method has confounders; limited use in patients who have visual impairment or who are unable to write
- Confusion assessment method (CAM): validated screening tool to evaluate for delirium
  - Pros: Validated tool to assess for delirium; takes less than 5 minutes; can be done at bed side; correlates with *DSM-IV* for delirium
  - Cons: does not assess severity of delirium
- Neuropsychological assessment: standardized clinical evaluation tool, which can assess cognitive performance and deficits. It can help differentiate between normal aging and dementia. The core part of neuropsychological assessment is the administration of neuropsychological tests.
  - Pros: comprehensive multimodal evaluation, with age-matched controls, which increases sensitivity and specificity of diagnosis; the psychologist gives specific feedback to patients and families on how to maintain function.
  - Cons: testing on average takes 3 hours and can be expensive.

Diagnostic Tests

- Laboratory tests:
  - Vitamin B_{12} and red blood cell (RBC) folate: Vitamin B_{12} and folate deficiency is a reversible cause of dementia corrected with supplements.
  - Thyroid function tests: Hypothyroidism and hyperthyroidism can cause confusion and apathy in the elderly; they are reversible causes of dementia.
  - Parathyroid hormone and calcium: Hypercalcemia in hyperparathyroidism can cause confusion.

- Rapid plasma reagin (RPR): Neuropsyphilis may manifests as dementia; treatment is required to prevent further deterioration.
- Urinalysis: Urinary tract infections are a common cause of confusion in the elderly.
- Comprehensive metabolic panel (CMP): Hyponatremia, uremia, metabolic alkalosis/acidosis, and hyperbilirubiemia can cause mental status changes.
- Complete blood count: Anemia and polycythemia may be the risk factors for developing dementia; vitamin B_{12}/folate deficiencies cause anemia.
- Cerebrospinal fluid analysis: useful for rapidly progressive dementias
- Oxygen saturation: Acute and chronic hypoxia may cause memory loss.
- Sleep study: indicated if there are signs and symptoms consistent with sleep apnea; one symptom of untreated sleep apnea is memory loss

■ Neuroimaging can be useful to support the clinical diagnosis of dementia or when the diagnosis is not certain
- Computerized tomography (CT) scan and MRI: consider if age is less than 65, acute neurologic change, concern for normal pressure hydrocephalus or mass lesion, history of head trauma, concern for cerebral infections and autoimmune diseases (i.e., lupus cerebritis), and concern for old strokes or white matter changes, which correlate with a clinical diagnosis of vascular dementia. Atrophy in the hippocampus region of the brain may support the diagnosis of AD. Frontal lobe atrophy may support the diagnosis of FT dementia.
- PET scan: sensitive and specific in differentiating AD from normal aging and other dementias (no current data comparing clinical diagnosis with imaging); Medicare may cover for atypical dementia or in frontotemporal dementia.

Helpful Hints

■ When evaluating a patient's baseline cognition, a detailed social history, which includes occupation, educational level, and level of ADLs independence should be obtained.
■ Literacy should be assessed.
■ If possible, patients should be evaluated with their assist devices (glasses, hearing aids, translators) in place.
■ Behavioral problems in dementia are best managed nonpharmacologically. Antipsychotics have not been shown to be effective in the treatment of dementia and have an increased risk of mortality in the elderly (Food and Drug Administration [FDA] black box warning).
■ Lewy body dementia patients may have paradoxical reactions to antipsychotics.

Suggested Readings

American Geriatric Society. *Geriatrics at Your Fingertips*. 13th ed. Philadelphia, PA: American Geriatric Society; 2011. www.nlm.nih.gov/medlineplus/dementia.html

Blennow K, deLeon MJ, Zetterberg H. Alzheimer's disease. *Lancet*. 2006;368(9533):387–403.

Geldmacher DS, ed. Dementia update: Overview from the first annual dementia congress. *J Am Geriatr Soc*. 2003;5(1, Suppl. 5):S281–S326.

McDonnell MN, Smith AE, Mackintosh SF. Aerobic exercise to improve cognitive function in adults with neurological disorders: A systematic review. *Arch Phys Med Rehabil*. 2011;92(7):1044–1052.

Petersen RC, Smith GE, Waring SC, et al. Mild cognitive impairment: Clinical characterization and outcome. *Arch Neurol*. 1999;56(3):303–308.

Examination: Musculoskeletal

Derek S. Buck MD DC

Description
The musculoskeletal examination of the geriatric patient requires special attention to certain areas, in addition to the standard examination.

History
- Recent hospitalizations and diagnoses
- Surgical history (especially joint replacement)
- Systemic disease (conditions causing joint dysfunction can include inflammatory arthropathies, connective tissue diseases, and autoimmune diseases)
- History of falls
- Work history (although many will be retired, their prior job may be a clue to musculoskeletal disease process as related to their chief complaint)

Inspection
- Apparent atrophy
- Joint deformity (symmetrical vs. asymmetrical)
- Posture
- Presence of tremor

Gait
- Width
- Clearance
- Stride length
- Presence of Trendelenburg sign
- Foot drop
- Steppage gait
- Festinating

Range of Motion
- Active versus passive
- Presence of crepitus
- Limitations (pain, deformity, weakness)

Manual Muscle Testing
- Focus on symmetry
- Proximal versus distal changes
- Consider noncontractile tissue limitations (e.g., bone against bone from osteoarthritis changes, frozen shoulder, or other conditions causing hard end feel in range of motion)

Reflexes
- 2+/4 motor stretch reflex in a geriatric patient may be hyperreflexic (as these reflexes decline in the normal geriatric patient).
- Look for symmetry.
- Achilles reflex may be absent without the presence of disease; if so, it should be absent bilaterally *not* unilaterally (unilateral absence is indicative of disease process, i.e., neurologic compromise).
- Consider history if changes are present (i.e., stroke, injury, etc.).

Spine
- Alignment (kyphosis, scoliosis, gibbus formation [sharp kyphotic angulation in the spine indicating vertebral body collapse])
- Cervical range of motion (presence of dizziness may indicate vertebral artery involvement)
- Lumbar range of motion (spine vs. hip movement)
- Loss of paraspinal musculature

Shoulder
- Evaluate muscle mass of rotator cuff
- Most common pathology in geriatric patient is acromioclavicular spurring and rotator cuff tear.

Impingement testing
- Neer impingement sign: Stabilize the scapula and passively flex the internally rotated arm forward to greater than 90°, eliciting pain. Pain indicates that the supraspinatus tendon is being compressed between the acromion and greater tuberosity.
- Hawkins impingement sign: Stabilize the scapula and passively forward flex (to 90°). Then, internally rotate the arm, eliciting pain. A positive test indicates that the supraspinatus tendon is being compressed against the cora coacromial ligament.
- Painful arc sign: Abducting the arm, with pain occurring roughly between 60 and 120°.

Rotator cuff testing
- Supraspinatus test: The arms are abducted to 90°, forward flexed to 30°, and internally rotated (thumb

pointing down). The patient resists downward pressure from the examiner. Pain and/or weakness are positive signs. In this position, the maximum amount of abduction is to 120°.
- Drop arm test: The arm is passively abducted. The patient is asked to lower the arm slowly. Inability to do so slowly with control, or without pain, is a positive finding and is suggestive of rotator cuff pathology.

Hands
- Presence of deformity: symmetric (systemic disease) versus asymmetric (degenerative process)
- Soft tissue changes
- Trigger finger: common in patients above age 40 and not gender specific. It is caused by repetitive trauma and inflammation of the tendon, which creates a nodule on the tendon. This nodule does not allow the tendon to glide properly through the pulley system. A nodule will be palpable and symptoms will be reproducible on repeated finger flexion.
- Dupuytren's contracture: Seen in males above age 40. It is caused by a thickening of the palmar fascia due to fibrotic proliferation. Painless nodules are found at the distal palmar crease. These nodules are initially nontender but may become tender as the disease progresses. The involved finger may be drawn into flexion as the nodules thicken and contract. Flexion is commonly seen at the metacarpophalangeal joint of the ring finger.

Hips
- Increased risk of fracture in the geriatric population (females greater than males) due to osteoporosis.
- Trochanteric bursitis: Pain over the greater trochanter made worse with direct palpation. It may be accompanied by "snapping hip."

Knees
- Ligamentous laxity: Varus and valgus stress testing. Laxity in the absence of trauma could indicate connective tissue disease or inflammatory arthritis (systemic lupus erythematosus [SLE], rheumatoid arthritis, etc.).
- Patellofemoral pain: may develop due to muscle weakness or bone spur formation related to osteoarthritis.

Feet
- Hallux valgus—lateral deviation of the great toe.
- Claw toe—characterized by extension of the metatarsophalangeal and flexion of the proximal and distal interphalangeal joints. Deformity is usually the result of incompetence of the foot intrinsic muscles, due to neurologic disorders affecting the strength of these muscles (i.e., diabetes, alcoholism, peripheral neuropathies, Charcot-Marie-Tooth disease, and spinal cord tumors).
- Hammer toe—flexion deformity of the proximal interphalangeal joints of the lesser toes. Passive extension of the metatarsophalangeal joint occurs on weight bearing.

Special Considerations
- Proximal muscle strength: assess deltoids (shoulder abduction) and hip flexor strength (raise knee against resistance), as well as hip extensors (sit to stand).
- Gait assessment: have patient walk in the clinic hall; assess with assistive device, if being used already.
- Balance (Romberg test with eyes open and closed)
- Cognition (as dementia can lead to motor retardation, elderly show slower motor processing normally; and poor cognition may cause worsening of motor control):
  – Proverb interpretation, serial seven's.
- Current functional level: abilities at home with personal care, cooking, shopping, distance able to ambulate regularly, and so on.

Helpful Hints
- Consider patient medications such as statins as a cause of myalgia, blood pressure medication for orthostasis and balance issues, and so on.
- If patient uses ambulatory aids, assess the appropriateness of use and fit.
- Consider nutritional status with findings such as loss or decreased proprioception or vibratory sense (Vitamins B_{12} and B_6).

Suggested Readings
Bickley LS. *Bates' Guide to Physical Examination and History Taking*. 10th ed. Philadelphia, PA: Lippincott, Williams & Wilkins; 2008.
Rubenstein LZ, Ganz D. *Falls and Their Prevention, an Issue of Clinics in Geriatric Medicine*. Philadelphia, PA: Saunders; 2010.
Sarwark J. *Essentials of Musculoskeletal Medicine*. 4th ed. Rosemont, IL: American Academy of Orthopaedic Surgeons; 2010.

Examination: Neurologic

Shadi R. Yaghi MD ■ Salah G. Keyrouz MD

Description
With the increasing prevalence of many neurologic ailments such as stroke and neurodegenerative diseases, the neurologic examination takes on an especially important role in the elderly. In this group of individuals, one should always consider the importance of testing items such as gait and tone that can further the ability to accurately diagnose a disorder. In addition, one should remember that certain findings encountered on examination do not necessarily signal the presence of a disease process but are regarded as age-related changes. It is sometimes difficult to determine whether a neurologic finding is the result of an acute process or is related to a remote, nondiscrete insult to the central or peripheral nervous system.

Mental Status Examination
The bedside examination of the mental state or sensorium is performed using short test batteries such as the minimental status examination (MMSE) or the Saint Louis University mental status examination (SLUMS). Below is a description of some important aspects of mental state examination.

Level of wakefulness
- Awake: sensorium fully intact
- Somnolent: arouses after normal stimuli; drifts back to sleep inappropriately
- Stupor: arouses to vigorous verbal stimuli
- Semicoma: arouses to painful stimuli
- Coma: no arousal

Alertness
- This is a measure of an individual's ability to remain attentive and to appropriately interact with the environment.
- An impaired attention span, as seen in delirium, is present when repeated reminders to the task at hand are needed.

Orientation
- Person: spouse, family members, examiner, or other individuals in the room
- Place: county, city, state, or country
- Time: date, day, month, year, or season
- In addition, orientation to famous individuals (e.g., President) and recent important events should be evaluated.

Memory
- Short term: registration and recall of three or more words after 5 minutes
- Long term: birth date, wedding date, or social security number

Cranial Nerve Examination
- Cranial nerve (CN) I (Olfactory): smell
- CN II (Optic): vision
- CN III (Oculomotor): elevates, extorts, and adducts the ipsilateral eye; constricts pupil and elevates upper eyelid
- CN IV (Trochlear): depresses and intorts ipsilateral eye
- CN V (Trigeminal): sensory perception over the face and anterior two thirds of the tongue; motor innervation to the muscles of mastication
- CN VI (Abducens): abducts ipsilateral eye
- CN VII (Facial): facial muscles (lifting eyebrows, closing eyes, smiling, and blowing cheeks), taste from anterior two thirds of the tongue
- CN VIII (Vestibulocochlear):
  – Vestibular: coordination and fine-tuning of head and eye movements; when function is disturbed, nystagmus may be present
  – Cochlear: response to whispering voice, Weber and Rinne Test
- CN IX (Glossopharyngeal): midline uvula, gag reflex, taste, and general sensation from posterior one third of the tongue
- CN X (Vagus): palate elevation
- CN XI (Spinal accessory): ipsilateral shoulder shrug and contralateral head turning
- CN XII (Hypoglossal): tongue bulk and strength (ask patient to push tip of the tongue against the inside of the cheek)

Motor Examination
- Muscle bulk: Atrophy of muscle groups should be evaluated by comparison and circumference measurement, when needed.
- Muscle tone: This reflects passive muscle contraction, without voluntary interference. Tone can be reduced (i.e., flaccidity) or increased (i.e., spasticity, plasticity, or rigidity). Special attention should be given to testing muscle tone. An abnormality such as spasticity could signal the presence of important and reversible pathologies such as cervical spine spondylosis. Examination of tone in the lower extremities should always be performed when lying down, while distracting the patient (to allow relaxation).
- Rigidity (seen in parkinsonism)
- Motor strength (Medical Research Council Scale)
  - 5: Full strength
  - 4: Good strength against resistance, yet not normal
  - 3: Good strength against gravity, but not against resistance
  - 2: Movement present, but not against gravity
  - 1: Flicker of contraction without generating movement
  - 0: No movement

Reflexes
- 0: Absent
- 1: Hypoactive
- 2: Normal
- 3: Hyperactive without clonus
- 4: Hyperactive with clonus

Pathologic Reflexes
- Babinski sign: Stroking the sole of the foot elicits extension of the big toe and fanning out of the remaining toes.
- While its presence is not specific for the presence of a certain disease, it signals impairment in the function of the corticospinal pathway.
- Hoffmann reflex: Flicking the fingernail of the middle finger causes the thumb, index, and ring fingers to flex.
- While its presence may signal a corticospinal tract pathology or cervical myelopathy, it can be found in 10% to 15% of normal individuals.
- Clonus should be checked at the ankles, knees, and wrists.
- Frontal release reflexes: These are central nervous system reflexes seen in normal infants. In older children and adults, they are inhibited by the frontal lobes, and therefore could reappear with frontal lobe pathology.
- Palmomental reflex: contraction of chin muscles when scratching the palm at the base of the thumb.
- Glabellar reflex: blinking in response to tapping on forehead. This pathologic reflex is uninhibited in individuals with parkinsonism.
- Snout reflex: pursing of the lips that is elicited by light tapping of the closed lips near the midline.
- Grasp reflex: flexion or clenching of the fingers or toes upon stimulation of the palm or sole; normal only in infancy.

Extrapyramidal System Examination
- Tremor: amplitude and frequency should be noted, as well as whether it is present at rest (Parkinson's disease), when one assumes a posture, or on intention (cerebellar disease).
- Dyskinesia: abnormal, involuntary, and nonpurposeful movements of the limbs, or of the neck and head. They can be intermittent or continuous.
- Dystonia: abnormal posture of a limb or head and neck caused by abnormal, sustained muscle tone.
- Myoclonus: intermittent, nonrhythmic jerky movements affecting certain muscles. Typically seen as a result of acute metabolic abnormalities (e.g., azotemia, hyperammonemia).
- Bradykinesia: the general paucity, and slowness, of movements; it is the hallmark of parkinsonism.

Sensory Examination
Face, trunk, and limbs should be tested for perception of the following:
- Pinprick
- Temperature
- Position
- Light touch
- Vibration

Decrease in vibration perception in the distal lower extremities is compatible with the aging process.

Cerebellar Examination
- Gait
- Posture while sitting (truncal ataxia may be the only finding suggestive of cerebellar dysfunction)
- Limb coordination
- Finger–nose–finger
- Heel–knee–shin
- Romberg's sign: Patient stands with feet together and is asked to close the eyes. A loss of balance upon eye closure is interpreted as indicative of abnormal proprioception.

Normal Findings on Neurologic Examination of the Elderly
- Decreased visual acuity
- Decreased hearing acuity
- Mild restriction in vertical ocular movements
- Mild decrease in bulk and strength of muscles
- Mild bradykinetic gait
- Mild decrease in coordination
- Decrease or absence of distal deep tendon reflexes
- Decreased distal proprioception
- Postural tremor
- Orthostatic hypotension

Helpful Hints
- Restriction of upward gaze can be a normal finding in the elderly
- Particular attention should be given to overall facial appearance: an expressionless or "poker" face is a hallmark feature of parkinsonism.
- Attention should be paid to the presence of chin or palatal tremors, typically seen in essential tremors or in Parkinson's disease.
- The jaw jerk is exaggerated when corticobulbar tract function is impaired.

Suggested Readings
Benassi G, D'Alessandro R, Gallassi R, et al. Neurological examination in subjects over 65 years: An epidemiological study. *Neuroepidemiology.* 1990;9:27–38.

DeMyer WE. *Techniques of the Neurological Examination.* 4th ed. New York, NY: Mcgraw Hill Professional; 1993.

Houten JK, Noce LA. Clinical correlations of cervical myelopathy and the Hoffmann sign. *J Neurosurg Spine.* 2008;9(3):237–242.

Electrodiagnosis: Nerve Conduction Studies

William L. Doss MD

Description
Nerve conduction studies are an evaluation of the integrity of the peripheral nervous system. An electrical stimulus is applied to a particular nerve, and the response of muscle or nerve at a distant point is recorded.

Key Principles
- Used to determine the presence of a peripheral neurologic disorder
- Used to determine the site of the peripheral neurologic disorder (anterior horn cell, nerve root, plexus, peripheral nerve).
- Used to determine the cause of nerve injury, based on the pattern of conduction of the peripheral nerves.
- Used to determine the severity and prognosis of nerve injury.

Features of the Nerve Conduction Study

Key terms
- *Latency*: This is the time it takes for an electrical impulse to travel from the stimulating electrode to the G1 (recording) electrode.
- *Compound motor action potential (CMAP)*: This is the motor action potential, the waveform depicted on the screen of the electromyography (EMG) machine. A supramaximal stimulus is applied to the nerve being studied, in order to stimulate all of the axons of that nerve. Each of these responses arrives at the G1 electrode at approximately the same time. The small electrical signals of the axons are summated, to generate the waveform. A similar response is possible for the sensory nerves, a *sensory nerve action potential.*
- *Nerve conduction velocity (NCV)*: This is the speed of the nerve impulse that is conducted from one point along the course of a nerve to another point. For example, the normal velocity (NCV) of the median nerve is approximately 50 m/s.
- *Mechanism of nerve conduction*: Nerve transmission occurs via saltatory conduction along the Nodes of Ranvier. This saltatory conduction allows the electrical impulse to travel quickly.
- Any time delays in the latency or slowing of the NCV suggest pathology of a nerve segment or the entire nerve; the greater the delay in the latency or the slower the NCV, the greater the pathology.

Indications
Diagnosis: A nerve conduction study is indicated when there is a suspected problem of the motor and/or sensory function of a nerve because of the history of physical examination findings. It can also be used to evaluate the function and integrity of muscles. Examples of diagnoses that can be made (in conjunction with the needle examination) are as follows:
- Carpal tunnel syndrome
- Cervical/lumbar radiculopathy

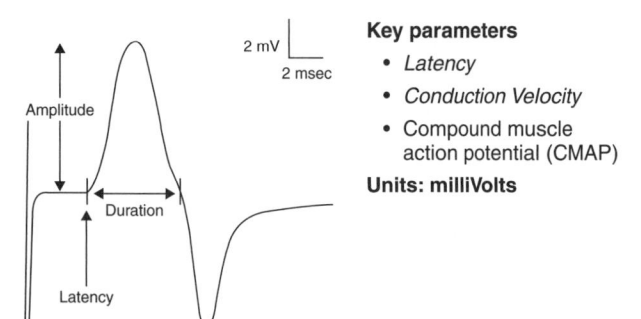

Key parameters
- *Latency*
- *Conduction Velocity*
- Compound muscle action potential (CMAP)

Units: milliVolts

Figure 1 Motor Nerve Conduction Study (NCS)

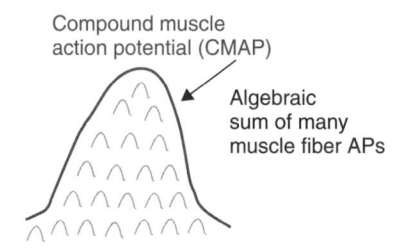

Figure 2 Compound motor action potential waveform

- Spinal stenosis
- Polymyositis
- Myasthenia gravis
- Amyotrophic lateral sclerosis (Lou Gehrig's disease)

Localization
- Another indication is to determine the location of a nerve injury due to trauma or entrapment. For example, if the median nerve is injured in the mid-forearm, the CMAP amplitude distal to this area will be normal; whereas, the proximal portion of the nerve will show a drop in CMAP amplitude (because not all of the axons are able to conduct the electrical impulse through the site of injury).

Prognosis
- This is usually determined over time, with a subsequent study compared to the initial study. If there is decrease of the latency or increased NCV from the initial study, this suggests a more favorable prognosis.

Determination of Normal Nerve Conduction Studies

Various methods can be used to determine whether a nerve conduction study is normal or abnormal.
- There are standard latencies and NCVs published for each nerve that is studied in the electrodiagnostic evaluation.
- A second method is to compare the site in question with the uninvolved extremity to see if there is a side-to-side difference. The involved side will have either a prolonged latency or decreased nerve conduction velocity compared to the uninvolved extremity.
- A third method in determining pathology is to compare segments along the course of a given nerve. Large segments can be compared, as can short segments ("inching technique").
- A fourth method of determining the state of a given nerve is by comparison with a different, but relatively similar nerve.

Nerve Anomalies
- One of the anomalies that can confound the nerve conduction study is the *Martin–Gruber Anastomosis*.
- This occurs when a portion of the median nerve crosses over to the ulnar nerve in the forearm.
- This can give the appearance that the distal CMAP amplitude is abnormal (smaller) compared with the proximal CMAP amplitude (larger).
- In actuality, this is a normal variant of the median nerve. An astute electromyographer must always be on the lookout for this, as well as other anomalous innervation patterns.

Contraindications
- Nerve conduction studies should not be performed immediately adjacent to a pacemaker or automatic implantable cardiodefibrillator (AICD) device, or near a potential source of electrical conduction to the heart, such as a central line.
- Should not be done over any open areas of skin

Anticipated Problems
- Patient may require repeated explanation of the purpose of the test.
- Difficulty in placing the patient in optimal position
- Patient's inability to tolerate full nerve conduction study
- Decreased temperature in the distal extremities, which will lead to erroneously prolonged distal latency and increased amplitude, due to temperature effects on the nerves
- Potential inability to obtain sensory responses in the elderly

Special Considerations in the Geriatric Population
- Sensory nerve action potentials may diminish in size with age, prolonged latency, or even absent responses, especially of the sural nerve; and do not necessarily indicate pathology in an otherwise normal neurologic examination.
- NCVs will decrease 1 to 2 m/s per decade with aging. For example, an individual with a peroneal NCV of 46 m/s at age 40 years would be expected to have a NCV of 40 m/s at age 70.
- The elderly may have concurrent electrodiagnostic findings during examination: diabetic neuropathy as well as Carpal Tunnel syndrome; this may confound the interpretation of the study.

Suggested Reading
Prahlow ND, Buschbacher RM. An introduction to electromyography: An invited review. *J Long-Term Effects Med Implants*. 2003;13(4):289–307.

Electrodiagnosis: The Needle Exam—Electromyography

William L. Doss MD

Description
- Electromyography (EMG), also known as the needle exam, is a complement to nerve conduction studies. It involves the insertion of a 35 to 75 mm pin or needle into the skeletal muscles.
- The activity of the muscle is recorded and is transmitted to the EMG machine.
- It is literally a "live" recording of muscle activity.
- The electrical activity is depicted as a visual "waveform" and in an auditory format, both of which have diagnostic value.
- Often the term EMG is used to refer to the entire electrodiagnostic study, including nerve conduction studies, as well as the needle exam.

Key Principles
- Used to determine the presence of muscle activity
- Used to determine the presence of muscle denervation, by recording abnormal waveforms, that is, positive sharp waves or fibrillation potentials
- "Positive" waves are initially downward deflections of the electrical activity of the muscle, which is opposite of the upward "negative" deflection of normal muscle.
- Used to determine the degree of muscle activation by having the patient recruit muscle activity through voluntary contraction of the muscle
- Used to determine the type of abnormality, that is, myopathic versus neuropathic process

Indications for an EMG Referral

Examples
- *Lumbar stenosis*: The geriatric patient will often have low back pain radiating down both legs, particularly with ambulation. Needle exam study will focus on both lower extremities, as well as the lumbar paraspinal muscles.
- *Neuropathy—especially diabetic*: The geriatric population will have comorbidities and may complain of neuropathic pain.
- *Inclusion body myositis*: This is the most common myopathy in men of 50 years of age or above. EMG findings will exhibit myopathic as well as neuropathic features.
- *Amyotrophic lateral sclerosis (ALS)*: This is not a common diagnosis, but should be investigated in any patient above 50 years of age with new bulbar symptoms (e.g., dysphagia) or insidious weakness and hyperreflexia that cannot be explained by cervical myelopathy and/or stenosis. Special attention on the needle exam should include evaluation of the bulbar muscles (e.g., facial, masseter, etc.), which are frequently involved in ALS. Also, the thoracic paraspinal muscles should be studied. These muscles in particular are usually involved in ALS.

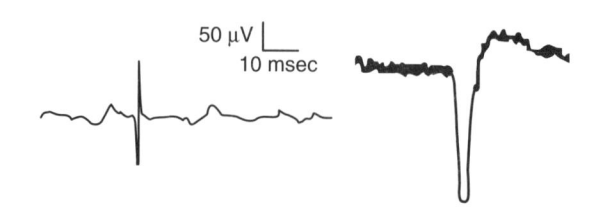

Figure 1 Increased Spontaneous Activity—Abnormal (Similar to Q Wave in ECG)

- Records the muscle at rest–spontaneous activity
- Records active/volitional activity–motor unit action potential (MUAP)

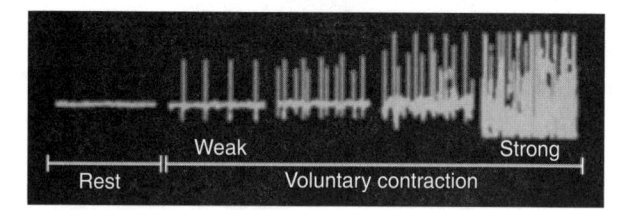

Figure 2 EMG—"Needle Exam"

Contraindications
- Found in individuals who have breast cancer and who have had lymph node dissection of one or both extremities (for fear of infection). This does not exclude all cancer patients, just those who have had lymph node dissection involving a particular extremity and in whom infection is a potential problem.
- Over any open wounds
- Can be done on patients taking Warfarin; however, special attention is needed for those patients who have excessive bleeding at a needle-insertion site. Certain sites where bleeding might be a particular problem may be avoided.

Special Considerations
- Caution should be exercised during the needle exam of muscles that are near the thorax—particularly in thin individuals—for fear of causing a pneumothorax.
- Such muscles include the following:
  - Serratus anterior, as it lies on top of the ribs
  - Rhomboid—deep muscle close to the chest wall
  - Supraspinatus—lies near apex of lung
  - Low cervical and thoracic paraspinals

Key Procedural Steps
- Needles that are smaller in length, that is, 25 to 37 mm gauge versus 50 to 75 mm needles, can be used to avoid pneumothorax, particularly in thin individuals; longer needles obviously need not be fully inserted.
- Skin can be stretched before needle insertion, in order to limit the degree of discomfort.
- The patient should be reassured that the test may be mildly to moderately uncomfortable; however, the discomfort should not last more than few minutes after the test.
- Examination of the lumbar paraspinal muscles may require a 75 mm needle in an obese patient.

Helpful Hints
- Motor unit action potential (MUAP) duration increases with age as motor units are slow to drop out.
  - Normal deltoid MUAP duration at age 20 to 29 is 9.5 to 13.2 ms.
  - Normal deltoid MUAP duration at age 70 to 79 is 13.7 to 17.7 ms.
- MUAP amplitude also increases as a result of normal motor unit drop out with resultant "normal" reinnervation.
- Increased polyphasic (excessively complex waveforms) potentials are to be expected in the elderly.

Suggested Readings
Dumitru D, Amato AA, Zwarts M. *Electrodiagnostic Medicine.* 2nd ed. Philadelphia, PA: Hanley & Belfus; 2001.

Preston DC, Shapiro B. *Electromyography and Neuromuscular Disorders: Clinical-Electrophysiologic Correlations.* Textbook with CD-ROM. 2nd ed. St. Louis, MO: Butterworth-Heinemann; 2005.

Sirven JI. *Clinical Neurology of the Older Adult.* 2nd ed. Philadelphia, PA: Lippincott Williams & Wilkins; 2008.

Tan, FC. *EMG Secrets.* Philadelphia, PA: Hanley & Belfus; 2003.

Evaluation of Balance and Mobility

Kevin M. Means MD

Key Principles
- Balance and mobility problems in the elderly are usually caused by or associated with multiple factors.
- Prudent assessment includes identification of potential contributing factors and assessment of the severity or risk of future balance dysfunction through
  - Careful clinical history
  - Physical examination
  - Diagnostic testing, as appropriate
  - Functional performance tests: This can be a helpful complement to the assessment process
- Many valid and reliable performance tests exist for use in a standardized balance and mobility assessment to compare patients with established performance "norms," or to compare an individual's subsequent performance with their baseline, for evaluating response to intervention.
- Most tests are quick to use (most take 2 or 3 minutes), require no special equipment, and can easily be incorporated into a clinical examination session.
- Balance tests variably measure the following:
  - Static standing balance
  - Dynamic standing balance
  - Adaptation to sensory alterations
  - Ability and stability during functional tasks
  Currently, there is no universally recognized gold standard measure for balance activity in patients.

Assessment Tools

One-leg stance test
- The patient is asked to stand unassisted on one limb of their choice; stance time is recorded from when the foot leaves the floor until it touches again.
- Score: stance greater than 30 seconds indicates very low fall risk; stance greater than 5 seconds is a good predictor of an injurious fall in the elderly.
- Need: watch or clock
- Good inter-rater reliability, but limited evidence for reliable measurement of change over time
- Pros: very simple and quick
- Cons: accurate but nonspecific; prolonged one-leg stance (OLS) not a functional activity

Sharpened (modified) Romberg test
- Measures static standing balance
- Length of time for which the patient can stand heel to toe with arms across the chest and eyes closed (up to 60 seconds × 4 trials).
- Perfect score is 4 × 60 = 240 sec.
- Equipment: stopwatch is optional.
- Limited reliability/validity data
- Pros: easy, inexpensive to administer, and timing adds objectivity
- Cons: nonspecific for a particular problem, pathway, or system; no functional information

Functional Reach: Appendix 1
- Tests active standing balance; mean from three trials used; reach of ≤6 in. predicts a fall
- Need: yardstick and mounting tape
- Good normative data, and inter-rater and test–retest reliability data; good criterion and concurrent validity data; sensitive to change over time
- Pros: simple and inexpensive; established reliability and validity; sensitive to change over time
- Cons: yields limited functional information

Get Up and Go/Timed Up and Go
- The patient is asked to rise from a chair, walk 3 m, then return; (1–5 qualitative scale; lower scores better); Timed Up and Go (TUG) version—timed performance of this task.
- Scoring (in seconds) implications
  - Less than 10 seconds—independent (IND)
  - 10 to 20 seconds—IND with transfers, stairs, and outdoors
  - 20 to 29 seconds—variable balance, gait speed, and functional capacity
  - ≥30 seconds—needs help with chair, toilet transfer, and stairs
- Need: watch and chair with arms
- Inter-rater and test–retest reliability, concurrent validity data available; limited predictive validity data
- Pros: simple, inexpensive to perform; can compare with other tools; and some functional task data
- Cons: not extensively tested and limited data on change sensitivity

Tinetti's Balance and Gait Index: Appendix 2
- Functional performance test
- Need: chair and unobstructed 10 to 20 ft. walkway
- Inter-rater and test–retest reliability; limited criterion validity or change sensitivity; and good predictive and concurrent validity
- Pros: simple, widely used, and some functional tasks
- Cons: subjective scoring and some nonfunctional tasks

Berg Balance Scale: Appendix 3
- Assesses the ability to stand and maintenance of standing, despite internally produced perturbations
- Items scored on 0 (unable) to 4 (safely done) scale (maximum score = 56)
- In elderly, a score of less than 45 correlates with a low fall risk.
- Change of eight points indicates a genuine function change for activity of daily living (ADL)-dependent older people
- Good inter-rater and intrarater reliability
- Pros: easy, quick (10–15 minutes), and familiar to most physical therapists
- Cons: frequent uncertainty between two close scores and low validity and sensitivity for nonambulatory stroke patients

Fullerton Balance Scale: Appendix 4

Computerized posturography
- Posturography is an alternative or complement to the functional balance and mobility tests listed above.
- Posturography—the use of computerized devices incorporating a force plate to measure balance
- Measurements:
  - Static posturography tracks and quantifies postural sway (movements of the center of mass during quiet standing).
  - Dynamic posturography quantifies multiple aspects of active postural control, including the use of sensory cues, voluntary weight shifting, and automatic postural reactions.
- Equipment: There are several manufacturers of posturography devices. The Smart Balance Master® (NeuroCom) and the Biodex Balance System® (Biodex Medical Systems, Inc.) are two examples in common use.

- Posturography advantages:
  - Provides automated, robust quantitative information about balance
  - Posturography has been most widely used in vestibular disorders.
  - Dynamic posturography can be used in testing and as a treatment modality.
  - Several testing and treatment protocols have been developed by the manufacturers.
- Disadvantages:
  - Dynamic posturography does not allow the clinician to identify the cause of dysfunction.
  - Published data on efficacy are limited.
  - Equipment is relatively expensive and operation requires some technical expertise.

Helpful Hints
- Examiner should be close enough to provide assistance as necessary during testing.
- Note: No single test measures all processes involved in balance and mobility in all situations.
- Consider digital video recording tests and storing as electronic clinical record.

Suggested Readings
Berg KO, Wood-Dauphinée SL, Williams JI, et al. Measuring balance in the elderly: Validation of an instrument. *Can J Public Health*. 1992;83(Suppl. 2):S7–S11.

Duncan PW, Weiner DK, Chandler J, et al. Functional reach: A new clinical measure of balance. *J Gerontol*. 1990;45:M192–M197.

Leddy AL, Crowner BE, Earhart GM. Functional gait assessment and balance evaluation system test: Reliability, validity, sensitivity, and specificity for identifying individuals with Parkinson disease who fall. *Phys Ther*. 2011;91:102–113.

Podsiadlo D, Richardson S. The timed "Up & Go": A test of basic functional mobility for frail elderly persons. *J Am Geriatr Soc*. 1991;39:142–148.

Tinetti ME, Williams TF, Mayewski R. Fall Risk Index for elderly patients based on number of chronic disabilities. *Am J Med*. 1986;80:429–434.

Tyson SF, Connell LA. How to measure balance in clinical practice. A systematic review of the psychometrics and clinical utility of measures of balance activity for neurological conditions. *Clin Rehabil*. 2009;23:824–840.

Yelnik A, Bonan I. Clinical tools for assessing balance disorders. *Clin Neurophysiol*. 2008;38:439–445.

Appendix 1: Functional Reach Test

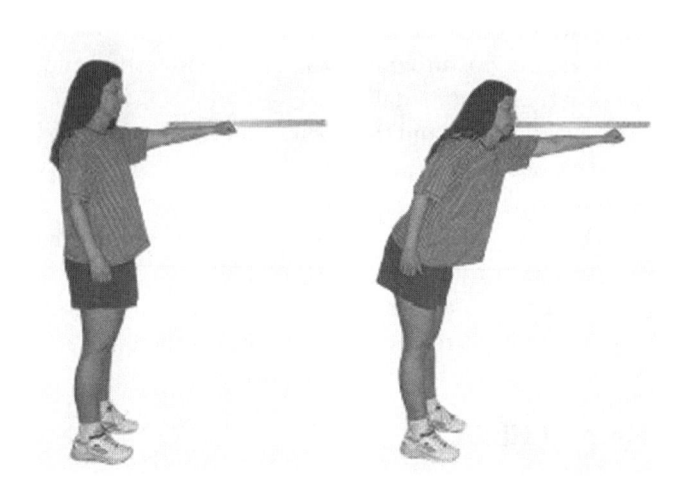

The functional reach test is a single-item test developed as a quick screen for balance problems in older adults.

Interpretation
A score of six or less indicates a significantly increased risk for falls.
A score between 6 and 10 inches indicates a moderate risk for falls.

Age related norms for the functional reach test

Age (years)	Men (in.)	Women (in.)
20–40	16.7 ± 1.9	14.6 ± 2.2
41–69	14.9 ± 2.2	13.8 ± 2.2
70–87	13.2 ± 1.6	10.5 ± 3.5

Requirements
The patient must be able to stand independently for at least 30 seconds without support, and be able to flex the shoulder to at least 90°.

Equipment and Set Up
A yard stick is attached to a wall at about shoulder height. The patient is positioned in front of this so that upon flexing the shoulder to 90°, an initial reading on the yard stick can be taken. The examiner takes a position 5 to 10 ft away from the patient, viewing the patient from the side.

Instructions
Position the patient close to the wall so that they may reach forward along the length of the yardstick. The patient is instructed to stand with feet–shoulder distance apart, then make a fist and raise the arm up so that it is parallel to the floor. At this time, the examiner takes an initial reading on the yard stick, usually spotting the knuckle of the third metacarpal. The patient is instructed to reach forward along the yardstick without moving the feet. Any reaching strategy is allowed, but the hand should remain in a fist. The therapist takes a reading on the yardstick of the farthest reach attained by the patient without taking a step. The initial reading is subtracted from the final to obtain the functional reach score.

Suggested Readings
Duncan PW, Studenski S, Chandler J, et al. Functional reach: Predictive validity in a sample of elderly male veterans. *J Gerontol.* 1992;47:M93.

Duncan PW, Weiner DK, Chadler J, et al. Functional reach: A new clinical measure of balance. *J Gerontol.* 1990;45:M192.

Mann GC, Whitney SL, Redfern MS, et al. Functional reach and single leg stance in patients with peripheral vestibular disorders. *J Vestib Res.* 1996;6:343.

Weiner DK, Bongiorni DR, Studenski SA, et al. Does functional reach improve with rehabilitation. *Arch Phys Med Rehab.* 1993;74:796.

Appendix 2: Tinetti's Balance and Mobility Assessment

I. Balance Tests

Initial Instructions: Subject is seated in a hard, armless chair. The following maneuvers are tested.

1. Sitting balance _____
   - 0 = Leans or slides in chair
   - 1 = Steady, safe

2. Arises _____
   - 0 = Unable without help
   - 1 = Able, uses arms to help
   - 2 = Able without using arms

3. Attempts to arise _____
   - 0 = Unable without help
   - 1 = Able, requires > 1 attempt
   - 2 Able to rise, 1 attempt

4. Immediate standing balance (first five seconds) _____
   - 0 = Unsteady (swaggers, moves feet, trunk sway)
   - 1 = Steady but uses walker or other support
   - 2 = Steady without walker or other support

5. Standing balance _____
   - 0 = Unsteady
   - 1 = Steady but wide stance (medial heels > 4 inches apart) and uses cane or other support
   - 2 = Narrow stance without support

6. Nudged _____
(subject at maximum stance position with feet as close together as possible, examiner pushes lightly on subject's sternum with palm of hand 3 times)
   - 0 = Begins to fall
   - 1 = Staggers, grabs, catches self
   - 2 = Steady

7. Eyes closed _____
(at maximum position, feet together)
   - 0 = Unsteady
   - 1 = Steady

8. Turning 360 degrees _____
   - 0 = Discontinuous steps
   - 1 = Unsteady (grabs, staggers)
   - 2 = Continuous

9. Sitting down _____
   - 0 = Unsafe (misjudged distance, falls into chair)
   - 1 = Uses arms or not a smooth motion
   - 2 = Safe, smooth motion

BALANCE SCORE: ___/16

II. Gait Tests

Initial Instructions: Subject stands with the examiner, walks down hallway or across room, first at usual pace, then back at rapid, but safe pace (usual walking aids).

10. Initiation of gait (immediately after told to go) _____
    - 0 = Any hesitancy or multiple attempts to start
    - 1 = No hesitancy

11. Step length and height
    a. Right swing foot _____
       - 0 = Does not pass left stance foot with step
       - 1 = Passes left stance foot
       - 0 = Right foot does not clear floor completely with step
       - 1 = Right foot completely clears floor.
    b. Left swing foot _____
       - 0 = Does not pass right stance foot with step
       - 1 = Passes right stance foot
       - 0 = Left foot does not clear floor completely with step
       - 1 = Left foot completely clears floor.

12. Step symmetry _____
    - 0 = Right and left step length not equal (estimate)
    - 1 = Right and left step appear equal

13. Step continuity _____
    - 0 = Stopping or discontinuity between steps
    - 1 = Steps appear continuous

14. Path _____
(Estimated in relation to floor tiles, 12-inch diameter; observe excursion of 1 foot over about 10 feet of the course)
    - 0 = Marked deviation
    - 1 = Mild/moderate deviation or uses walking aid
    - 2 = Straight without walking aid

(continued)

(*continued*)

15. Trunk
    0 = Marked sway or uses walking aid
    1 = No sway but flexion of knees or back pain or spreads arms out while walking
    2 = No sway, no flexion, no use of arms, and no use of walking aid

16. Walking stance
    0 = Heels apart wide base
    1 = Heels almost touching while walking.

GAIT SCORE: ___/12

BALANCE AND GAIT SCORE: ___/18

Risk Indicators

Risk of Falls

≤18—High
19–23—Moderate
≥24—Low

Source: This document can be found on the web at AROM.com—the web address for physical therapy.

Appendix 3: Berg Balance Scale

Description
14-item scale designed to measure balance of the older adult in a clinical setting.

Equipment Needed
Ruler, 2 standard chairs (one with arm rests, one without). Footstool or step, Stopwatch or wristwatch, 15-ft walkway.

Completion
Time: 15–20 minutes
Scoring: A five-point ordinal scale, ranging from 0–4. "0" indicates the lowest level of function and "4" the highest level of function. Total Score = 56
Interpretation: 41–56 = low fall risk
21–40 = medium fall risk
0–20 = high fall risk

Criterion Validity
"Authors support a cut off score of 45/56 for independent safe ambulation."
Riddle and Stratford, 1999, examined 45/56 cutoff validity and concluded:
- Sensitivity = 64% (Correctly predicts fallers)
- Specificity = 90% (Correctly predicts non-fallers)
- Riddle and Stratford encouraged a lower cut off score of 40/56 to assess fall risk.

Comments
Potential ceiling effect with higher level patients. Scale does not include gait items.

Norms
Lusardi MM. Functional performance in community living older adults. *J Geriatr Phys Ther.* 2004;26(3):14–22.
Table A1 Berg Balance Scale Scores: Means, Standard Deviations, and Confidence Intervals by Age, Gender, and Use of Assistive Device

Table A1. Berg Balance Scale Scores: Means, Standard Deviations, and Confidence Intervals by Age, Gender, and Use of Assistive Device

Age (years)	Group	N	Mean	SD	CI
60–69	Male	1	51.0	–	35.3–66.7
	Female	5	54.6	0.5	47.6–61.6
	Overall	6	54.0	1.5	52.4–55.6
70–79	Male	9	53.9	1.5	48.7–59.1
	Female	10	51.6	2.6	46.6–56.6
	Overall	19	52.7	2.4	51.5–53.8
80–89	Male	10	41.8	12.2	36.8–46.8
	Female	24	42.1	8.0	38.9–45.3
	No Device	24	46.3	4.2	44.1–48.5
	Device	10	31.7	10.0	28.3–35.1
	Overall	34	42.0	9.2	38.8–45.3
90–101	Male	2	40.0	1.4	28.9–51.1
	Female	15	36.9	9.7	32.8–40.9
	No Device	7	45	4.2	40.9–49.1
	Device	10	31.8	7.6	28.4–35.2
	Overall	17	37.2	9.1	32.5–41.9

Berg Balance Scale

Item description	*Score (0–4)*
Sitting to standing	_____
Standing unsupported	_____
Sitting unsupported	_____
Standing to sitting	_____
Transfers	_____
Standing with eyes closed	_____
Standing with feet together	_____
Reaching forward with outstretched arm	_____
Retrieving object from floor	_____
Turning to look behind	_____
Turning 360 degrees	_____
Placing alternate foot on stool	_____
Standing with one foot in front	_____
Standing on one foot	_____
Total	_____

(continued)

(*continued*)

General instructions

Please document each task and/or give instructions as written. When scoring, please *record the lowest response category that applies* for each item.

In most items, the subject is asked to maintain a given position for a specific time. Progressively more points are deducted if:

- The time or distance requirements are not met
- The subject's performance warrants supervision
- The subject touches an external support or receives assistance from the examiner

Subject should understand that they must maintain their balance while attempting the tasks. The choices of which leg to stand on or how far to reach are left to the subject. Poor judgment will adversely influence the performance and the scoring.

Equipment required for testing is a stopwatch or watch with a second hand, and a ruler or other indicator of 2, 5, and 10 inches. Chairs used during testing should be of reasonable height. Either a step or a stool of average step height may be used for item #12.

Berg Balance Scale

Sitting to standing

Instructions: Please stand up. Try not to use your hand for support.
- ( ) 4 Able to stand without using hands and stabilize independently
- ( ) 3 Able to stand independently using hands
- ( ) 2 Able to stand using hands after several tries
- ( ) 1 Needs minimal aid to stand or stabilize
- ( ) 0 Needs moderate or maximal assist to stand

Standing unsupported

Instructions: Please stand for two minutes without holding on.
- ( ) 4 Able to stand safely for 2 minutes
- ( ) 3 Able to stand 2 minutes with supervision
- ( ) 2 Able to stand 30 seconds unsupported
- ( ) 1 Needs several tries to stand 30 seconds unsupported
- ( ) 0 Unable to stand 30 seconds unsupported

If a subject is able to stand 2 minutes unsupported, score full points for sitting unsupported. Proceed to item #4.

Sitting with back unsupported but feet supported on floor or on a stool

Instructions: Please sit with arms folded for 2 minutes.
- ( ) 4 Able to sit safely and securely for 2 minutes
- ( ) 3 Able to sit 2 minutes under supervision
- ( ) 2 Able to able to sit 30 seconds
- ( ) 1 Able to sit 10 seconds
- ( ) 0 Unable to sit without support 10 seconds

Standing to sitting

Instructions: Please sit down.
- ( ) 4 Sits safely with minimal use of hands
- ( ) 3 Controls descent by using hands
- ( ) 2 Uses back of legs against chair to control descent
- ( ) 1 Sits independently but has uncontrolled descent
- ( ) 0 Needs assist to sit

Transfers

Instructions: Arrange chair(s) for pivot transfer. Ask subject to transfer one way toward a seat with armrests and one way toward a seat without armrests. You may use two chairs (one with and one without armrests) or a bed and a chair.
- ( ) 4 Able to transfer safely with minor use of hands
- ( ) 3 Able to transfer safely definite need of hands
- ( ) 2 Able to transfer with verbal cuing and/or supervision
- ( ) 1 Needs one person to assist
- ( ) 0 Needs two people to assist or supervise to be safe

Standing unsupported with eyes closed

Instructions: Please close your eyes and stand still for 10 seconds.
- ( ) 4 Able to stand 10 seconds safely
- ( ) 3 Able to stand 10 seconds with supervision
- ( ) 2 Able to stand 3 seconds
- ( ) 1 Unable to keep eyes closed 3 seconds but stays safely
- ( ) 0 Needs help to keep from falling

Standing unsupported with feet together

Instructions: Place your feet together and stand without holding on.
- ( ) 4 able to place feet together independently and stand 1 minute safely
- ( ) 3 able to place feet together independently and stand 1 minute with supervision
- ( ) 2 able to place feet together independently but unable to hold for 30 seconds
- ( ) 1 needs help to attain position but able to stand 15 seconds feet together
- ( ) 0 needs help to attain position and unable to hold for 15 seconds

Reaching forward with outstretched arm while standing

Instructions: Lift arm to 90 degrees. Stretch out your fingers and reach forward as far as you can. (Examiner places a ruler at the end of fingertips when arm is at 90 degrees. Fingers should not touch the ruler while reaching forward. The recorded measure is the distance forward that the fingers reach while the subject is in the most forward lean position. When possible, ask subject to use both arms when reaching to avoid rotation of the trunk.)

( ) 4 Can reach forward confidently 25 cm (10 inches)
( ) 3 Can reach forward 12 cm (5 inches)
( ) 2 Can reach forward 5 cm (2 inches)
( ) 1 Reaches forward but needs supervision
( ) 0 Loses balance while trying/requires external support

Pick up object from the floor from a standing position

Instructions: Pick up the shoe/slipper, which is placed in front of your feet.

( ) 4 Able to pick up slipper safely and easily
( ) 3 Able to pick up slipper but needs supervision
( ) 2 Unable to pick up but reaches 2–5 cm (1–2 inches) from slipper and keeps balance independently
( ) 1 Unable to pick up and needs supervision while trying
( ) 0 Unable to try/needs assist to keep from losing balance or falling

Turning to look behind over left and right shoulders while standing

Instructions: Turn to look directly behind you over toward the left shoulder. Repeat to the right. Examiner may pick an object to look at directly behind the subject to encourage a better twist turn.

( ) 4 Looks behind from both sides and weight shifts well
( ) 3 Looks behind one side only other side shows less weight shift
( ) 2 Turns sideways only but maintains balance
( ) 1 Needs supervision when turning
( ) 0 Needs assist to keep from losing balance or falling

Turn 360 degrees

Instructions: Turn completely around in a full circle. Pause. Then turn a full circle in the other direction.

( ) 4 Able to turn 360 degrees safely in 4 seconds or less
( ) 3 Able to turn 360 degrees safely only one side in 4 seconds or less
( ) 2 Able to turn 360 degrees safely but slowly
( ) 1 Needs close supervision or verbal cuing
( ) 0 Needs assistance while turning

Place alternate foot on step or stool while standing unsupported

instructions: Place each foot alternately on the step/stool. Continue until each foot has touched the step/stool four times.

( ) 4 Able to stand independently and safely and complete 8 steps in 20 seconds
( ) 3 Able to stand independently and complete 8 steps in >20 seconds
( ) 2 Able to complete 4 steps without aid with supervision
( ) 1 Able to complete >2 steps needs minimal assist
( ) 0 Needs assistance to keep from falling/unable to try

Standing unsupported one foot in front

Instructions (demonstrate to subject): Place one foot directly in front of the other. If you feel that you cannot place your foot directly in front, try to step far enough ahead that the heel of your forward foot is ahead of the toes of the other foot. (To score 3 points, the length of the step should exceed the length of the other foot and the width of the stance should approximate the subject's normal stride width.)

( ) 4 Able to place foot tandem independently and hold 30 seconds
( ) 3 Able to place foot ahead independently and hold 30 seconds
( ) 2 Able to take small step independently and hold 30 seconds
( ) 1 Needs help to step but can hold 15 seconds
( ) 0 Loses balance while stepping or standing

Standing on one leg

Instructions: Stand on one leg as long as you can without holding on.

( ) 4 Able to lift leg independently and hold >10 seconds
( ) 3 Able to lift leg independently and hold 5–10 seconds
( ) 2 Able to lift leg independently and hold ≥ 3 seconds
( ) 1 Tries to lift leg unable to hold 3 seconds but remains standing independently.
( ) 0 Unable to try or needs assist to prevent fall

TOTAL SCORE = ___/56

Appendix 4: Fullerton Advanced Balance Scale

1. Stand with feet together and eyes closed
( ) 0   Unable to obtain the correct standing position independently
( ) 1   Able to obtain the correct standing position independently but unable to maintain the position or keep the eyes closed for more than 10 seconds
( ) 2   Able to maintain the correct standing position with eyes closed for more than 10 seconds but less than 30 seconds
( ) 3   Able to maintain the correct standing position with eyes closed for 30 seconds but requires close supervision
( ) 4   Able to maintain the correct standing position safely with eyes closed for 30 seconds

2. Reach forward with outstretched arm to retrieve an object (pencil) held at shoulder height
( ) 0   Unable to reach the pencil without taking more than two steps
( ) 1   Able to reach the pencil but needs to take two steps
( ) 2   Able to reach the pencil but needs to take one step
( ) 3   Can reach the pencil without moving the feet but requires supervision
( ) 4   Can reach the pencil safely and independently without moving the feet

3. Turn 360 degrees in right and left directions
( ) 0   Needs manual assistance while turning
( ) 1   Needs close supervision or verbal cueing while turning
( ) 2   Able to turn 360 degrees but takes more than four steps in both directions
( ) 3   Able to turn 360 degrees but unable to complete in four steps or fewer in one direction
( ) 4   Able to turn 360 degrees safely taking four steps or fewer in both directions

4. Step up onto and over a 6-inch (15 cm) bench
( ) 0   Unable to step up onto the bench without loss of balance or manual assistance
( ) 1   Able to step up onto the bench with leading leg but trailing leg contacts the bench or swings around the bench during the swing-through phase in both directions
( ) 2   Able to step up onto the bench with leading leg, but trailing leg contacts the bench or swings around the bench during the swing-through phase in one direction
( ) 3   Able to correctly complete the step up and over in both directions but requires close supervision in one or both directions
( ) 4   Able to correctly complete the step up and over in both directions safely and independently

5. Tandem walk
( ) 0   Unable to complete 10 steps independently
( ) 1   Able to complete the 10 steps with more than five interruptions
( ) 2   Able to complete the 10 steps with three to five interruptions
( ) 3   Able to complete the 10 steps with one to two interruptions
( ) 4   Able to complete the 10 steps independently and with no interruptions

6. Stand on one leg
( ) 0   Unable to try or needs assistance to prevent falling
( ) 1   Able to lift leg independently but unable to maintain position for more than 5 seconds
( ) 2   Able to lift leg independently and maintain position for more than 5 but less than or equal to 12 seconds
( ) 3   Able to lift leg independently and maintain position for more than 12 but less than 20 seconds
( ) 4   Able to lift leg independently and maintain position for the full 20 seconds

7. Stand on foam with eyes closed
( ) 0   Unable to step onto foam or maintain standing position independently with eyes open
( ) 1   Able to step onto foam independently and maintain standing position but unable or unwilling to close eyes
( ) 2   Able to step onto foam independently and maintain standing position with eyes closed for 10 seconds or less
( ) 3   to step onto foam independently and maintain standing position with eyes closed for more than 10 seconds but less than 20 seconds

( ) 4   Able to step onto foam independently and maintain standing position with eyes closed for 20 seconds

Do not perform test item 8 if score is 2 or lower on test item 4. Also do not introduce test item 8 if test item 4 was not performed safely and/or it is contraindicated to perform this test-item (review test administration instructions for contraindications). Give test item 8 a score of 0 and proceed to test item 9.

8. Two-footed jump
( ) 0   Unable to attempt or attempts to initiate jump but one or both feet do not leave the floor
( ) 1   Able to initiate jump with both feet but one foot either leaves the floor or lands before the other
( ) 2   Able to perform jump with both feet but unable to jump farther than the length of feet
( ) 3   Able to perform jump with both feet and achieve a distance greater than the length of feet
( ) 4   Able to perform jump with both feet and achieve a distance greater than twice the length of feet

Evaluating risk for falls

Long Form Fullerton Advanced Balance (FAB) scale Cut-Off Score: ≤ 25/40 Points
Short-Form Fullerton Advanced Balance (FAB) scale Cut-Off Score: ≤ 9/16 Points

Evaluation of Depression

Kevin M. Means MD

Description

- Many older patients in the outpatient rehabilitation setting with somatic complaints, such as fatigue or pain, and problems that are difficult to diagnose or successfully treat, may be depressed.
- Depressed older rehabilitation inpatients may have symptoms that are masked by communication or physical impairment.
- Psychiatric consultation may not always be available or necessary.
- Numerous screening measures have been specifically designed to detect depression in older patients.
- Physicians can select screening assessments that are appropriate for their patients and clinical setting, and for monitoring change in patients being treated for depression.
- Self-report measures that can be quickly completed and scored are available.
- Interviewer-administered assessments that require more time may be necessary for cognitively impaired patients.

Table 1 summarizes information on seven commonly used and validated assessments for screening in adults aged above 60.

Table 1 Depression Screening Assessments

Instrument	Spanish version available?	# of items	Time to administer (in min)
GDS	Yes	30	10–15
GDS-short	Yes	15	5–10
GDS-5	No	5	Less than 5
CSDD	No	19	10 for patient, 20 with caregiver
BDI	Yes	21	5–10
CES-D	Yes	20	5–10
Zung DRS	No	20	5–10

Assessment Instruments

Geriatric Depression Scale (not shown)

- A 30-item assessment specifically developed for use in cognitively intact geriatric patients; contains fewer somatic items than other instruments; and can be self-administered.
- A 15-item shortened version of the Geriatric Depression Scale (GDS-short) has been validated and requires less administration time.
- More recently, an even shorter five-item version (GDS-5) has also been developed and used.
- The GDS, GDS-short, and GDS-5 formats frame questions within the past week and require a simple "yes" or "no" response for easy comprehension.

GDS-short

Choose the best answer for how you have felt over the past week:

Are you basically satisfied with your life? Yes/*No*
Have you dropped many of your activities and interests? *Yes*/No
Do you feel that your life is empty? *Yes*/No
Do you often get bored? *Yes*/No
Are you in good spirits most of the time? Yes/*No*
Are you afraid that something bad is going to happen to you? *Yes*/No
Do you feel happy most of the time? *Yes*/No
Do you often feel helpless? *Yes*/No
Do you prefer to stay at home, rather than going out and doing new things? *Yes*/No
Do you feel you have more problems with memory than most? *Yes*/No
Do you think it is wonderful to be alive now? Yes/*No*
Do you feel pretty worthless the way you are now? *Yes*/No
Do you feel full of energy? Yes/*No*
Do you feel that your situation is hopeless? *Yes*/No
Do you think that most people are better off than you are? *Yes*/No

Answers indicating depression are bold and italicized and count for 1 point each; a score of 5 to 9 indicates a strong probability of depression; a score of 10 or more almost always indicates depression.

GDS-5 scale
Positive screen is indicated by two or more bold and italicized responses.

Are you basically satisfied with your life? Yes/**No**
Do you often get bored? **Yes**/No
Do you often feel helpless? **Yes**/No
Do you prefer to stay at home rather than going out and doing new things? **Yes**/No
Do you feel pretty worthless the way you are now? **Yes**/No

Cornell scale for depression in dementia
- A 19-item interviewer-administered assessment. Rate the patient over the past week in the following areas:
  A. Mood-related signs:
    1. Anxiety feelings (expression, ruminations, worrying)
    2. Sadness (sad expression, sad voice, tearfulness)
    3. Lack ability to enjoy pleasant events and persons
    4. Irritability (easily annoyed, short tempered)
  B. Behavioral disturbances:
    1. Agitation (restlessness, handwringing, hair pulling)
    2. Retardation (slow movements, slow speech, slow reactions)
    3. Multiple (new) physical complaints (indigestion, pains, hyperventilation, etc.)
    4. Acute loss of interest in usual activities
  C. Physical signs:
    1. Appetite loss
    2. Weight loss
    3. Lack of energy (recent easy fatigability or inability to sustain activities)
  D. Cyclic functions
    1. Diurnal (day or night) variation of mood
    2. Difficulty falling asleep (later than usual)
    3. Multiple awakenings during sleep
    4. Early morning awakenings (earlier than usual)
  E. Ideational disturbances:
    1. Suicide (has suicidal wishes or makes suicide attempt)
    2. Self-deprecation (self-blame, poor self-esteem, feelings of failure)
    3. Pessimism (anticipation of the worst)
    4. Mood-congruent delusions (delusions of poverty, illness, or loss)
- The CSDD is more appropriate than GDS to assess depressive symptoms in cognitively impaired patients, who may lack insight to provide reliable responses.
- Validated with both cognitively intact and impaired patients
- Easy to administer and uses responses from both the patient and the primary caregiver; requires more time to administer; however, both tests are more appropriate than self-report instruments for cognitively impaired older patients.
- Scoring (based on symptoms/signs occurring during the week prior to testing): a = unable to evaluate; 0 = absent; 1 = mild or intermittent; 2 = severe
  - The item scores are added. Scores above 10 indicate a probable major depression.
  - Scores above 18 indicate a definite major depression.
  - Scores below 6 as a rule are associated with the absence of significant depressive symptoms.
- Higher scores are not diagnostic of depression, but indicate a greater need for further evaluation.

Beck depression inventory (not shown)
- The BDI (now replaced by the BDI®-II) is a 21-item test that is either self-administered or verbally administered by staff for the assessment of depression symptoms and their intensity. Questions are based on the activities 2 weeks prior to the assessment.
- A new seven-item version of the BDI®-II is now available—the BDI®-FastScreen.
  - The BDI®-II and the BDI®-FastScreen are available for purchase at http://psychcorp.pearsonassessments.com/pai/ca/cahome.htm

Center for epidemiological studies depression scale
- Rates depression symptoms experienced over the past week
- Recommended for cognitively intact older adults
- Scoring: Indicates how often each symptom was experienced during the past week; rarely or none of the time (less than 1 day); some or a little of the time (1–2 days); occasionally/moderate amount of time (3–4 days); and most or all of the time (5–7 days). Range varies from rarely = 0 to most or all = 4; with maximum total score = 60.
- Higher scores indicate more depression symptoms.
- Four items (#4, 8, 12, and 16) are reverse scored as follows:
  - Rarely or none of the time (less than 1 day) = 3
  - Some or little of the time (1–2 days) = 2
  - Occasionally or more moderate amount of the time (3–4 days) = 1
  - More or all of the time (5–7 days) = 0
- Once you have assigned a value for each item, compute a total, adding the values for each of the 20 items. The resulting score should range between 0 and 60. Do

not compute a total if there is more than one answer missing.
- Questions:
  1. I was bothered by things that usually do not bother me.
  2. I did not feel like eating; my appetite was poor.
  3. I felt that I could not shake off the blues even with help from my family or friends.
  4. I felt I was just as good as other people.
  5. I had trouble keeping my mind on what I was doing.
  6. I felt depressed.
  7. I felt that everything I did was an effort.
  8. I felt hopeful about the future.
  9. I thought my life had been a failure.
  10. I felt fearful.
  11. My sleep was restless.
  12. I was happy.
  13. I talked less than usual.
  14. I felt lonely.
  15. People were unfriendly.
  16. I enjoyed life.
  17. I had crying spells.
  18. I felt sad.
  19. I felt that people dislike me.
  20. I could not get "going."

Zung Self-Rating Depression Scale (not shown)
- A 20-item, self-administered survey about depression symptoms
- Answers were scored on a 1 to 4 Likert scale; minimal: none or little of the time; severe: most or all of the time.
- Raw score is converted to a 100-point scale; score less than 50: normal; score less than 60: mild depression; score 60 to 70: moderate or marked major depression; score less than 70: severe or extreme major depression.
- Available at http://healthnet.umassmed.edu/mhealth/ZungSelfRatedDepressionScale.pdf

Helpful Hints
- Depression screening measures do not diagnose depression. They do confirm the presence of depression symptoms and indicate the severity of symptoms.
- All measures have a statistically predetermined cutoff score at which depression symptoms are considered significant.
- When using depression screening instruments with elderly patients, the presence and degree of cognitive impairment and visual deficits should be considered.
- Some depression screening instruments have questionable validity on patients with a minimental state examination score of 15 or less because some of the symptoms of depression and dementia are similar, and because people with dementia may have difficulty explaining how they feel.
- For aged patients with depression who present with unexplained somatic symptoms and may deny sadness or loss of pleasure, clinical judgment may be more helpful than screening measures.

Suggested Readings
Hoyt MT, Alessi CA, Harker JO, et al. Development and testing of a five item version of the Geriatric Depression Scale. *J Am Geriatr Soc*. 1999;47:873–878.

Radloff LS. The CES-D scale: A self-report depression scale for research in the general population. *Appl Psychol Meas*. 1977;1:385–401.

Sharp LK, Lipsky MS. Screening for depression across the lifespan: A review of measures for use in primary care settings. *Am Fam Physician*. 2002;66:1001–1009.

Sheikh JI, Yesavage A. Geriatric Depression Scale (GDS): Recent evidence and development of a shorter version. In: Brink TL, ed. *Clinical Gerontology: A Guide to Assessment and Intervention*. New York, NY: Haworth; 1986:165–172.

Evaluation of Function

Jamie Harrison MD

Description
A person with functional impairment has difficulty performing, or requires assistance by another person in performing, activities of daily living (ADLs) or instrumental activities of daily living (IADLs). Having the ability to perform special tests that assess functional capabilities in older persons allows for successful planning and delivery of needed care for these persons.

ADLs—The Essential Activities of Self-Care
- Bathing and showering
- Bowel and bladder management
- Dressing
- Eating
- Feeding
- Functional mobility
- Personal hygiene and grooming

IADLs—More Complex Tasks Required for Independent Living in the Community
- Administering medication
- Grocery shopping
- Preparing meals
- Using the telephone
- Driving and transportation
- Handling finances
- Housekeeping and laundry
- Pet care

Epidemiology
- Functional impairment increases with age.
- One half of community-dwelling persons living in the United States and above the age of 65 have limitations in their ability to perform ADLs.
- Approximately 15% of persons above age 75 are home bound.

Natural History
- As one's ability to perform ADLs and IADLs declines, the risk of adverse outcomes such as depression, falls, poor hospital outcomes, institutionalization, and death increases.
- In contrast, as one's number of medical conditions increases, there is not always a direct decline in the ability to perform ADLs and IADLs.

ADL Rating Scales
- Katz ADL Scale
- Lawton IADL Scale
- Barthel Index
- Physical Self-Maintenance Scale
- Stanford Health Assessment Questionnaire (HAQ)
- Functional Independence Measure

Functional Assessments
- Gait and balance
  - "Get Up and Go" test
  - Functional reach test
- Nutrition
  - Weight
  - Body mass index (BMI)
  - Mini Nutritional Assessment Short Form (MNA-SF)
- Mood and depression
  - Yesavage Geriatric Depression Scale
- Memory and cognition
  - Folstein Minimental State Questionnaire (MMSE)
- Home environment and home layout
- Vision screening
  - Snellen acuity chart
- Hearing screening
  - Whisper test
  - Formal audiometric testing

Suggested Readings
Fleming KC, Evans JM, Weber DC, et al. Practical functional assessment of elderly persons: A primary-care approach. *Mayo Clin Proc.* 1995;70:890–910.

Hazzard William, Blass JP, Halter JB, et al. *Principles of Geriatric Medicine and Gerontology.* 5th ed. New York, NY: McGraw-Hill; 2003.

Leukoff SE, Chee YK, and Noguchi S. *Aging in Good Health Multidisciplinary Perspectives.* New York, NY: Springer; 2001.

Spirduso WW, Francis KL, MacRae PG. *Physical Dimensions of Aging.* 2nd ed. Champaign, IL: Human Kinetics; 2005.

Evaluation of Osteoporosis: Detection of Significant Bone Loss

Vikki Stefans MD

Detection and Diagnosis of Significant Bone Loss

- The World Health Organization defines osteopenia as a bone mineralization *T*-score between −1.0 and −2.5 standard deviations and osteoporosis as a *T*-score −2.5 standard deviations or lower. The *T*-score is a comparison to the healthy young adult female at peak bone mass (age 18–30).
- *Z*-scores, comparing age-matched individuals, are more appropriate for pediatric assessments, where weight- or size-adjusted norms for age are more applicable to actual fracture risk.
- *T*-scores are most strongly correlated with fracture risk in the elderly.
- Current recommendations for screening the elderly have recently been expanded by the National Osteoporosis Foundation (NOF) and the United States Preventive Services Task Force (USPSTF) to include younger women (age 50 or at the age of menopause) with the risk equivalent of the average 65-year-old Caucasian female with no additional risk factors, which is about 9.3% for the subsequent 10 years. This can be assessed via the FRAX or similar tool, available at the website: www.shef.ac.uk/FRAX or www.nof.org.
- Routine screening for men at average risk has not been specifically recommended.
- The preferred method of screening and measurement is dual energy X-ray absorptiometry (DEXA); alternatives such as quantitative computerized tomography (QCT) scan and peripheral ultrasound exist, but may not correlate well. This is particularly true of ultrasound.
- Applicability of serum and urine markers of bone collagen turnover (serum and urinary c- and n-telopeptides) has not been established for screening purposes in the general population.
- DEXA involves a low radiation dose (0.08–4.6 microSv), which compares favorably to standard lateral radiographs or QCT (25–360 microSv).
- Densitometry can be repeated after 9 to 24 months to detect a meaningful change in response to treatment.

Suggested Readings

U.S. Preventive Services Task Force. Screening for osteoporosis: Recommendations from the U.S. Preventive Services Task Force [published online ahead of print January 17, 2011]. *Ann Intern Med.* 2011;154:1–40. http://www.annals.org/content/154/5/356.full?sid=c8552006-4b5c-4b8f-bc31-4a21f847807b.

NOF clinician's guide to prevention and treatment of osteoporosis. http://.nof.org/sites/default/files/pdfs/NOF_ClinicanGuide2009_v7.pdf

II

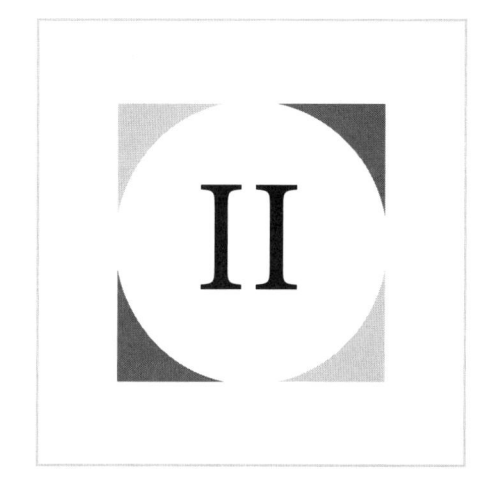

Organ System Diseases and Disorders

Anemia

Konstantinos Arnaoutakis MD

Description
Anemia is defined as a reduction in the number of circulating red cells below the normal range. The usual criteria are hemoglobin under 12 g/dL or hematocrit under 36% for women, and hemoglobin under 14 g/dL or hematocrit under 41% in men.

Etiology/Types
- The three most common causes of anemia are as follows:
  - Blood loss
  - Excessive red cell destruction (hemolytic anemia)
  - Impaired red cell formation
- Anemia can be also classified by morphology:
  - Microcytic
  - Macrocytic
  - Normocytic
- The most common causes of anemia in elder community dwellers are as follows:
  - Iron deficiency anemia
  - Anemia of chronic disease
  - Megaloblastic anemia
  - Unexplained anemia of the elderly

Epidemiology
- The prevalence of anemia in people aged 61 and 75 years is 8% and 25%, respectively.
- Prevalence increases by 16% to 26% for patients aged above 75.

Pathogenesis
- Depends on the underlying cause
- The most common pathogenesis is decreased red blood cell (RBC) production (hypoproliferative anemia).
- The mechanisms of the unexplained anemias remain elusive. Possible causes include
  - Failure of precursor cells
  - Decline of erythropoietin and testosterone
  - Inflammation
  - Declining renal function
  - Myelodysplastic syndromes

Risk Factors
- Nutritional deficiencies (e.g., iron, vitamins B_{12}, and folate)
- Renal disease
- Hypothyroidism
- Gastrectomy
- Alcohol abuse
- Family history of anemia

Clinical Features
Symptoms of anemia are a function of the following:
- Severity
- Rapidity of onset
- Age of the patient
  Acute clinical manifestations include those typical of hypovolemia such as
- Pallor
- Tachycardia
- Hypotension
- Visual impairment
- These symptoms require urgent attention.
  Other symptoms include
- Shortness of breath
- Palpitations
- Ankle edema
- Angina
- Dizziness and confusion
- Depression or apathy
- Agitation
- Headache
- Fatigue

Diagnosis

Differential diagnosis
- Bleeding
- Hemolysis
- Iron deficiency
- Vitamin B_{12} deficiency
- Folic acid deficiency
- Anemia of chronic disease
- Hypothyroidism

- Chronic liver disease
- Chronic renal disease
- Myelodysplasia

History
- Time course of onset
- Potential source of blood loss
- History of colonoscopy
- Transfusion history
- Past blood count measurements
- Complete list of medications, including herbal remedies and supplements
- History of alcohol use
- Family history
- Dietary habits

Examination
- Pallor, especially the color of the buccal and lingual mucosae and the nail beds
- Integument:
  - Tongue, often smooth and pale
  - Angular cheilosis (i.e., cracks/lesions in the corners of the mouth)
  - Koilonychias (i.e., abnormal fingernails; spoon shaped)
- Cardiac: forceful apical pulse, wide pulse pressure, tachycardia, flow murmurs

Laboratory tests
- Complete blood count (CBC) with special attention to mean corpuscular volume (MCV), and to white cell and platelet counts
- Reticulocyte count
- Peripheral smear, to evaluate for dysplasia/signs of myelodysplasia
- Blood urea nitrogen (BUN), creatinine, and urinalysis (to evaluate for occult blood loss)
- Serum iron, total iron binding capacity, and ferritin
- Serum B_{12} and folate
- Bilirubin and lactate dehydrogenase (LDH)
- Occult blood stool test

Pitfalls
- Iron deficiency is a symptom and not a disease. Physicians should ask why the patient is iron deficient.

Red flags
- A bone marrow biopsy may be indicated for worsening or unexplained anemias, especially if associated with other cytopenias.

Treatment

Medical
Depends on the cause of anemia:
- Iron supplementation for iron-deficiency anemia
- Erythropoietin for anemia of renal disease
- Red cell transfusion may be needed for some patients when anemia is severe, acute, or if significant symptoms are present, especially in the face of limited cardiac reserve.

Surgical
- Rarely needed for acute bleeding

Consults
- Hematology

Complications of treatment
- Potential side effects from blood transfusion include
  - Volume overload
  - Urticaria
  - Anaphylaxis
  - Infection
  - Hemolysis
  - Fever
  - Iron overload

Prognosis
- Depends on the cause. However, the presence of anemia is associated with impaired functional and cognitive performance.
- Mortality in older anemic patients is approximately twice that of older nonanemic patients.

Helpful Hints
- With the data obtained from one tube of blood (i.e., CBC, MCV, reticulocytes, and peripheral smear), anemia can be well characterized.

Suggested Readings
Arenson C, Busby-Whitehead J, Brummel-Smith K, et al. *Reichel's Care of the Elderly: Clinical Aspects of Aging*. 6th ed. New York, NY: Cambridge University Press; 2009.

Cashen A, Wildes T, eds. *The Washington Manual Hematology and Oncology Subspecialty Consult*. 2nd ed. Philadelphia, PA: Lippincott Williams & Wilkins; 2008.

Hillman R, Ault K, Leporrier M, et al. *Hematology in Clinical Practice*. 5th ed. New York, NY: Lange/McGraw-Hill Professional; 2010.

Tallis R, Fillit H. *Brocklehurst's Textbook of Geriatric Medicine and Gerontology*. 6th ed. London: Churchill Livingstone; 2003.

Blood Disorders

Issam Makhoul MD

Description
Contrary to a commonly held belief, physiologic changes related to aging in the hematologic system are rare, if any.

Hematologic changes associated with normal aging
- The marrow cellularity and the number of stem cells decline, while the prevalence of myeloid dysplasia and coagulation markers (D-dimers in the circulation) increase
- Incorporation of iron (Fe) in the elderly marrow cells is less responsive to erythropoietin
- Hemoglobin and hematocrit values decline slightly but remain within normal limits
- Mean corpuscular volume (MCV) increases slightly
- Red blood cell (RBC) content of 2,3-diphosphoglycerate decreases
- RBC osmotic fragility increases
- No significant changes are noted in white blood cells (WBC) or platelets

Etiology/Types

Red blood cell
- Decreased (anemia)
  - Bleeding or hemolysis
  - Iron-deficiency anemia (IDA)
  - Anemia of chronic disease (ACD)
  - Nutritional deficiencies (B_{12} and folate deficiency)
  - Myelodysplastic syndrome (MDS)
- Increased
  - Polycythemia Vera (PV)

White blood cell
- Decreased
  - Drugs
  - B_{12} or folate deficiency
  - MDS
  - Acute leukemia (AL); acute myeloid leukemia—(AML); acute lymphoid leukemia—(ALL)
- Increased
  - Infection and inflammation
  - Chronic myeloid leukemia (CML; myeloid cells)
  - Chronic lymphocytic leukemia (CLL; lymphocytes)

Platelets
- Decreased
  - B_{12} or folate deficiency
  - Immune thrombocytopenic purpura (ITP)
  - Drugs
- Increased
  - Essential thrombocythemia (ET)

Plasma cells
- Increased
  - Multiple myeloma (MM)

Bleeding and hypercoagulability
- Bleeding is often associated with drugs such as antiplatelet agents (Aspirin, Plavix), Coumadin, or heparin.
- Hypercoagulability is often acquired due to blood vessel injury and a bed-ridden state.

Epidemiology
- Anemia is common in the elderly, with increasing incidence with age from 1 in 10 between ages 65 and 75 to 1 in 4 after age 85.
- Males are more commonly affected than females and blacks more commonly than whites.
- IDA and ACD are the most common causes of anemia in the elderly.
- MDS and polypharmacy are the most common causes of leucopenia and thrombocytopenia in the elderly.
- CLL is the most common cause of chronic leukemia in the elderly.
- More than 50% of patients diagnosed with AL and 70% of those who die of AL are 65 or older.
- MM is a disease of the elderly, as most patients are older than 65.

Pathogenesis
- Anemia in the elderly is multifactorial
  - Nutritional (decreased intake or absorption of B_{12}, folate, and Fe)
  - Blood loss
  - Malabsorption of Fe due to celiac disease
  - Multiple comorbidities (chronic illnesses, inflammation)
  - Polypharmacy

- MDS is believed to be related to life-long exposure to different environmental factors that lead to DNA damage and ultimately to the emergence of leukemia.
- The cause of CML is a reciprocal translocation between chromosomes 9 and 22, leading to the formation of the fusion gene BCR-ABL.
- The causes of CLL and MM are not known, but the weakening of the immune system with age may allow for the survival of aberrant clones of the progenitor lymphoid cells that ultimately lead to these disorders.

Risk Factors
- Poor nutrition
- Multiple comorbidities (renal, heart, or liver failure; chronic infections; chronic inflammatory diseases—rheumatoid arthritis, etc.)
- Polypharmacy

Clinical Features

Anemia
- Asymptomatic, if mild
- Decreased oxygenation
  - Exertional dyspnea
  - Dyspnea at rest
  - Fatigue
  - Bounding pulses
  - Lethargy, confusion
- Decreased blood volume
  - Fatigue
  - Muscle cramps
  - Postural dizziness
  - Syncope

Neurologic symptoms of B_{12} deficiency
May occur without anemia or with mild anemia
- Paresthesias of the fingers and toes
- Reduced vibration sense (256 Hz) and proprioception
- Ataxia (combined system disease)
- Perversion of taste and smell
- Optic atrophy
- Dementia, memory loss, and depression
- "Megaloblastic Madness"—paranoid schizophrenia

Leucopenia
- Asymptomatic, if mild
- Frequent infections, if severe

Platelets
- Asymptomatic
- Bleeding (usually mucocutaneous with purpura or petechiae), if severely decreased
- Thrombosis if elevated

Coagulation disorders
- Hemoptysis, upper or lower gastrointestinal bleeding, hematuria
- Ecchymoses, nose bleeds
- PV may lead to visceral and peripheral vein thromboses or arterial thromboembolic events.

Multiple myeloma
- Bone pain
- Hypercalcemia
- Pathologic fractures
- Renal insufficiency

Natural History
- If untreated, anemia will have deep consequences in the elderly (decreased functional status in general, with multiple comorbidities).
- Severe anemia by itself may increase the mortality of the elderly.
- Neurologic symptoms associated with B_{12} deficiency may not regress, despite correcting B_{12} levels.
- CML, if untreated, progresses from a chronic phase, to an accelerated phase, then to a blast crisis over the course of 2 to 3 years.
- CLL is usually an indolent disease and may remain stable for years. Richter's transformation, bulky lymphadenopathy, severe anemia, or thrombocytopenia may occur and require treatment.
- AL progresses toward death in a few weeks to months.
- Bleeding disorders may lead to chronic blood loss and IDA if mild, or to death within hours to days, if severe.
- MM leads to bone and kidney disease and multiple cytopenias. Hypercalcemia is a common complication of MM.

Diagnosis

History and examination
- Full drug history and physical comorbidities

Testing
- Complete blood count (CBC)/differential/platelets, reticulocyte, and peripheral blood smear
- Fe/total iron binding capacity (TIBC), ferritin, and soluble transferrin receptor
- B_{12}, folate (RBC level). In borderline cases, methylmalonic acid (MMA; elevated only in B_{12} deficiency), and serum homocysteine (elevated in both)
- Chemistry panel (creatinine clearance)
- Fecal occult blood testing
- Serum erythropoietin, thyroid stimulating hormone (TSH), serum testosterone, erythrocyte sedimentation

rate (ESR), C-reactive protein (CRP), interleukin-6 (IL-6)
- Bone marrow aspiration and biopsy, cytogenetics, and JAK2 mutation
- Serum protein electrophoresis (SPEP), urine protein electrophoresis (UPEP), and serum protein immunofixation
- Prothrombin time (PT), partial thromboplastin time (PTT), fibrinogen, and platelet function tests
- Specific magnetic resonance imaging (MRI) abnormalities of B_{12} deficiency: contrast enhancement of the posterior and lateral columns of the spinal cord, mainly of the cervical and upper thoracic segments

Red Flags
- Fe deficiency in the elderly should always prompt an evaluation for a source of blood loss, which very commonly is a gastrointestinal source.
- Hemoptysis and hematuria should always prompt an investigation for a primary cancer of the lung or urinary tract, respectively.

Treatment

Medical
- Nutritional deficiencies should be corrected (B_{12}, 1000 mcg daily sublingual; ferrous sulfate 325 mg three times a day × 2 months, then twice daily until ferritin exceeds 50 mcg/L; folate 1 mg a day)
- Recombinant human erythropoietin is very effective in treating anemia related to chronic kidney disease.
- ACD, treatment of the cause
- MDS: referral to hematology for demethylating agents, transfusion support, and Fe chelation
- CML: imatinib is the treatment of choice
- CLL: if mild and early stage, no need for treatment. Treatment is indicated only if there is transformation, significant anemia or thrombocytopenia, or bulky lymphadenopathy
- AL: referral to hematology for induction chemotherapy and supportive measures
- MM: referral to hematology for induction and autologous bone marrow transplant.
- PV: referral to hematology for phlebotomy (hematocrit goal less than 45% for males, less than 42% for females)
- Bleeding disorders: anticoagulant agents should be discontinued, if possible. Clotting times should be corrected with fresh frozen plasma and vitamin K (in the case of Warfarin toxicity).

Consults
- Hematology
- Nephrology for renal insufficiency
- Rheumatology for chronic connective tissue diseases
- Gastroenterology for evaluation of a gastrointestinal bleeding source and a small bowel biopsy (celiac disease)

Complications of treatment
- None for nutritional replacements
- Multiple end-organ damage from chemotherapy
- Side effects from medications

Prognosis
- Nutritional deficiencies are easily corrected, but B_{12} deficiency-related neurologic symptoms may persist.
- The prognosis of MDS is variable, and some patients progress to AL. The prognosis of CML and CLL is excellent.
- The prognosis of PV is very good when phlebotomy is pursued regularly after reaching the hematocrit goal.
- MM has a good prognosis in general, but there are forms that progress quickly to death.

Helpful Hints
- Anemia in the elderly is not a part of normal aging.
- Look always for correctable causes, such as nutritional deficiencies (one third of the causes of anemia in the elderly), kidney failure, and polypharmacy.

Suggested Readings
Balducci L, Ershler W, De Gaetano G. *Blood Disorders in the Elderly*. 1st ed. New York, NY: Cambridge University Press; 2008.

Guralnik JM, Eisenstaedt RS, Ferrucci L, et al. Prevalence of anemia in persons 65 years and older in the United States: Evidence for a high rate of unexplained anemia. *Blood*. 2004;104(8):2263–2268.

Zakai NA, Katz R, Hirsch C, et al. A prospective study of anemia status, hemoglobin concentration, and mortality in an elderly cohort. The Cardiovascular Health Study. *Arch Intern Med*. 2005;165:2214–2220.

Cancer

Gayle R. Spill MD ■ Gail L. Gamble MD

Description
Geriatric cancer rehabilitation can be defined as any rehabilitation assessment and intervention addressing the physical, cognitive, psychological, and social issues that can cause functional impairment in geriatric patients diagnosed with cancer.

Etiology/Types

Direct tumor involvement
- Pathologic fracture
- Spinal cord compression
- Brain metastases

Tumor obstruction of organ systems
- Lymphedema
- Hydrocephalus
- Urinary retention
- Bowel obstruction

Remote tumor effects
- Paraneoplastic syndromes
- Hypercalcemia

Treatment related
- Chemotherapy-induced peripheral neuropathy (CIPN)
- Radiation myelitis
- Chemotherapy-related cardiotoxicity
- Surgical effects

Other cancer-related issues
- Cancer-related fatigue
- Deconditioning
- Debility
- Psychological and emotional distress

Epidemiology
- Cancer incidence increases significantly with age.
- In all 60% of all malignancies occur in people aged above 65.
- In all 65% of people with cancer live 5 years or more after diagnosis.
- Approximately 50% of geriatric cancer patients have difficulty with basic activities of daily living, and 75% have difficulty with instrumental activities of daily living.
- Those aged 70 years or above with cancer require an average of 10 hours of informal caregiver support per week compared to less than 7 hours per week for those without cancer.

Pathogenesis
A combination of pre-existing functional problems; age-related medical comorbidities; cancer type, location, and grade; treatment effects; psychosocial support; and personal coping styles influences cancer-related debility.

Risk Factors for Complications
- CIPN is seen in treatment with taxanes, vinca alkaloids, and platinum compounds; increased risk is seen in those with
  - Diabetes
  - Renal failure
  - Peripheral and other nerve disorders
- Cardiomyopathy is seen in treatment with anthracyclines; increased risk is seen in those with
  - Pre-existing cardiac disease
  - History of chest radiation
- Osteoporosis/osteopenia is seen in treatment with steroids and aromatase inhibitors; increased risk is seen in those with
  - Poor baseline bone health
- Pulmonary debility is seen in treatment with antitumor antibiotics, methotrexate, alkylating agents, and nitrosureas; increased risk is seen in those with
  - Chronic obstructive pulmonary disease (COPD)
  - Pre-existing pulmonary disease
- Functional impairment is seen in those with critical illness and cancer-related fatigue; increased risk is seen in those with
  - Pre-existing stroke
  - Osteoarthritis
  - Diabetes
  - Vision/hearing loss
- Lymphedema is increased with
  - Surgical lymph node dissection in the axilla or groin
  - Radiation therapy
  - Trauma
  - Infection/inflammation
  - Weight gain since surgery

Clinical Features

Primary and metastatic brain tumors
- Physical and/or cognitive impairments can mimic complications of traumatic brain injury or stroke.

Spinal cord injury: complete or partial
- Cord compression by primary or metastatic tumors
- Radiation myelitis can be seen as a late effect of radiation therapy.
- Metastatic leptomeningeal disease
- Pathologic spine fracture with or without compression

Chemotherapy-induced peripheral neuropathy
- Commonly a symmetric sensory neuropathy
- Dose dependent
- Less common motor involvement occurs at higher doses
- Platinum compound related form can occur weeks after the last dose.

Chemo-brain
- Mild encephalopathy is possible during chemotherapy.
- More severe metabolic encephalopathy
  - Can be seen as a side effect of chemotherapy (vomiting, poor oral intake, infection)
  - Elderly patients are at high risk.
- Radiation-related encephalopathy
  - Late-effect of brain radiation
  - Dose dependent
  - More common with whole brain radiation

Lymphedema
- Can be seen in the upper or lower extremities, face, trunk, and genitalia

Cancer fatigue, pain, and weakness
- Poor activity level in acute care hospital
- Cardiopulmonary and musculoskeletal deconditioning
- No referral for rehabilitation interventions

Diagnosis

Medical and cancer history
- Surgeries
- Chemotherapy regimens
- Radiation sites
- Comorbid chronic health issues

Comprehensive general medical and neuromuscular examination

Testing
- Electrodiagnosis
- Neuroimaging—helpful for neuropathic etiology
- Bedside cognitive tests are useful to screen for dementia.

Pitfalls
- Patients minimize functional deficits in order to
  - Qualify for more chemotherapy
  - Avoid loss of independence
- Cancer-related pain affects physical examination findings such as
  - Functional status
  - Mood
  - Cognition

Red flags
- Polypharmacy is common and can worsen mild impairment.
- Depression, dementia, and delirium, the 3Ds of geriatrics, are *always* in the differential of the patient with new functional deficits.

Treatment

Exercise
Regardless of age and disease stage, patients benefit from rehabilitation.
- Acute care—the patient should get up, stretch, perform a range of motion exercises, and ambulate; decreases morbidity
- Inpatient rehabilitation—focus should be on attainable short-term goals, pain management, nutrition, and conditioning
- Outpatient therapy—focus should be on independent function, a patient-driven program, and community re-entry
- Home therapy/life style change—exercise programs can reduce recurrence in some cancers, as well as reduce morbidity.

Goal setting
Goal setting should be individualized.
- Disease stage, trajectory of disease (stable or rapid progression), patient comorbidity, and frailty must be considered.
- In advanced disease, the patient goals may be limited to help with transfers, home management, support services, and adaptive equipment.
- Family training may be an important goal.

Palliative rehabilitation and symptom management
Palliative care can be offered to all patients who need it.
- Function, not just pain management, should be addressed.

- Rehabilitation modalities, spinal orthoses, adaptive equipment, and braces/orthoses can be considered.
- Compression wrapping to manage uncomfortable edema may be useful.
- Positioning evaluations can be performed to improve comfort in the bed and in a chair.
- Patient priorities and family priorities must align.

Prognosis

Functional prognosis for geriatric cancer patients is often tied to cancer prognosis, but, in general, rehabilitation can help improve the quality of life for patients at every stage of cancer.

Helpful Hints

- Communication with a patient's oncologist and primary physician is a *must*, and can help clarify goals of care.
- Maintenance of functional independence and not "being a burden" are two of the most common wishes of advanced cancer patients, often more important than prolonging life. Rehabilitation interventions are key.
- In brain tumor involvement, edema reduction via steroids can lead to significant rapid symptom improvement in some cases.

Suggested Readings

Buschbacher RM, Paul K. Cancer rehabilitation: Increasing awareness and removing barriers. *Am J Phys Med Rehabil.* 2011;90(5, Suppl. 1):S1–S4.

Cancer supportive and survivorship care. www.cancersupportivecare.com

Care during chemotherapy and beyond. www.chemocare.com

Cheville A. Cancer rehabilitation. *Semin Oncol.* 2005;32:219–224.

Lee TY, Ganz SB. Geriatric issues in cancer rehabilitation. In: Stubblefield MD, O'Dell MW, eds. *Cancer Rehabilitation: Principles and Practice.* New York, NY: Demos Medical Publishing; 2009:869–880.

Nussbaum NJ. Rehabilitation and the older cancer patient. *Am J Med Sci.* 2004;327(2):86–90.

Scialla S, Cole R, Scialla T, et al. Rehabilitation for elderly patients with cancer asthenia: Making a transition to palliative care. *Palliat Med.* 2000;14:121–127.

Cardiovascular: Amputation

Heikki Uustal MD

Description
Surgical removal of any segment of a limb due to ischemia, infection, deformity, or trauma. Most commonly, amputation occurs in the distal lower limb due to the complications of diabetes and dysvascular disease.

Etiology/Types
- Peripheral arterial disease (atherosclerosis) causing ischemia
- Diabetes with macrovascular and microvascular disease
- Infection (cellulitis, osteomyelitis)
- Deformity (Charcot joint)
- Trauma
- Most common levels of amputation include
  - Toe amputation
  - Trans-metatarsal (TMA): distal to mid-metatarsal level with a plantar flap
  - Trans-tibial (TTA): 4 to 6 in. of tibial bone length with good gastrocnemius flap
  - Trans-femoral (TFA): distal third of femur (but above femoral condyles) with myodesis from quadriceps to hamstring muscles

Epidemiology
- 130,000 amputations per year in the United States (all levels and ages)
- 80,000 to 100,000 major amputations per year (two third below knee and one third above knee)
- 82% are dysvascular (97% lower limb)
- 16% are trauma (68% upper limb)
- Of the 1.6 million amputee survivors, only 32% are dysvascular; due to higher morbidity and mortality, they have a relatively short lifespan after amputation.

Pathogenesis
- Typically, a sensory impaired and dysvascular limb suffers a minor insult or injury (rubbing from shoe, infected toenail) as the inciting event.
- Poor perfusion does not allow adequate healing, due to poor delivery of oxygen and antibiotics.
- Gangrene/necrosis develops in the wound as metabolic demand exceeds the capacity of the delivery system (circulation).
- The involved segment must be amputated to avoid sepsis.

Risk Factors
- Poor footwear
- Little or no social support system
- Cognitive or vision impairment
- Severe neuropathy (sensory loss)
- Severe peripheral arterial disease
- Severe cardiovascular disease
- Poor compliance with medical management (particularly diabetes)

Clinical Features
- The energy cost of ambulation increases with increasing level of amputation (trans-tibial, 40% increase; trans-femoral, 60% increase; bilateral amputation, 100% increase)
- Pain (residual limb, phantom pain, opposite limb, and back)
- Skin breakdown from prosthesis or delayed healing of wound
- Hip and knee flexion contractures from delayed mobilization

Natural History
- Typically starts with a complication/progression of diabetes and peripheral arterial disease
- There is commonly a slow deterioration in ambulation and function prior to amputation.
- Limb salvage/revascularization and then amputation surgery leads to a prolonged period of immobility and hospitalization, causing further deconditioning and functional decline.
- Generally, patients never regain all previous function after amputation.
- Better outcomes occur with shorter periods of immobility and with early prosthetic fitting and rehabilitation.

Diagnosis

History
- Functional level and ambulation prior to and after amputation
- Onset of problem and duration of treatment
- Review of all procedures performed before and after amputation
- Level of pain before and after amputation, including phantom pain
- Prosthetic devices used, other assistive devices needed

Examination
- Residual limb level of amputation, bone length, and quality of soft tissue coverage
- Status of the other foot (skin, pulses)
- Range of motion and strength at critical muscles and joints:
  - Lower limb: hip extensors, hip abductors, and knee extensors
  - Upper limb: hand dexterity, grip, triceps, and shoulder depressors
- Gait assessment, with or without prosthesis, as appropriate
- Evaluation of prosthesis for fit, function, and component wear and tear

Testing
- Echocardiogram for ejection fraction and electrocardiogram (ECG) for arrhythmias to help predict functional level and write precautions for therapy program
- Arterial Doppler studies of opposite limb for the evaluation of claudication/ischemia

Red Flags
- Dependency in self-care and mobility prior to amputation indicates poor prognosis for use of prosthetic device.
- Failure to progress in therapy
- Limited use of prosthesis at home
- Flexion contractures of hip or knee
- Impairment of cognition, vision, and hand function
- Previous stroke
- Renal failure with hemodialysis: causes volume changes in limb
- Severe cardiopulmonary disease or nonambulator prior to amputation has poor prognosis for prosthetic use.

Treatment

Preprosthetic care
- Education, early mobilization, range of motion/strength, desensitization, pain control, ace-wrapping for edema control (shrinker after sutures removed), proper footwear for the other foot, and psychological support

Prosthetic fitting
- Initial prosthesis is usually fitted 4 to 6 weeks after surgery, if the wound is healed.
- Rigid dressing and/or immediate postoperative prosthesis (IPOP; in ideal setting)
- Trans-tibial design: patellar-tendon-bearing socket with single-axis foot
- Trans-femoral design: Ischial containment socket with stance control knee and single-axis foot
- Permanent prosthesis components are based on medicare functional level:
  1—Transfers or limited household ambulator
  2—Household and limited community ambulator
  3—Unlimited community ambulator
  4—High-energy activities

Prosthetic training/rehabilitation
- Trans-tibial amputee: 4 to 8 weeks of outpatient therapy
- Trans-femoral amputee: 6 to 12 weeks of outpatient therapy
- Slowly progress both the wearing time and ambulation, based on skin integrity and overall medical status.

Follow-up
- Physician/physiatrist follow-up weekly for preprosthetic phase, monthly for prosthetic phase, and 1 to 2 visits annually after permanent prosthesis is fitted and checked-out.

Prosthetic gait troubleshooting
- Trunk lean:
  - Check prosthetic limb length
  - Check hip abductor strength
- Asymmetrical step length:
  - Check for hip flexion contracture
  - Painful socket
- Lateral/medial thrust of TTA socket:
  - Inset/outset prosthetic foot
- Early/late heel rise of TFA foot:
  - Check flexion/extension resistance of prosthetic knee

Complications
- Falls with or without prosthesis
- Depression
- Pain
- Skin breakdown
- Neuroma
- Phantom pain

Prognosis
The *50/50 rule* states that *50%* of geriatric amputees will die within 5 years, and *50% of the survivors* will have a second major amputation.
- Perioperative survival: TTA—94%, TFA—83%
- 1-year survival: TTA—74%, TFA—50%
- 5-year survival: TTA—48%, TFA—22%
- Approximately, 75% of geriatric lower limb amputees are fitted with a prosthesis, but only 50% walk with a prosthesis after 1 year.

Helpful Hints
- Early mobilization minimizes morbidity and mortality.
- Careful management of medical problems, such as diabetes, minimizes complications, and helps with wound healing
- Lightweight and comfortable prosthesis is more essential than heavier and more complex prosthesis.

Appropriate rehabilitation/therapy and follow-up are important to ensure maximum function and to manage complications and problems as they arise.

Suggested Readings
Cumming JC, Barr S, Howe TE. Prosthetic rehabilitation for older dysvascular people following a unilateral transfemoral amputation. *Cochrane Database Syst Rev.* 2006;(4):CD005260.

Goldberg T. Postoperative management of lower extremity amputations. *Phys Med Rehabil Clin N Am.* 2006;17(1):173–180, vii.

Kulkarni J, Pande S, Morris J. Survival rates in dysvascular lower limb amputees. *Int J Surg.* 2006;4(4):217–221.

Uustal H. Prosthetic rehabilitation issues in the diabetic and dysvascular amputee. *Phys Med Rehabil Clin N Am.* 2009;20:689–703.

Van Velzen JM, van Bennekom CA, Polomski W, et al. Physical capacity and walking ability after lower limb amputation: A systematic review. *Clin Rehabil.* 2006;20(11):999–1016.

Cardiovascular: Peripheral Arterial Disease

Deepthi S. Saxena MD

Definition
- Peripheral arterial disease (PAD) is a compromise to the blood flow in the extremities, presenting as pain in one or more muscle groups or no pain.
- PAD is defined by ankle-brachial index (ABI) less than 0.9.
- PAD, a significant predictor of mortality, is associated with limitations in physical function and reduced health-related quality of life (QOL).

Epidemiology
- In the Cardiovascular Health Study, the prevalence of ABI less than 0.9 increased to about 30% in men and 40% in women, at 85 years.
- The National Health and Nutrition Examination Survey (NHANES) of 2,174 individuals reported a 14.5% prevalence of PAD in those aged 70 years or above.
- PARTNERS program: The prevalence of PAD in 7,000 patients, aged ≥70 years and aged 50 to 69 years with a history of cigarette smoking was 29%.
- In this study, PAD alone was seen in 13%, and PAD + cardiovascular disease (CVD) was seen in 16%.

Risk Factors
- Smoking
- Diabetes mellitus
- Hypertension
- Chronic kidney disease
- Elevated C-reactive protein (CRP)
- Dyslipidemia
- Metabolic syndrome

Etiology
- PAD occurs in the aorta and its branches, exclusive of coronary arteries, due to
  - Stenosis
  - Occlusion
- Arterial occlusion can occur due to
  - Emboli from a distant source, such as cardiac emboli due to
    . Atrial fibrillation
    . Myocardial infarction
    . Endocarditis
    . Valvular disease
    . Prosthetic valves
  - Arterial thrombosis due to
    . Atherosclerosis
    . Vascular grafts
    . Hypercoagulable state
  - Direct arterial trauma

Pathogenesis
- Claudication occurs when skeletal muscle oxygen demand exceeds the oxygen supply.
- During intermittent claudication, blood flow and oxygen consumption in the leg are normal at rest, but the metabolic needs of the exercising muscle are not met due to single or multiple occlusive lesions in the arteries of the limb.
- Patients with critical limb ischemia typically have multiple occlusive lesions, due to which even the resting blood supply diminishes and cannot meet the nutritional needs of the limb.

Clinical Features

PAD of lower extremities
- Intermittent claudication
- Atypical leg pain
- Asymptomatic functional impairment (decreased function even in the absence of claudication)
- Skin changes related to chronically impaired circulation
- Critical limb ischemia (in advanced cases; rest pain, ulcers, or gangrene)

Abdominal aortic aneurysms
- Asymptomatic in early stages

- As the aneurysm enlarges: abdominal pulsations, back pain, abdominal discomfort, bruits over the renal and/or femoral arteries, diminished or absent peripheral pulses, skin changes, and, less commonly, neurologic symptoms arises.

Diagnosis

History
- Walking impairment
- Symptoms of claudication
- Ischemic rest pain
- Nonhealing wounds

Screening
- Abdominal ultrasound indicated for 60-year-old men with family history of abdominal aortic aneurysms (AAA) or 65- to 75-year-old smokers/ex-smokers.

Testing
- The ABI, an objective assessment of PAD, is calculated by dividing the ankle systolic pressure by the higher brachial systolic pressure.
- ABI less than 0.9 is up to 95% sensitive, 99% specific, and has 98% accuracy.
- A low ABI is predictive of an increased risk of mortality.

Localization of lesion for revascularization procedures
- Segmental limb pressure, pulse-volume recording
- Duplex ultrasonography
- Magnetic resonance (MR) and conventional angiography

Differential diagnosis
- Spinal stenosis
- Osteoarthritis
- Deep venous thrombosis (DVT)
- Musculoskeletal disorders
- Venous claudication
- Peripheral neuropathy

Classification of PAD
Fontaine's stages: I to IV:
 I—Asymptomatic
 IIa—Mild claudication
 IIb—Moderate to severe claudication
 III—Ischemic rest pain
 IV—Ulceration or gangrene
Rutherford's categories: 0 to 6:
 0—Asymptomatic
 1—Mild claudication
 2—Moderate claudication
 3—Severe claudication
 4—Ischemic rest pain
 5—Minor tissue loss
 6—Major tissue loss

Treatment

Risk factor modification
- Smoking cessation
- Maintain low density lipoprotein (LDL) cholesterol at less than 100 mg/dl.
- Maintain glycosylated hemoglobin at less than 7%
- Maintain blood pressure at less than 130/85
- Angiotensin-converting enzyme (ACE) inhibition
- Antiplatelet therapy

Rehabilitation
- *Cochrane Database Systematic Review*, 2000: Exercise is an inexpensive, low-risk option for intermittent claudication; benefits more than angioplasty at 6 months.
- Study of 156 patients with 81% asymptomatic PAD, with an ABI ≤0.95: Exercise increased walking distance in 6-minute walk test, compared with those in the placebo group.

Exercise prescription
- Supervised physical therapy (PT) 45 to 60 minutes/session, with the goal of "symptom-limited claudication"; treadmill or track starts at 35 minutes and increases at 5 minutes/session for 50 minutes. In all three sessions/week for more than 12 weeks.

Pharmacologic therapy
- Vasodilation and suppressing platelet aggregation can give symptomatic relief and slowdown the disease progression.
- **Antiplatelets**: for secondary prevention of *cerebrovascular accident* (CVA) and coronary artery disease (CAD). Drugs of choice: Aspirin, 75 mg/d to 162 mg/d and Clopidogrel, 75 mg/d.
- **Cilostazol**: phosphodiesterase inhibitor used to increase maximal and pain-free walking distances. Trial: 3 to 6 months, 100 mg BID. Contraindicated: heart failure.

It is used selectively due to cost and modest clinical benefit.
- Pentoxifylline: American College of Cardiology (ACC)/American Heart Association (AHA): Second-line agent to Cilostazol to improve the walking distance.

American College of Chest Physicians (ACCP) recommends against it.
- Ginkgo/vasodilators/vitamin E/prostaglandins: ACC/AHA: not established or recommended

Revascularization

Criteria
- Severe disability that limits the patient's ability to work or perform activities of daily living (ADLs) and instrumental activities of daily living (IADLs) or other function.
- Failure to respond to rehabilitation and pharmacologic management.

Benefits
- Reduces symptoms and the likelihood of subsequent amputation.

Types
- Percutaneous
- Surgical

Indications for AAA Repair
- Symptoms
- Rapid dilatation
- Aneurysms ≥5.5 cm in diameter

Natural History
Patients with PAD are at increased risk of
- CAD
- Cerebrovascular disease

Outcomes in 5 Years in Patients With Claudication
- Worsening claudication: 10% to 20%
- Critical limb ischemia: 1% to 2%

Outcomes in 1 Year in Patients With Critical Limb Ischemia
- Amputation: 25%
- Cardiovascular mortality: 25%

Consults
- Internal medicine
- Infectious disease
- Cardiology
- Podiatry
- Cardiovascular surgery

Helpful Hints
- Intermittent claudication is reproducible, and is not affected by body position, unlike spinal stenosis and degenerative joint disease (DJD).
- It is *quickly* relieved by rest.

Suggested Reading
Salameh MJ, Ratchford EV. Update on peripheral arterial disease and claudication rehabilitation. *Phys Med Rehabil Clin N Am.* 2009;20:627–656.

Yazdanyar N. The burden of cardiovascular disease in the elderly: Morbidity, mortality and costs. *Clin Geriatr Med.* 2009;25(4):563–577.

Cardiovascular: Syncope and Orthostatic Hypotension

Deepthi S. Saxena MD

Description
Syncope is a sudden, transient loss of consciousness and postural tone, not due to trauma, followed by complete recovery.

Etiology/Types
In older adults, the cause of syncope is often multifactorial. The cause is unknown in one-third cases.
- Vasovagal syncope is the most common cause, occurring in more than 30% of patients aged above 65.
- Cardiac causes are the second most common, with bradycardia being the single most common cardiac cause.
- Other causes include neurologic problems, such as seizures, stroke, and transient ischemic attacks.

Epidemiology
- The incidence of syncope increases with age, with over 80% of patients hospitalized for syncope being above the age of 65.

Pathogenesis
Vasovagal and cardiac
- Reduced cerebral perfusion causing syncope is due to
  - A decrease in systemic blood pressure (BP) or
  - An increase in cerebral vascular resistance
- When a person assumes the standing position, gravity causes up to one third of the blood volume to pool in the legs; reducing venous return, decreasing cardiac output (CO), and lowering cerebral BP.
  - To compensate, carotid and aortic baroreceptors increase autonomic sympathetic tone, which also activates the renin-angiotensin system (RAS), retaining sodium to maintain the extracellular fluid volume.
  - Additionally, the postural response of a reduction in atrial natriuretic factor further facilitates vasoconstriction.
- The autonomic and endocrine reflex pathways that cause rapid compensation of these effects become less responsive with age.
- The cardiac response to beta-adrenergic stimulation decreases, resulting in a less effective baroreflex, causing little increase in heart rate (HR) and vasoconstriction; thus, making it difficult to maintain postural BP.
- Additionally, comorbid conditions affecting postural responses, such as diabetes mellitus and medications such as alpha, beta, and calcium channel blockers, can impair postural reflexes.

Risk Factors
- Age
- Increased alcohol intake
- Diabetes
- History of arrhythmia
- Abnormal electrocardiogram (ECG)
- History of heart failure (congestive heart failure [CHF])
- History of stroke
- Transient ischemic attacks
- Hypertension
- Lower body mass index

Clinical Features
- Syncope in sitting or supine suggests a profound hemodynamic disturbance, as in cardiac arrhythmia.
- Myocardial ischemia or aortic stenosis can occur during physical exertion.
- Syncope after turning motions of the head occurs in carotid sinus hypersensitivity.
- Diaphoresis, presyncope, and gastrointestinal symptoms, such as nausea or vomiting, can be associated with vasovagal syncope.
- Generally, patients with cardiac syncope are flaccid and motionless while unconscious, unless the event lasts for more than 15 seconds, when myoclonic jerks and truncal extension can be seen. In contrast, increased body motion, tone, and head turning to one side with loss of consciousness are more indicative of seizures.
- Syncope can be a cause of falls.

Natural History
- Predictors of poor outcome (San Francisco Syncope Rule):
  - Systolic BP lower than 90 mmHg
  - Complaints of dyspnea
  - History of CHF
  - ECG—new changes or rhythm other than sinus
  - Hematocrit lower than 30

Diagnosis

Differential diagnosis
- Neurocardiogenic
- Carotid sinus hypersensitivity
- Orthostasis:
  - Volume loss and gastrointestinal bleeding
  - Prolonged bed rest and deconditioning
- Medication
- Pulmonary embolus
- Cardiovascular syncope:
  - Arrhythmia
  - Ischemia
  - Myocardial infarction

History
- A point score to identify cardiac syncope has been developed with two multicenter cohorts. Scores of three or more were associated with cardiac syncope:
  - Palpitations preceding syncope: 4
  - Heart disease and/or abnormal ECG: 3
  - Syncope during effort: 3
  - Syncope while supine: 2
  - Precipitating factors: −1
  - Prodrome (nausea/vomiting): −1

Examination
- Cardiovascular examination
- Neurologic examination
- Postural or orthostatic hypotension is diagnosed when, within 2 to 5 minutes of quiet standing, after a 5-minute period of supine rest, one or more of the following is present:
  - A total of 20 mmHg fall in systolic pressure
  - A total of 10 mmHg fall in diastolic pressure
  - Increase in HR of 20 beats/minute or more.
  - Cerebral hypoperfusion symptoms.

Testing
The cause of syncope being multifactorial, tests have a low yield, unless clinical findings suggest a particular cause. Some tests that can be considered include
- Ambulatory ECG
- Implantable loop recorders
- Echocardiography
- Electrophysiologic studies
- Tilt-table testing
- Neurological tests: computerized tomography (CT), magnetic resonance imaging (MRI), and electroencephalography (EEG).

Treatment

Medical
- Often requires treatment of multiple possible underlying causes in geriatric patients.
- In cardiac causes, it is important to focus therapeutic interventions on a single underlying cause.
- Avoidance of vasovagal triggers, vasodilators, and postprandial hypotension
- Reducing or discontinuing diuretics
- Ensuring adequate fluid volume
- Liberalizing salt intake
- Waist-high compression stockings providing 20 to 30 mm pressure
- Sleeping in a head-up position
- Caffeine and midodrine: increase HR
- Fludrocortisone: expands plasma volume

Rehabilitation
- Counterpressure maneuvers, including leg crossing and handgrip and arm tensing, can reduce syncope burden in patients with recurrent syncope.

Consults
- Internal medicine
- Cardiology
- Neurology

Prognosis
- The prognosis depends on the underlying cause.
- The one-year mortality for patients with syncope due to cardiac causes is 18% to 33%, with deaths being due to the cardiac disease rather than syncope.
- The one-year mortality with noncardiac causes of syncope is about 6%.
- Since vasovagal syncope in older adults is frequently associated with comorbid illness that can increase overall mortality, it may not be as benign as in younger patients.

Suggested Reading
Moya A, Sutton R, Ammirati F, et al. Guidelines for the diagnosis and management of syncope. *Eur Heart J.* 2009;30:2631–2671. www.americangeriatrics.org, guidelines and recommendations.

Cardiovascular: Thromboembolic Disease

Carlo E. Adams MD

Description
Deep venous thrombosis (DVT) is a blood clot in the deep venous system that usually affects the lower extremities or pelvic veins. Venous thrombi may dislodge from their distal site and travel proximally, embolizing to the pulmonary arteries causing pulmonary embolism (PE). Venous thromboembolism (VTE) causes significant morbidity and mortality in the geriatric population.

Etiology/Types
- Virchow's Triad: contributors to thrombus formation
  - Abnormal vessel wall trauma
  - Hypercoagulable state
  - Venous stasis
- Other sources of embolism include the following:
  - Air
  - Fat
  - Tumor
  - Amniotic fluid
  - Arthroplasty cement
  - Sepsis
- Hypercoagulability may also be genetically predisposed (factor V Leiden mutation).

Epidemiology
- DVT is the third most common cardiovascular disease, following myocardial infarction and stroke.
- DVT was found in 16% of postacute care patients by Doppler ultrasound.
- The risk of VTE in older, acute medical patients without prophylaxis is 10% to 15%.
- VTE is five to six times more common in the elderly compared to younger patients.
- Fatal PE is seen in 10% to 20% of autopsy-confirmed geriatric unit deaths.

Pathogenesis
- Deep proximal veins of the lower extremity are the most common clot-formation areas.
- Platelets release vasoactive agents, which impairs gas exchange, increases vascular resistance, and leads to pulmonary edema.
- Elevated pulmonary vascular resistance promotes right heart wall dysfunction and ultimately left heart failure.

Risk Factors
- Advanced age
- Family or past history of VTE
- Poor mobility
- Hospitalization/surgery
- Heart and respiratory failure
- Current or previous malignancy
- Genetic factors (factor V Leiden mutation, elevated factor VIII levels, activated protein C resistance)

Clinical Features
- DVT
  - Extremity pain
  - Swelling
  - Erythema
- PE
  - Dyspnea
  - Tachypnea
  - Pleuritic pain
  - Cough
  - Hemoptysis and signs of right heart dysfunction

Natural History
- Rates of VTE increase with age, with rates in those aged above 65 more than three times their younger counterparts.
- Men have higher rates of VTE above age 75.
- Cancer, hospitalization, and postoperative state are frequently associated with VTE.
- The 1-month VTE mortality may range up to 11%, with a yearly recurrence of 7.7% in acute medical patients.

Diagnosis

Differential diagnosis
- DVT
  - Superficial thrombophlebitis
  - Chronic venous insufficiency
  - Cellulitis
  - Fracture
  - Arterial ischemia
  - Hematoma
  - Lymphedema
  - Heterotopic ossification
  - Muscle tear
- PE
  - Aortic stenosis
  - Atrial fibrillation
  - Myocardial infarct
  - Pneumonia
  - Pneumothorax
  - Musculoskeletal
  - Pleuritis
  - Chronic obstructive pulmonary disease (COPD)
  - Costochondritis

History
- Often, acute medical patients with cardiac and/or lung disease, who may have cancer, stroke, systemic lupus erythematosus (SLE), or who recently had a major surgery.
- Idiopathic causes results in as many as half of DVT patients.

Examination
- Homan's sign—pain in the calf region, while the knee is flexed to 90° and the ankle actively dorsiflexed
- Nonspecific for lower extremity DVT
- Both dyspnea and tachypnea are the most frequent symptoms of PE.

Imaging
- Doppler ultrasound (DVT) and spiral chest computed tomography (PE) use is increasing due to their speed, sensitivity, and non-invasiveness
- Plethysmography, pulmonary angiograpy, and V/Q scan continue to play a diagnostic role when PE is suspected, but computed tomography cannot be performed.

Pitfalls
- Presenting symptoms may be insidious
- PE often mimics other cardiopulmonary diseases
- As much as 70% of PEs are diagnosed at autopsy.

Red flags
- Syncope, hypotension, and cyanosis may indicate massive PE

Treatment
- Pharmacologic, mechanical (sequential compression devices), and inferior vena cava filter can be used for prophylaxis.
- Elastic compression stockings should be used only in low-risk patients.
- Heparin products (unfractionated and low molecular weight) and Warfarin have been shown to be effective in the initial and long-term treatment of VTE.
- Intensity and duration of therapy depends on the individual patient, but should last at least 3 months.
- Some patients with thrombophilias may require lifetime anticoagulation.
- PE can be treated similar to DVT.
- Initial inpatient treatment is recommended for PE due to risk of cardiovascular instability.
- In-hospital-monitored thrombolysis can be used in patients with massive PE.
- Some newer anticoagulant medications may also be beneficial.
- Geriatric patients have an increased bleeding tendency, but benefits may outweigh risks for pharmacologic VTE treatment.

Helpful Hints
- A low threshold of suspicion of thromboembolic disease is important. Waiting until the clinical diagnosis is obvious before initiating evaluation and treatment can result in patient death.

Suggested Readings

Cushman M. Deep vein thrombosis and pulmonary embolism in 2 cohorts: The longitudinal investigation of thromboembolism etiology. *Am J Med*. 2004;117:19–25.

Geerts WH. Prevalence of venous thromboembolism: American College of Chest Physicians evidenced-based clinical practice guidelines (8th edition). *Chest*. 2008;133(Suppl. 6):381S–453S.

Heit JA. The epidemiology of venous thromboembolism in the community: Implications for prevention and management. *J Thromb Thrombolysis*. 2006;21:23–29.

Lee J. Prevention and clinical outcomes in older inpatients with suspected venous thromboembolism. *J Gerontol Nurs*. 2010;36:40–48.

Sellier E. Risk factors for DVT in older patients: A multicenter study with systematic compression ultrasonography in post-acute care facilities in France. *J Am Geriatr Soc*. 2008;56:224–230.

Spyropoulos AC. Management of VTE in the elderly. *Drugs Aging*. 2006;23:651–671.

Depression

Kevin M. Means MD

Description
Depression is a syndrome complex characterized by mood disturbance in addition to cognitive, psychological, and vegetative disturbances.

Etiology/Types

Types
- Major depression
- Minor depression
- Dysthymic disorder
- Bipolar disease

Common depression triggers
- Rejection or abandonment
- Anniversary of a negative event
- Death/major illness of loved one
- Loss of a pet
- Medication noncompliance
- Arguments with friends/relatives
- Chronic disabling illness, recent major physical illness, and age-related illness
- Substance use
- Medications that can lead to depression
  - Benzodiazepines
  - Propranolol
  - Corticosteroids
  - Estrogen
  - Progesterone
  - Chemotherapy agents
  - Psychostimulants
  - Cimetidine
  - Clonidine
  - Hydralazine
  - Alpha-methyldopa
  - Digitalis

Epidemiology
- 2 million Americans above age 65 have clinically significant depression.
- 29% prevalence is reported in the geriatric outpatient rehabilitation setting.
- Over 25% prevalence in long-term care settings.
- 40% prevalence is found among hospitalized elderly.
  - Over 8% to 25% have minor depression
  - 10% to 45% have major depression
- In all 3% to 16% prevalence is found in community-dwelling elderly.
  - A ratio of 2:1 female-to-male incidence
  - Greater prevalence among the oldest is due to higher proportion of women, more physical disability, more cognitive impairment, and lower socioeconomic status.
  - Similar prevalence among white and African Americans
  - 14% prevalence within 2 years after death of a spouse
  - 15% prevalence in medically ill elderly
- Under 20% of elderly with depression are treated.
- Direct and indirect costs: $43 billion annually in United States.

Pathogenesis
Many biopsychosocial etiologies and risk factors for late-life depression have been proposed:
- Elevated stress levels, decreased norepinephrine and/or serotonin
- Cerebrovascular disease with frontal lobe hypoperfusion
- Deep white matter hyperintensity
- Hypersecretion of corticotropin-releasing factor (CRF)
  - May explain sleep and appetite disturbances, reduced libido, and psychomotor changes
- Low levels of dehydroepiandrosterone sulfate (DHEA-S)

Risk Factors
- Biological/genetic factors
  - High prevalence in first-degree relatives
  - High concordance with monozygotic twins
  - Short allele of serotonin-transported gene
- Medical illness
  - Parkinson's disease, Alzheimer's disease, cancer, diabetes, or stroke

- Vascular changes in the brain
- Chronic or severe pain
- Previous history of depression
- Substance abuse
- Urinary incontinence
- Diastolic hypotension
- Male veterans hospitalized during World War II for head injury
- Social factors
  - Loneliness, isolation, and bereavement
  - Lack of social supports
  - Decreased mobility (illness or nondriving)
  - Religious practice
- Psychological factors
  - Role changes
  - Frequent or severe negative life events or daily hassles
  - Traumatic experiences, abuse, or neglect
  - Loss of body image
  - Fear of death
  - Frustration with memory loss

High-Risk Elderly
- Recently bereaved
- Diagnosis of dementia, Parkinson's disease, or stroke
- Significant somatic concerns
- Refusal to eat or neglect of personal care
- Recurrent or prolonged hospitalization
- Recent placement in a nursing home

Clinical Features
- Depression is a major problem among older patients.
- Depression in older patients is often missed because typical symptoms may be masked and because patients may not spontaneously describe emotional difficulties.
- Depression in late life is frequently comorbid with other physical and psychiatric conditions, especially in the oldest.
- Depression is a barrier to rehabilitation. Addressing the illness and injury as well as the depression is important to prevent further debility in the elderly.
- Depression can decrease motivation and participation in rehabilitation, resulting in slow progress, delayed discharge, and lower functional outcomes.
- Successful depression treatment can improve motivation and rehabilitation outcomes.
- Elderly people with depression are more likely to
  - Have somatic complaints (hypochondriasis in 65% of depressed elderly)
  - Minimize expressing their depressed mood to others
  - Hide their feelings of guilt
- Elderly persons under-report depression due to
  - Aphasia, hearing impairment
  - Dementia
  - Depression thought to be "normal"
  - Symptoms "masked" by comorbid illness

Natural History
- Historical studies conducted before the availability of electroconvulsive therapy found that approximately half of the patients with untreated major depression eventually recovered, although, often after long periods (about 18 months) of morbidity.
- Few double-blind placebo-controlled trials involving patients aged above 65 comparing tricyclic antidepressants found that drugs are superior to placebo with about 50% improvement in depression scale scores versus 20% to 25% improvement on placebo.

Diagnosis

Differential
- Includes other psychiatric disorders
  - Dysthymia
  - Bipolar disorder
- Central nervous system (CNS) diseases
  - Parkinson's disease
  - Neoplastic lesions
- Endocrine disorders
  - Hyperthyroidism
  - Hypothyroidism
- Drug-related conditions
  - Cocaine abuse
  - Side effects of beta-blockers
- Infectious diseases
  - Syphilis
  - Sleep-related disorders

History
- Psychiatric history
- Previous similar episodes
- Drug or alcohol abuse
- Thoughts of suicide

Examination
- Neurologic examination
  - Mental status
  - Lateralization

- Tremor
- Changes in muscle tone
- Slowed reflexes

Testing
- Complete blood count
- Basic metabolic profile
- Thyroid studies
- Vitamin B_{12} level (methylmalonic acid and homocystine levels, if vitamin B_{12} is in the low-normal range)
- Radiologic imaging
  - Brain imaging (computerized tomography [CT] or magnetic resonance imaging [MRI]) indicated whether the neurologic examination is abnormal.
  - Or, if cerebrovascular abnormality is suspected

Criteria for major depression (Diagnostic and Statistical Manual, Fourth edition)
- Criteria for major depression include occurrence of five or more of the following:
  - Depressed mood
  - Diminished interest or pleasure
  - Significant decrease or increase in weight or appetite
  - Insomnia or hypersomnia
  - Psychomotor agitation or retardation
  - Fatigue or loss of energy
  - Feelings of worthlessness or inappropriate guilt
  - Diminished energy to concentrate
  - Recurrent thoughts of death or suicidal ideas
    The above symptoms present for two or more weeks; change from previous functioning.

Criteria for minor depression (DSM-IV)
- Criteria for minor depression include the following:
  - The presence of either one of the core symptoms (depressed mood or lack of interest)
  - One to three additional symptoms (listed above for major depression)
- Minor depression has been associated with the following:
  - Impairment similar to that of major depression (impaired physical functioning, disability days, poorer self-rated health)
  - Use of psychotropic medications
  - Perceived low social support
  - Female gender and being unmarried

Criteria for dysthymic disorder
- A long-lasting, chronic mood disturbance
- Less severe than major depression
- Lasts for 2 years or longer

Screening assessments
- Several screening instruments exist to aid accurate diagnosis of depression in the elderly (see chapter on Evaluation of Depression)

Treatment
The following treatments have been successfully used to treat depression in elderly patients:
- Medications
- Electroconvulsive therapy (ECT)
- Behavioral psychotherapy

Antidepressant medications
- Selective serotonin reuptake inhibitors (SSRIs)
  - Fluvoxamine, citalopram, sertraline, escitalopram, fluoxetine, and paroxetine
- Tricyclic antidepressants (TCAs)
  - Amitriptyline, desipramine, and nortriptyline
- Monoamine oxidase inhibitors (MAOIs)
- Other agents
  - Venlafaxine, buproprion, moclobemide, mirtazapine, and trazodone
    - Minimal interference with other medications
- Potential adverse effects
  - SSRIs can cause
    - Hyponatremia
    - Extrapyramidal symptoms
- TCAs
  - Have anticholinergic side effects
  - Known to increase risk of falls and should be used with caution
- MAOIs can cause hypotension.
- Bupropion can cause tremor and visual hallucinations.

Guidelines for antidepressant therapy: "start low, go slow"
- In the elderly, start at half the dose of younger people.
- Aim to reach an average dose at 1 month.
- An adequate antidepressant trial is 2 months.

Other effective depression treatments
- Psychological treatments
  - Cognitive behavior therapy (less effective for stroke patients)
  - Psychodynamic psychotherapy
  - Reminiscence and life review therapy
- ECT (under extreme circumstances)

When to refer to the psychiatrist
Patients are referred to psychiatrists if they have the following:
- Psychotic depression

- Bipolar disorder
- Depression with suicidal ideation or intent
- Comorbid substance abuse
- Severe major depressive episode
- Comorbid dementia

Prognosis
- Elderly depressed outpatients without significant comorbid medical illness or dementia, and who are treated optimally, may exhibit a much better outcome, with over 80% recovering and remaining well throughout follow-up.
- Elderly depressed patients with limited social support, comorbid illness or disability, and poor self-rated health experience a longer time to remission.
- In a recent systematic review
  - One third of treated patients developed a chronic course or a fluctuating course of depression.
  - Prognostic indicators for persistent depression include higher baseline depression level, older age, somatic comorbidity, functional limitations, and external locus of control (a belief that one's environment, some higher power, or other people controlling a person's decisions and their life).

Helpful Hints
- Depression is common in older adults in the rehabilitation setting and is a treatable source of disability in this population.
- Effective pharmacologic and psychosocial therapies exist for older adults.
- A combination of pharmacologic and psychosocial therapies is likely to be more effective than either one alone in treating and preventing depression.

Suggested Readings
Blazer DG. Depression in late life: Review and commentary. *Focus.* 2009;7:118–136.

Cully JA, Gfeller JD, Heise RA, et al. Geriatric depression, medical diagnosis, and functional recovery during acute rehabilitation. *Arch Phys Med Rehabil.* 2005;86:2256–2260.

Frazer CJ, Christensen H, Griffiths KM. Effectiveness of treatments for depression in older people. *Med J Aust.* 2005;182:627–632.

Nelson JC. Diagnosing and treating depression in the elderly. *J Clin Psychiatry.* 2001;62(Suppl. 24):18–22.

Licht-Strunk E, van der Windt DAWM, van Marwijk HWJ, et al. The prognosis of depression in older patients in general practice and the community. A systematic review. *Fam Pract* 2007;24:168–180.

Diabetes Mellitus

Monica Agarwal MD ■ Vitaly Kantorovich MD ■ Debra L. Simmons MD MS FACE FACP

Description
Diabetes mellitus is a chronic metabolic disease that requires a multidisciplinary approach. The natural history of diabetes can vary widely. Progression depends on etiology, as well as genetics and environmental factors. Early diagnosis and treatment can prevent long-term microvascular and macrovascular complications. Low density lipoprotein (LDL) cholesterol and blood pressure control help decrease the risk of cardiovascular disease.

Etiology/Types
- The pathogenesis of diabetes is complex and is an active area of research for basic understanding and drug discovery.
- Type 1 diabetes mellitus (T1DM) is an autoimmune disease resulting in absolute insulin deficiency. People with T1DM always need insulin.
- Type 2 diabetes mellitus (T2DM) results from insulin resistance, beta cell dysfunction, and increased hepatic glucose production. Those with advanced beta cell failure may require insulin-like T1DM.
- Other types of diabetes include medication induced (i.e., steroids), exocrine pancreatic disease (i.e., cystic fibrosis and pancreatitis), endocrinopathies (i.e., Cushing's syndrome), genetic defects (i.e., maturity-onset diabetes of the young), and so on.
- Gestational diabetes (GDM) is diabetes first diagnosed during pregnancy, other than those diagnosed by screening at the first prenatal visit due to risk factors.
- Prediabetes is not a clinical identity, but a category of hyperglycemia above normal but below that for diagnosis of diabetes. It is associated with an increased risk of developing diabetes and/or cardiovascular disease.

Epidemiology
- Diabetes is the seventh leading cause of death in the United States.
- Cardiovascular disease is the leading cause of death for people with diabetes.
- Diabetes affects 25.8 million people, 8.3% of the U.S. population.
- Among U.S. residents aged 65 years and above, 10.9 million or 26.9% had diabetes in 2010.

Risk Factors
- Age less than 45 years
- Overweight (body mass index [BMI] less than 25 kg/m2)
- Physical inactivity
- First-degree relative with diabetes
- High-risk race/ethnicity
- Women who delivered a baby less than 9 lb or who had GDM
- Hypertension (less than 140/90 mmHg or on therapy)
- High density lipoprotein (HDL) cholesterol less than 35 mg/dL and/or triglycerides less than 250 mg/dL
- Polycystic ovarian syndrome
- Cardiovascular disease
- Impaired fasting glucose or impaired glucose tolerance or A1C less than 5.7%
- Acanthosis nigricans and other conditions associated with insulin resistance

Clinical Features
- Prediabetes and diabetes are common in the elderly population.
- Frequent comorbidities are obesity, dyslipidemia, hypertension, cardiovascular disease, and depression, which can contribute to problems with polypharmacy.
- Patients may have unrecognized, advanced microvascular disease such as retinopathy, nephropathy, neuropathy, and/or macrovascular disease such as coronary artery disease and peripheral vascular disease.
- Diabetes is associated with increased prevalence of cognitive dysfunction.
- Diabetes is a major contributor to functional impairment, falls, and fractures.
- Hypoglycemia related to treatment can lead to significant morbidity and mortality.

Diabetes Mellitus

Diagnosis

Diagnostic criteria
- Diabetes is diagnosed by criteria as outlined in Table 1. All tests need to be repeated on a separate day unless there is unequivocal hyperglycemia.

Differential diagnosis
- Polyuria and polydipsia—diabetes insipidus and psychogenic polydipsia
- Weight loss—malignancy, hyperthyroidism, and depression

History
- Type and duration of diabetes, acute and chronic complications, vascular disease, hypertension, and hyperlipidemia
- Previous eye and foot examinations
- Pertinent review of systems
  - Weight loss
  - Polyuria, polyphagia, and polydipsia
  - Vision changes
  - Vaginitis
  - Erectile dysfunction
  - Symptoms of peripheral neuropathy, that is, burning and numbness

Examination
- Weight, BMI
- Orthostatic vital signs
- Dilated funduscopic examination
- Cardiovascular examination
- Skin and joints
- Injection sites
- Comprehensive foot examination

Laboratory tests
- A1C
- Fasting blood glucose
- Basic metabolic panel
- Estimated glomerular filtration rate
- Urine microalbumin-to-creatinine ratio
- Thyroid stimulating hormone (TSH) and free T4
- Lipid panel
- Liver function tests
- Serum and urine ketones (during hyperglycemic crisis)

Pitfalls
- Misdiagnosing diabetes by point-of-care testing for A1C or glucose
- Anemia can result in a falsely low A1C.
- Not recognizing mild hyperglycemia as diabetes

Table 1 Diagnostic Criteria for Diabetes

	A1C[a]	Fasting blood glucose (less than 8 hr fast)	Glucose 2 hr post 75-gram glucose load
Prediabetes	5.7%–6.4%	100–125 mg/dl	140–199 mg/dl
Diabetes	>6.5%	>126 mg/dl	>200 mg/dl

Random plasma glucose of >200 mg/dl during classic symptoms (polyuria, polydipsia, polyphagia, and weight loss) or hyperglycemic crisis

Note. For nonpregnant adults.
[a] A1C should be performed in a laboratory using a method that is National Glycohemoglobin Standardization Program (NGSP) certified and standardized to the Diabetes Control and Complications Trial (DCCT) assay.

- Not diagnosing T1DM in older people
- Assuming signs and symptoms are due to inevitable complications of diabetes rather than evaluating for other etiologies
- Fatigue and poor exercise tolerance may represent cardiac ischemia or congestive heart failure.

Treatment

Goals of therapy
- Overall A1C less than 7%, higher for frail adults
- Avoidance of severe hyperglycemia or hypoglycemia
- Individualize toward functional and psychosocial capacity (see Figure 1)

Overall approach to treatment of diabetes
- Team approach—patient, physical therapist, physician, nutritionist, and nursing staff
- Patient education
  - Skills for self-management of diabetes
  - Tailor to the patient and family/caregiver/caregivers needs
- Blood glucose monitoring
  - Frequency should match the goals for glucose control and therapy
  - Multiple insulin injections or insulin pump—check before meals and at bedtime
  - Oral agents—check once or twice daily, alternate times (fasting + premeal or bedtime)
  - At risk for hypoglycemia—check before and after activity
- Education for hypoglycemia management to patients and their families

Most intensive	Less intensive	Least intensive
6.0%	7.0%	8.0%

Psychosocioeconomic considerations

Highly motivated, adherent, knowledgeable, excellent self-care capacities, and comprehensive support systems		Less motivated, nonadherent, limited insight, poor self-care capacities, and weak support systems

Hypoglycemia risk

Low	Moderate	High

Patient age, y

40	45	50	55	60	65	70	75

Disease duration, y

5	10	15	20

Other comorbid conditions

None	Few or mild	Multiple or severe

Established vascular complications

None	Cardiovascular disease	
None	Early microvascular	Advanced microvascular

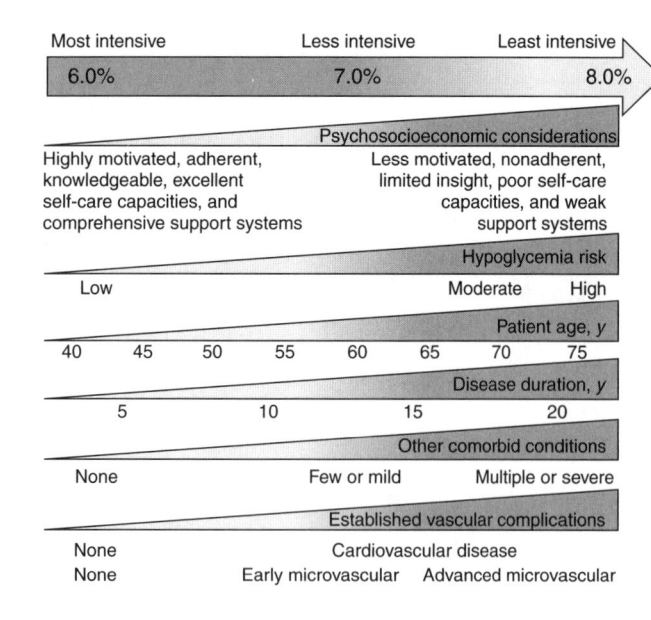

Figure 1 Framework to Assist in Determining Glycemic Treatment Targets in Patients With Type 2 Diabetes

Reprinted with permission from Faramarz Ismail-Beigi, MD, PhD, et al. Individualizing glycemic targets in type 2 diabetes mellitus: Implications of recent clinical trials. *Ann Intern Med.* 2011;154.

Medical nutrition therapy
- The elderly may suffer from overnutrition or undernutrition.
- Healthy meal choices
- Lifestyle changes
- Weight management
- Physical activity

Exercise
- Regular exercise may prevent T2DM in high-risk individuals.
- Aerobic exercise and resistance training can be beneficial.
- Careful clinical judgment when recommending exercise with attention to
  - Cardiovascular disease (clinical and subclinical)
  - Peripheral neuropathy
  - Autonomic neuropathy
- Pre-exercise and postexercise blood glucose monitoring may be needed for optimization of medication and diet with exercise.

Pharmacological therapy
Oral agents
- Lower risk of hypoglycemia—metformin, dipeptidyl peptidase-4 inhibitors (DPP-IV), thiazolidinediones (TZDs), alpha-glucosidase inhibitors, bromocriptine, and colesevelam
- Higher risk of hypoglycemia—sulfonylureas and meglitinides

Noninsulin injectables
- Glucagon-like peptide-1 (GLP-1) agonists and pramlintide

Insulins
- Rapid-acting insulin—aspart, lispro, and glulisine (administered with meals)
- Short-acting insulin—regular (administered 20 to 30 minutes before meals)
- Intermediate-acting insulin—neutral protamine Hagedorn (NPH) insulin (administered once or twice daily)
- Long-acting insulin—glargine and detemir (administered once or twice daily)
- Premixed insulins are administered twice daily, with or before morning and evening meals.
- Consider dose delivery methods (insulin pen, insulin syringes) in patients with impaired vision, dexterity, or cognition

Consults
- Diabetes education
- Endocrinology
- Ophthalmology
- Podiatry
- Nephrology
- Physical therapy
- Cardiology
- Vascular surgery
- Mental health

Complications of treatment
- Weight gain
- Lipoatrophy and/or lipohypertrophy
- Hypoglycemia on many oral diabetes medications and injectables
- Insulin is a high-alert medication.
- Vitamin B_{12} deficiency may be more common with metformin.

Hypoglycemia
- Ranges from a mild to a life-threatening complication of diabetes therapy
- Risk of hypoglycemia needs to be weighed carefully with potential benefits of intensive control.
- Hypoglycemic awareness (ability to sense hypoglycemia) should be assessed.
- Hypoglycemic awareness may be impaired or absent in patients with frequent hypoglycemia and advanced long-standing diabetes.
- Patient and family/caregiver(s) should be educated about hypoglycemia management.

- Hypoglycemic events should be corrected and blood glucose testing should be repeated in 15 minutes.
- Intravenous dextrose and intramuscular glucagon can be used for management of severe hypoglycemia.
- Adjustment of oral and/or injectable diabetes regimen should occur after hypoglycemic episodes.
- Assess for underlying causes
  - Increased physical activity
  - Decreased oral intake
  - Liver and/or renal dysfunction (decreased metabolism or clearance of medications)
  - Other endocrine disease: hypothyroidism or adrenal insufficiency

Prognosis
- Early diagnosis and management of T2DM can prevent and delay complications.
- Good control of glucose increases the life span and decreases the complications in T1DM patients.

Helpful Hints
- Onset at a young age and thin habitus is more likely to be associated with T1DM but can occur at any age.
- A1C goal should be individualized.
- Simple insulin regimen (once or twice daily) in patients with multiple comorbidities is preferred.
- Hypoglycemia is associated with morbidity and mortality and should be avoided.
- Education for hypoglycemia management is important.
- Periodic examination for monitoring of microvascular and macrovascular complications is important.

Suggested Readings

American Diabetes Association. Diagnosis and classification of diabetes mellitus. *Diabetes Care*. 2012;35(Suppl. 1):S64–71.

American Diabetes Association. Standards of medical care in diabetes-2012. *Diabetes Care*. 2012;35(Suppl. 1):S11–63.

De Paula FJA, et al. Novel insights into the relationship between diabetes and osteoporosis. *Diabetes Metab Res Rev*. 2010;26:622–630.

Ismail-Beigi F, et al. Individualizing glycemic targets in type 2 diabetes mellitus: Implications of recent clinical trials. *Ann Intern Med*. 2011;154:554–559.

Strachan MWJ, et al. Cognitive function, dementia and type 2 diabetes mellitus in the elderly. *Nat Rev Endocrinol*. 2011;7:108–114.

Viljoen A, Sinclair AJ. Diabetes and insulin resistance in older people. *Med Clin N Am*. 2011;95:615–629.

Diabetes: The Diabetic Foot

Ruth Thomas MD

Description
Many patients with diabetes develop sensory, motor, and autonomic neuropathy, most commonly manifested as pain and deformity in their feet.
- Patients with diabetes are at increased risk for ulceration that can lead to amputation.

Etiology/Types
Neuropathic problems likely result from a combination of the following:
- Metabolic factors
  - Glycosylation of proteins (affects myelin)
  - Nerve growth factor depletion
  - Autoimmune response, with antibodies leading to autonomic neuropathy
- Microvascular insufficiency
  - Endothelial cell hyperplasia and basement membrane thickening due to high glucose
  - Focal mononeuropathies from microvascular insult

Epidemiology
- Almost 10% of the U.S. population has diabetes and this percentage is increasing.
- Foot disease is the most common complication.
- The risk of amputation is
  - About 15 times higher in diabetics with an ulcer than with no ulcer
  - About 10 times higher than in the nondiabetic population
  - Twice as high in men as in women
  - About 2.7 times higher in Native Americans and 1.8 times higher in Mexican Americans than in Caucasians
- About 60% of patients with diabetic ulcers have evidence of peripheral vascular disease.

Pathogenesis
- About 70% of diabetics have sensory neuropathy.
- Loss of sensation leads to untreated foot trauma.
- Motor neuropathy leads to atrophy of the foot intrinsic muscles and forefoot deformities.
- Tendo-Achilles shortening is common, increasing the forefoot and midfoot plantar pressures.
- Charcot neuroarthropathy can lead to bone fractures and foot collapse.
- Autonomic neuropathy causes dry, hyperkeratotic skin, which fissures and ulcerates more easily.
  - Loss of sensation plus deformity equals pressure, which can lead to ulceration.

Risk Factors
- Poor diabetic control
- Length of time for diagnosis of diabetes
- Poor nutrition
- Skin trauma
- Poor footwear
- Poor skin care
- Vascular disease
- Poor diabetic education/compliance
- Smoking
- Acquired deformity of the foot and ankle

Clinical Features
- Early
  - Decreased sensation
  - Clawing of toes
  - Dry cracked skin
  - Pressure points from shoewear
- Later
  - Loss of protective sensation
  - Diminished pulses
  - Loss of ankle dorsiflexion
  - Poor skin turgor
  - Fissures between toes
  - Ulcerations at points of pressure

Natural History
- About 15% of diabetics will develop a foot ulcer at some time during the disease course.
- Diabetic patients who develop Charcot neuroarthropathy that results in deformity of the foot and ankle have increased risk of weight-bearing pressure ulcers that can lead to amputation.
- The causes of diabetic foot problems progress over time, and require aggressive preventative management.

Diagnosis

History
- Loss of sensation
- History of skin and nail changes
- Prior ulcer history
- Course of diabetes: length of time, level of control, and past complications

Examination
- Protective sensory loss diagnosed with Semmes–Weinstein monofilament test: The test is abnormal when the patient cannot perceive a 5.07 monofilament, applied perpendicular to the plantar skin.
- Motor involvement is apparent with the development of claw toes and equinus contracture of the Achilles tendon.
- Autonomic neuropathy manifests as dry skin subject to cracks and fissures.
- Vascular examination includes palpation of the dorsalis pedis and posterior tibialis pulses.
- Absence of hair on the feet and toes is often associated with ischemia.
- If ulceration is present, it should be described as to size, location, and depth to allow comparison over time; signs of infection or gangrene should be noted.

Testing
- Sensory loss; Semmes–Weinstein monofilament test
- Vascular compromise
  - Ankle-brachial index (ABI) with toe pressures (blood pressure measured in the toes) performed in a vascular lab using Doppler ultrasonography
  - Transcutaneous oxygen tension less than 40 mmHg is considered hypoxia.
  - Arteriography
- Evaluation of bone deformity and/or presence of ulceration
  - X-rays—three views of the foot and/or ankle as indicated.
  - Nuclear Medicine Studies may be helpful in differentiating between soft-tissue infection, osteomyelitis, and Charcot arthropathy. Bone scan alone can be misleading in both osteomyelitis and Charcot arthropathy and usually must be combined with an Indium white blood cell (WBC) study. Indium WBC study with colloid can be even more useful when underlying bone deformity is present. Single-photon emission computed tomography (SPECT) is a three-dimensional study that can improve specificity.
  - Magnetic resonance imaging (MRI)—may not be able to differentiate between Charcot arthropathy and infection.
- Laboratory testing
  - Complete blood count, erythrocyte sedimentation rate, C-reactive protein, glucose, hemoglobin A1C, and albumin
- Electrodiagosis is useful in diagnosing peripheral neuropathy, but may not be sensitive in small axonal disease.

Pitfalls
- In all 67% of ulcers that can be probed to the bone have underlying osteomyelitis.
- Callus may hide underlying ulcer and should be removed during foot examination.
- Missing a deep infection can be limb or life–threatening.

Red flags
- Foot infections in diabetics are emergencies.
- Only minor soft-tissue infections should be treated on an outpatient basis with oral antibiotics and close medical monitoring.
- Significant cellulitis with or without an associated ulcer should be admitted for intravenous (IV) antibiotics and surgical evaluation.
- Before initiating the antibiotic treatment for a diabetic ulcer, an appropriate culture specimen should be obtained by biopsy, ulcer curettage, or aspiration (rather than a wound swab).

Treatment

Medical
- Any diabetic foot with loss of protective sensation and deformity needs protective footwear, including extra-depth soft leather shoes with custom molded plastazote/poron/pelite liners.
- Ulcer management includes the following:
  - Sharp debridement of necrotic tissue, leaving a healthy base
  - Elimination of all pressure from the ulcer site
  - Nonweight-bearing on the affected extremity using crutches or a walker
  - Wound care providing a moist environment using a dressing that absorbs exudates and provides a protective barrier
  - A total contact cast applied by an experienced cast technician and changed weekly or every 2 weeks, as indicated by patient tolerance

- Ulcer healing requires adequate vascularity (ABI greater than 0.45 and toe pressures greater than 40 mmHg), elimination of external pressure, serum albumin level of at least 3.0 g/dL, and total lymphocyte count greater than 1500/mm3.

Surgical
- Surgical management, when indicated, includes the following:
  - Drainage of deep infections and removal of infected bone
  - Correction of deformity

Consults
- Orthopaedic foot and ankle surgery
- Vascular surgery
- Wound management clinic
- Prosthetics and orthotics vendor
- Occupational or physical therapy

Prognosis
- In all 70% of healed ulcers will recur within 5 years.
- In all 30% of amputees will lose the opposite limb within 3 years.

Helpful Hints
- Prevention is the key in managing diabetic foot problems.
- Diabetics at risk for foot ulcers must be taught a self-management program.
- The American Diabetes Association reports that diabetes-related lower extremity amputations can be reduced by half with comprehensive patient education and multidisciplinary foot-care programs.

Suggested Reading
Berlet GC, Philbin TM. The diabetic foot and ankle. *AAOS Comprehensive Rev.* 2009;2:1217–1224.

Functional Decline: Deconditioning

Patrick M. Kortebein MD

Description
In the rehabilitation vernacular, deconditioning (i.e., hospital-associated deconditioning) may be defined as the functional decline of an individual due to the cumulative effects of a prolonged or complicated hospitalization. In a more general sense, deconditioning has been defined as the multiple changes in organ system physiology that are induced by inactivity and reversed by activity. This loss of function should not be due to a specific neurologic or orthopedic disorder. This chapter will discuss hospital-associated deconditioning; see chapters Functional Decline: Frailty and Functional Decline: Sarcopenia for information regarding community-dwelling individuals.

Etiology/Types
Deconditioning is a multifactorial disorder influenced by the following:
- Premorbid (prehospitalization) function
- Bed rest/immobility
- Medical/surgical treatment and complications
- Inflammation, generalized (e.g., elevated tumor necrosis factor-α, TNF-α, interleukin-6 [IL-6])
- Compromised nutrition, especially protein
- Anemia
- Pain
- Sleep deprivation
- Fatigue
- Depression

Epidemiology
- Due to the lack of discrete diagnostic criteria and a consistent diagnostic terminology (e.g., debility, generalized weakness, asthenia), the specific incidence and prevalence of deconditioning are unknown.
- In the acute rehabilitation setting approximately 5% to 13% of patients are admitted for deconditioning, and approximately 20% of rehabilitation consultations in the acute hospital setting may have deconditioning.

Pathogenesis
- See the section on Etiology above. The specific contribution of each of these factors is not presently known.

Risk Factors
In studies examining functional decline during acute hospitalization, the following factors were identified as risk factors:
- Age above 80 years
- Deficits in basic or instrumental activities of daily living (IADL)
- Cognitive deficits
- Use of a gait aid

Clinical Features
- Decline in physical function from baseline that occurs during an acute care hospitalization.
- Manifest as an inability to perform
  - Basic physical functions such as bed mobility, transfers, ambulation, and activities of daily living (ADL, e.g., dressing, bathing) without assistance
  - Generalized muscle weakness is typically present, although strength may be normal when considering associated general muscle atrophy.
  - No focal neurologic deficits should be present.

Natural History
Frequently deconditioned patients cannot be discharged to their homes due to functional compromise. Discharge locations include
- Inpatient rehabilitation
  - Approximately 70% discharged to home
  - About 12% to 20% readmitted to acute hospital
- Skilled nursing facility/subacute rehabilitation
- Long-term acute care (LTAC)
- Home with home health care therapies

Diagnosis

Differential diagnosis
- Critical illness myopathy/polyneuropathy
- Myopathies, including steroid-induced form
- Cervical myelopathy
- Neuromuscular junction disorders (e.g., myasthenia gravis)
- Neuromuscular disorders (e.g., amyotrophic lateral sclerosis, ALS)

History
- Prior level of function, including the use of gait aids or adaptive equipment and assistance from spouse/family/friends should be assessed.
- Current level of function (often from therapy and nursing evaluations) should be assessed.
- Medications should be reviewed for adverse effects (e.g., corticosteroids, cholesterol-lowering agents).
- Systems should be reviewed to exclude other medical conditions that would explain the functional decline.

Examination
No discrete diagnostic criteria exist; however, the following have been proposed:
- Muscle atrophy, generalized
- Muscle weakness, generalized (Grade 4/5 symmetric bilateral)
- Sit to stand; unable or requiring assistance
- Gait; unable or requiring assistance/gait aid
- No focal/asymmetric neurologic findings

Testing
- Orthostatic hypotension evaluation
- Short physical performance battery

Red Flags
- Increased risk of venous thromboembolism
- Orthostatic hypotension/falls
- Pressure ulcers/breakdown
- Constipation
- Compromised nutrition

Treatment

Medical
- Nutrition; optimization of protein and caloric intake via dietary consultation
- Anabolic agents (e.g., topical testosterone enanthate, creatine phosphate)

Exercise

Physical therapy
- Bed mobility/transfers
- Gait and balance training
- Ambulatory endurance with/without gait aid
- Stair climbing
- Muscle strength and endurance training (especially hip/knee extensors)

Occupational therapy
- ADL training, including fine motor skills and adaptive equipment needs
- IADL/homemaking/community survival skills
- Upper-extremity muscle strength and endurance training (e.g., shoulder and elbow groups, and fine motor/grip strength)
- Energy conservation and joint-protection principles
- Cognitive and safety awareness evaluation and training

Prognosis
- Patients with hospital-associated deconditioning have increased risk of mortality and nursing home institutionalization.

Helpful Hints
- Other, potentially treatable, causes of weakness and loss of function should be evaluated and ruled out.
- Deconditioning puts the person at risk for other medical comorbidities.
- Deconditioning can be treated with rehabilitation.

References
Gill TM, Allore HG, Holford TR, et al. Hospitalization, restricted activity, and the development of disability among older persons. *JAMA* 2004;292:2115–2124.

Herridge MS, Cheung AM, Tansey CM, et al. One-year outcomes in survivors of the acute respiratory distress syndrome. *N Engl J Med* 2003;348:683–693.

Hirsch CH, Sommers L, Olsen A, et al. The natural history of functional morbidity in hospitalized older patients. *J Am Geriatr Soc* 1990;38:1296–1303.

Killewich LA. Strategies to minimize postoperative deconditioning in elderly surgical patients. *J Am Coll Surg* 2006;203:735–745.

Kortebein P. Rehabilitation for hospital associated deconditioning. *Am J Phys Med Rehabil* 2009;88:66–77.

Kortebein P, Granger CV, Sullivan DH. A comparative evaluation of inpatient rehabilitation for older adults with debility, hip fracture, and myopathy. *Arch Phys Med Rehabil* 2009;90:934–938.

Raj G, Munir J, Ball L, et al. An inpatient rehabilitation service for deconditioned older adults. *Top Geriatr Rehabil* 2007;23:126–137.

Sager MA, Franke T, Inouye SK, et al. Functional outcomes of acute medical illness and hospitalization in older persons. *Arch Intern Med* 1996;156:645–652.

Walter LC, Brand RJ, Counsell SR, et al. Development and validation of a prognostic index for 1-year mortality in older adults after hospitalization. *JAMA* 285:2987–2994.

Functional Decline: Frailty

Jordan Tate MD MPH ■ Dale Strasser MD

Description
Frailty is defined as a clinically recognizable state of increased vulnerability. Frail elders represent a high-risk subset of the patient population, who are more susceptible to major health changes caused by minor stressing events.
- Identification and classification of frailty in the clinical setting is an important means for prevention of comorbid geriatric syndromes, disability, institutionalizations, and death.
- Once recognized, interventions can be initiated to target frailty and to improve the patient's clinical condition.

Etiology/Types
Diagnosis of frailty is made through clinical assessment. While consensus on the method of diagnosis and classification has not been made, two models of diagnosis have been proposed:
- Physical phenotype: the Fried model
  - Utilization of this model allows for classification of elders into three clinical stages: nonfrail, prefrail, and frail.
- Multidomain phenotype: the Frailty Index (FI)
  - Diagnosis of frailty via this model is dependent on the presence of certain physical, psychological, and social domains.

Epidemiology
- In the United States, frailty is estimated to be present in
  - About 7% to 12% of community-dwelling adults above age 65
  - About 3.9% of those aged 65 to 75 years
  - About 25% of those 85 and above
- African American elders have twice the risk of diagnosis of frailty.

Pathogenesis
Detrimental and cumulative interaction of age-related changes in multiple systems leads to frailty. A cycle of frailty has been suggested:
- Chronic malnourishment → weight loss → sarcopenia → decreased strength, decreased basal metabolic rate, and exhaustion → decrease in walking speed, impaired balance, and falls → decreased activity → disability and dependency.

Risk Factors
- Advancing age
- Decreased social resources
- Decrease in "Life-Space" (a measure of social interactions and physical movement)
- Reduced functional reserve
- Sarcopenia (loss of skeletal muscle mass)
- Anorexia
- Osteoporosis
- Medical comorbidities

Clinical Features
- Weakness is the most common initial manifestation.
- Weakness, slowness, and low physical activity precede exhaustion and weight loss in 76% of baseline nonfrail women in the Women's Health and Aging Studies (WHAS II).

Natural History
- The natural loss of muscle strength and bulk, beginning in midlife, initiates the frailty cycle.
- Two thirds have slow progression; one third have rapid progression from nonfrailty to frailty.
- Those presenting with exhaustion or weight loss progress to frailty more rapidly.
- One study revealed that 35% of the sample population without specific intervention progressed from frail to prefrail stage in 18 months. The same study revealed that a transition from frail to nonfrail stage was rare.

Diagnosis

Physical phenotype: the Fried model
It is based on the clinical presence of five criteria:
  0 criteria present: Nonfrail stage
  1–2 criteria present: Prefrail stage
  3–5 criteria present: Frail
Criteria are as follows:
- Weakness, assessed via dynamometer for low grip strength

- Exhaustion, self-reported on the Center for Epidemiologic Studies Depression Scale
- Slowness, 15-foot walk test, scoring less than the 20th percentile, stratified for sex and height
    Low energy expenditure: defined as either complete inactivity or performing low-intensity activities less than 1 hour per week (males: less than 383 kcal/week, females: less than 270 kcal/week)
- Unintentional weight loss
    - Body mass index (BMI) less than 18.5
    - Weight loss of more than 10 pounds in the past year
    - Greater than 10% loss of weight from the patient's baseline at age 60

Multidomain phenotype: FI
- Scored by the presence of deficits accumulated over time in the following domains:
    - Disability
    - Disease
    - Physical impairment
    - Cognitive impairment
    - Psychosocial risk factors (e.g., depression, low socioeconomic status, isolation)
    - Geriatric syndromes (e.g., falls, delirium, incontinence, pressure sores)
- Various scales exist in the literature. A 30-item scale and a 70-item scale are the most commonly encountered FIs.

Red Flags
- Malignancy, thyroid and other metabolic disorders, neurologic, and orthopedic disorders need to be ruled out by thorough investigation. Frailty is a diagnosis of exclusion.

Treatment
Interventions targeted at nutrition, physical rehabilitation, and pharmacological means such as anabolic steroids have been studied.

- Good evidence exists that physical rehabilitation in both individual and group settings improves the functional status of frail elders.

Prognosis
- A greater severity of deficits is associated with a worse prognosis.
- Frailty leads to worsening activities of daily living, increased hospitalizations, and death.
- Slow gait speed has been shown to be the most predictive indicator of frailty.
- Identifying patients at risk for frailty or those in the prefrail stage, and modifying the risk factors delays the development of severe stages of frailty.

Helpful Hints
- Clinical screening of all elderly patients for frailty may allow for earlier detection and prevention of deterioration of clinical and functional status.

Suggested Readings
Bakker FC, Robben SHM, Olde Rikkert MGM. Effects of hospital-wide interventions to improve care for the frail older inpatients: A systematic review. *BMJ Qual Saf.* 2011;20:680–691.

Clegg A, Young J. The frailty syndrome. *Clin Med.* 2011;11:72–75.

Rothman MD, Leo-Summers L, Gill TM. Prognostic significance of potential frailty criteria. *J Am Geriatr Soc.* 2008;56(12):2211–2116.

Van Kan G, Rolland Y, Houles M, et al. The assessment of frailty in older adults. *Clin Geriatr Med.* 2010;26:275–286.

Wells JL, Seabrook JA, Stolee P, et al. State of the art in geriatric rehabilitation. Part I: Review of frailty and comprehensive geriatric assessment. *Arch Phys Med Rehabil.* 2003;84:890–897.

Xue Q-L. The frailty syndrome: Definition and natural history. *Clin Geriatr Med.* 2011;27:1–15.

Functional Decline: Sarcopenia

Patrick M. Kortebein MD

Description
Sarcopenia is not a disease per se but is a term initially used in 1989 to describe the age-related loss of skeletal muscle. More recently, some authors have expanded the use of this term to include age-related loss of strength and function.

Etiology/Types
The specific etiology of sarcopenia is not known; however, it is felt to be a multifactorial disorder with an overall decline in anabolic factors and increased catabolic factors. The available data support the following as contributors:
- Neurologic—loss of alpha motor neurons with aging
- Hormonal dysfunction—decline in testosterone, growth hormone (GH)/insulin-like growth factor 1 (IGF-1), and estrogen
- Metabolic dysfunction—decreased muscle protein synthesis (controversial)
- Nutritional dysfunction—decline in calorie/protein intake
- Inflammation, generalized—elevated interleukin (IL)-6, IL-1, and tumor necrosis factor-α (TNF-α)
- Renin angiotensin aldosterone system dysfunction
- Physical inactivity

Epidemiology
- There is no agreed upon definition or measurement technique for sarcopenia; thus, the reported prevalence varies depending upon the method of measuring muscle mass. In general, the muscle mass of older individuals is compared to that of younger adults in a manner similar to bone density measurements (e.g., more than 2 standard deviations below the sex/ethnic specific means of young adults).
- Measurement instruments include: dual-energy X-ray absorptiometry (DEXA), magnetic resonance imaging (MRI), and computed tomography (CT).
- Prevalence rates
  - United States/Europe: 5% to 13% of 60- to 70-year-olds and 11% to 50% of those above age 80
  - Asia: 8% to 22% of females and 6% to 23% of males

Pathogenesis
See the section on Etiology above. The specific contribution of each of these factors is presently unknown.
- Muscle mass losses are generally approximately 1% to 2% per year after age 50, while strength declines around 1% to 3% per year after 40 to 50 years of age, with a more accelerated decline of both parameters in older individuals (above age 70).

Risk Factors
- Physical inactivity; especially lack of resistance exercise
- Poor protein/calorie intake

Clinical Features
- Low muscle mass (e.g., more than 2 standard deviations below the mean of young adults of the same sex/ethnicity)
- Low gait speed (less than 0.8 m/sec for 4-m walk; proposed)

Natural History
- Sarcopenia appears to be a progressive phenomenon that is more pronounced after the age of approximately 70 years.

Diagnosis

Differential diagnosis
- Frailty syndrome (characteristics: weakness, slow gait speed, weight loss, exhaustion, and physical inactivity)
- Cachexia
- Malignancy
- Myopathies
- Cervical myelopathy
- Neuromuscular junction disorders (e.g., myasthenia gravis)
- Neuromuscular disorders (e.g., amyotrophic lateral sclerosis, ALS)
- Medication side effects (e.g., corticosteroids, cholesterol-lowering agents)

Functional Decline: Sarcopenia

History
- Current level of function, including ambulation, use of gait aids, or adaptive equipment, and assistance from spouse/family/friends
- Medication review (e.g., corticosteroids)
- Systems review to exclude other medical conditions (e.g., malignancy)

Examination
- Muscle atrophy, generalized
- Muscle weakness, generalized
- Sit to stand; unable or requiring assistance
- Gait; unable or requiring assistance/gait aid
- No focal/asymmetric neurologic findings

Testing
- Short physical performance battery (SPPB; chair rise/gait speed/balance)
- Muscle mass measurement (data available if normative); DEXA, MRI, and CT

Red Flags
- Falls
- Pressure ulcers/breakdown

Proposed Treatment

Medical
- Nutrition; optimize protein (1.2–1.5 gm/kg/d) and caloric intake; possible vitamin D supplementation
- Anabolic agents; testosterone enanthate (topical/intramuscular) and creatine phosphate
- Angiotensin-converting enzyme (ACE) inhibitors

Exercise

Resistance training
- Major muscle groups of the upper and lower extremities. Recommended: 8 to 10 exercises, two to three sets of each, with 8 to 12 repetitions at 70% to 80% of the one-repetition maximum amount (the maximum weight that can be lifted one time), or exercise at a rating of perceived exertion of 14 to 15 out of 20.

Investigational
- Myostatin antagonists
- Selective androgen receptor antagonists (SARMs)

Prognosis
- Sarcopenia does not appear to be lethal in and of itself, but likely contributes to the overall functional decline with aging, and perhaps even an increased risk of institutionalization/death.

Suggested Readings

Burton LA, Sumukadas D. Optimal management of sarcopenia. *Clin Interv Aging.* 2010;5:217–228.

Cruz-Jentoft AJ, et al. Sarcopenia: European consensus on definition and diagnosis. *Age Ageing.* 2010;39:412–423.

Doherty TJ. Invited review: Aging and sarcopenia. *J Appl Physiol.* 2003;95:1717–1727.

Roubenoff R. Sarcopenia: Effects on body composition and function. *J Gerontol A Biol Sci Med Sci.* 2003;58A:1012–1017.

Waters DL, Baumgartner RN, Garry PJ, et al. Advantages of dietary, exercise-related, and therapeutic interventions to prevent and treat sarcopenia in adult patients: An update. *Clin Interv Aging.* 2010;5:259–270.

Gastrointestinal: Constipation

Reginald D. Talley MD

Description
Constipation is the most common digestive complaint in the general population. Based upon the epidemiologic studies in the United States and the United Kingdom, constipation has been defined as a stool frequency of less than three per week. It is to be noted that constipation is a symptom, not a disease.

Etiology/Types
- Specific diseases or conditions, including neurologic, metabolic, and endocrine disorders, such as stroke, spinal cord injury, Parkinson's disease, diabetes mellitus, and hypothyroidism
- Lack of physical activity (especially in the elderly)
- Medications (examples include narcotics, antidepressants, anticonvulsants, iron supplements, calcium channel blockers, and aluminum-containing antacids)
- Not enough fiber in the diet
- Problems with the colon and rectum, including colorectal cancer, hemorrhoids, or fissures
- Psychological conditions such as anxiety and depression
- Abuse of laxatives
- Dehydration
- Ignoring the urge to have a bowel movement
- Lactose intolerance
- Problems with intestinal function (chronic idiopathic constipation)
- In the elderly, constipation is categorized as
  - Normal-transit constipation
  - Slow-transit constipation
  - Obstructed defecation
  - Irritable bowel syndrome (IBS): A chronic disorder characterized by episodes of cramping, abdominal pain, bloating, constipation, and diarrhea.

Epidemiology
- For patients of age 65 years or above, approximately 26% of men and 34% of women complain of constipation.
- There is a positive correlation between constipation and decreased calorie intake.

Pathogenesis
- Colonic motility dysfunction, or dysmotility, is failure of coordinated motor activity to move the stool through the colon. Examples include
  - Dysfunction of the autonomic nervous system
  - Disruption in the enteric nervous system
  - Disruptions in the neuroendocrine system
  - Colonic myopathy
- Pelvic floor dysfunction or disorders of the anorectum and pelvic floor result in outlet dysfunction and an inability to adequately evacuate rectal contents. Examples include
  - Dyschezia
  - Pelvic dyssynergia.
- Both mechanisms can coexist in some patients.

Risk Factors
- Pathophysiologic changes with aging (decreased cholinergic myenteric activity that can cause smaller contractions and impaired peristalsis)
- Gender: female (hormonal and structural changes)
- Low fiber diet
- Neuromuscular or metabolic disease
- Medications/undergoing chemotherapy
- History of sexual abuse (extreme stress and psychiatric problems)
- Depressive symptoms
- Low income (associated with poor lifestyle choices)
- Less than 12 years of education (associated with poor lifestyle choices)

Clinical Features
- Abdominal pain
- Nausea and/or vomiting
- Loss of appetite
- Abdominal distension
- Acute mood changes
- Pain upon defecation

Natural History
- For most patients, constipation becomes a chronic problem with continual expenses and decreased quality of life.

- Complications can include, but are not limited to, the following:
  - Diverticulosis
  - Fecal impaction
  - Rectal prolapse
  - Rectocele
  - Enterocele
  - Overflow of fecal incontinence.
- The risk for colorectal cancer is increased.

Diagnosis

Most physicians use the Rome III criteria for diagnosing functional constipation, which includes two or more of the following fulfilled for the last 3 months, with symptom onset at least 6 months prior to diagnosis:

(i) Fewer than three bowel movements per week
(ii) Straining (≥25% of defecations)
(iii) Lumpy or hard stools (≥25% of defecations)
(iv) Sensation of incomplete evacuation (≥25% of defecations)
(v) Sensation of anorectal obstruction or blockage (≥25% of defecations)
(vi) Manual maneuvers to facilitate a bowel movement (≥25% of defecations)

Differential diagnosis
- Colon cancer
- Abdominal hernias
- Inflammatory bowel disease
- Anxiety or depression
- Hypothyroidism
- Intra-abdominal ischemia
- Rectal outlet obstruction (anatomic alterations such as rectocele responsible for incomplete evacuation of fecal contents from rectum)

History
- History can include the following:
  - Decrease in stool frequency
  - Excessive straining
  - Feeling of incomplete evacuation
  - Recent changes in diet
  - Change in physical activity
- Recent medication changes (as stated above)
- Past medical history of neurologic, metabolic, or gastrointestinal diseases

Examination
- Skin examination: Identify skin changes such as pallor and edema that may suggest a secondary cause, such as hypothyroidism.
- Abdominal examination can identify problems such as
  - Distension
  - Masses
  - Surgical scars
- Rectal examination (including rectal sensation) can identify problems such as
  - Hemorrhoids
  - Rectal prolapse
  - Fissures
  - Dyssynergia

Testing
- Thyroid function tests
- Basic metabolic panel (electrolytes, blood urea nitrogen/creatinine, glucose)
- Complete blood count
- Calcium
- Colorectal cancer screening (fecal blood stool or colonoscopy) may be needed for alarming symptoms, such as rectal bleeding.
- In resistant cases of constipation, the following can be considered:
  - Defecography—X-ray test that shows the rectum and anal canal as they change during defecation: used to investigate conditions such as rectocele or enterocele.
  - Colon transit studies—X-ray test to determine how well food moves through the colon: used to investigate slow-transit constipation.
  - Anorectal manometry—measures pressures and electrical activity of the anal sphincter muscles and the sensation in the rectum: used to investigate constipation (functional type) or fecal incontinence. This can have therapeutic benefits (see below).

Pitfalls
- Many patients may feel that they are constipated due to minor changes in bowel function when in fact they are not; therefore, the diagnosis must be confirmed by the history and examination; patient education is very important.
- Irritable bowel syndrome is a diagnosis of exclusion.

Red flags
- The elderly patient who presents with rectal bleeding (or positive fecal occult blood test), unexplained weight loss, family history of bowel cancer, or inflammatory bowel disease must be suspected of having bowel cancer, until proven otherwise.

Treatment

Medical
- Initial management consists of maintaining daily fiber intake around (20 g/day) and water intake of at least 2 L/day.
- If no response within 3 to 4 weeks, stool softeners such as docusate (colace) by mouth may be used for the short term. Excessive use can lead to electrolyte abnormalities, most notably hypokalemia.
- Alternative treatments are osmotic agents, such as lactulose, sorbitol, magnesium hydroxide, and polyethylene glycol that act by retaining water in the intestinal lumen and accelerating intestinal transit. Such agents are to be used for the short term and have side effect profiles, including electrolyte abnormalities, diarrhea, or abdominal bloating.
- Stimulants such as bisacodyl and senna act by stimulating peristalsis, along with water and electrolyte secretion. They usually work within hours and can cause abdominal cramps, among other side effects.
- Enemas are usually used if oral agents have not been effective. Examples include soapsuds, mineral oil, tap water, and phosphate. They work to soften and lubricate stool. The least side effect profile is seen with tap water and soapsuds enema.
- Other drugs used include
  - Lubiprostone (Amitiza): activates type 2 chloride channels and increases fluid secretion with no significant systemic absorption; selected for patients with chronic idiopathic constipation and IBS (constipation predominant)
  - Tegaserod (5-HT4 receptor agonist): improves constipation in women with IBS
  - Colchicine (microtubule-formation inhibitor): can be effective for patients with refractory constipation
  - Misoprostol (prostaglandin E1 analog): side effect is diarrhea
  - There is limited study of colchicine and misoprostol in the elderly population.

Exercises
- Encouraging physical activity as simple as walking can help regulate bowel movements.
- Biofeedback therapy for patients with pelvic floor dyssynergia using an anorectal electromyography or manometry has had long-lasting benefits and success rates of around 70%.

Consults
- Gastroenterology
- Nutrition

Complications of treatment
- Medications used for constipation have side effects such as
  - Fluid and electrolyte disturbances
  - Abdominal bloating and cramps
  - Diarrhea

Prognosis
- Although many cases of constipation can lead to chronic problems, with proper treatment, most patients can expect a full recovery and return to normal bowel function.

Helpful Hints
- Surgery is usually indicated for those selected patients with conditions such as
  - Intra-abdominal ischemia
  - Rectal outlet obstruction (see above)
  - Refractory slow-transit constipation (subtotal colectomy is effective, provided that pelvic floor dysfunction has been excluded or treated).

Suggested Readings
Lacy BE, Cole MS. Constipation in the older adult. *Clin Geriatr.* 2008;16(1):44–54.

McCrea GL, Miaskowski C, Stotts NA, et al. Pathophysiology of constipation in the older adult. *World J Gastroenterol.* 2008;14(17):2631–2638.

Talley NJ, Fleming KC, Evans JM, et al. Constipation in an elderly community: A study of prevalence and potential risk factors. *Am J Gastroenterol.* 1996;91:19.

Gastrointestinal: Fecal Incontinence

Tanya Cabrita MD ■ Dale Strasser MD

Description
Recurrent inability to control passage of fecal material for at least 1-month duration.
- Fecal incontinence (FI) is a challenging condition of diverse etiology with devastating psychosocial impact. It is the leading cause of nursing home placement, a marker of poor health, and is associated with increased morbidity and mortality. Inpatient rehabilitation settings have a 10-fold decrease in community discharges in patients with FI. It is important to understand that FI is not uncommon and can often be successfully treated.

Etiology/Types
Often due to multiple mechanisms such as the following:
- Overflow: abnormal capacity or compliance; commonly associated with rectal surgery, radiation, inflammatory bowel disease, or other conditions causing scarring and decreased compliance of the rectum.
- Loose feces: altered consistency; caused by medications, lactose intolerance, neoplasia, colitis, infections, and other food sensitivities.
- Functional incontinence: restricted mobility.
- Cognition related: uninhibited rectal contraction due to dementia and frontal lobe lesions.
- Anorectal incontinence: pelvic floor or anal sphincter dysfunction and weak external sphincter due to trauma, surgery, and radiation.
- Comorbidity: stroke, diabetes mellitus, spinal cord injuries (SCIs)/plexus injuries, degenerative disorders, idiopathic bowel disease, colon cancer, thyroid disorders, depression, and hemorrhoids.

Epidemiology
- FI is estimated to affect 18 million U.S. adults, approximately 1 in 12.
- Prevalence estimates vary from 2% to 24%, depending on definition, frequency, and clinical setting.

Prevalence
- General population: 2% to 3%, community: 6% to 12% of those above age 65, 18% to 29% of those above age 80
- Nursing home residents: 37% to 54%

Pathogenesis
- Bowel control requires cognition, along with structural and functional integrity of the nerves and muscles of the anus and rectum.
- Age-related factors include
  - Decreased strength of the external anal sphincter (EAS) causing weak anal squeeze
  - Increased rectal compliance
  - Decreased resting tone of the internal anal sphincter (IAS)
  - Lower rectal volumes relax the internal sphincter, cause perianal descent at rest, decrease colonic motility, slow pudendal conduction, and decrease anorectal sensation.

Risk Factors
- Urinary incontinence; 50% to 70% coexistence
- White race
- Male sex (traditionally higher in females, new studies show higher in males)
- Age above 65 years
- Anal sphincter injury
- Chronic constipation
- Major depression
- Neurologic diseases
- Degenerative diseases
- Dementia
- Restricted mobility
- Polypharmacy/drug side effects
- Poor general health

Clinical Features
- Repeated underwear soiling
- Diarrhea
- Constipation
- Gas
- Abdominal pain
- Disordered urination

Natural History
- Variable, depends on the cause and whether it is treatable
- At risk for skin breakdown, social isolation, and depression

Diagnosis

Differential diagnosis
- Chronic constipation
- Diarrhea
- Fecal impaction
- Gastroenteritis
- Anal tumor
- Sphincter defects
- Pelvic floor dysfunction
- Rectal nerve damage
- Perianal fistula
- Rectal prolapse
- Rectocele
- Inflammatory bowel diseases
- Neurologic diseases
- Pelvic fracture
- Vertebral fracture
- Herniated disc
- Dementia
- Seizure
- Drug intoxication

History
Good rapport should be established with the patient. Individuals are reluctant to admit symptoms due to incontinence stigma and embarrassment.
- All patients with diarrhea, constipation, or anorectal problems should be asked about FI.
- Detailed clinical history; including anorectal trauma, surgery, pelvic radiation, hygiene, and obstetric history (for women).
- Description of FI, including onset, stool type, bowel habits, frequency of episodes, associated symptoms, and impact on patient's quality of life.
- Identification of evacuation difficulties; urgency, delay, straining, incomplete evacuation, and pain.
- Review of medications, supplements, dietary habits, and toxin exposure.
- Review of systems eliciting comorbid systemic medical conditions.
- Assessment of functional status: ambulation, communication, assistance, and access to facilities.
- Prior FI modifications and treatments.
- FI surveys can be given to quantify and qualify the severity: Incontinence Quality of Life Scale provided in Rockwood et al (2000) and FI Questionnaire provided in Reilly et al (2000).

Examination
- Abdomen: assessment of bowel sounds, tenderness, and fullness.
- Neurologic: mental status and gait/mobility
- Gastrointestinal/genitourinary: inspection of perineal, vaginal, and anal anatomy; evaluation for sphincter defects, hemorrhoids, anal fissures/fistula-in ano, scars, absence of perianal creases, rectal prolapse, abscess, dermatitis, and poor hygiene.
- Perianal sensation; anocutaneous reflex: absence of reflex contraction of EAS suggests disruption of spinal arc.
- Digital rectal examination: assessment of resting tone, anal sphincter and levator ani tone, length of canal, anorectal angle, resistance, masses, and blood.
  - Sensitivity, specificity, and positive predictive value of the digital examination as an objective test to evaluate the anal sphincter is low.

Testing
No single test is confirmatory; a combination of tests along with clinical evaluation is the most helpful in diagnosis.

Laboratory
- Electrolytes
- Thyroid stimulating hormone (TSH)
- Calcium
- Complete blood count (CBC)
- *Clostridium difficile* toxin

Imaging studies
- Kidney, ureter, and bladder (KUB) X-ray: to identify intestinal distention, feces, obstruction, and masses.
- Endoanal ultrasonography: The IAS is seen clearly; diagnostic evaluation of anal sphincters, anorectal angle, defects, and perineal descent.
- Magnetic resonance imaging (MRI): The EAS is seen clearly; comparable to ultrasonography.
- Cinedefecography: Rectal contrast imaging to observe process, rate, and evacuation.

Diagnostic procedures
- The clinical history and physical examination can provide insight into the cause of fecal incontinence, thus, allowing focused diagnostic testing. It is recommended that patients with symptoms have inspection of the distal colon and anus with flexible sigmoidoscopy and anoscopy, if the anus is not well visualized. Patients with diarrhea can additionally have stool studies and full colonoscopy. Colonoscopy can identify and exclude bleeding, mucosal disease, polyps, ulcers, and cancer.
- Anal ultrasound: Ultrasound uses sound waves that bounce and reflect off tissue to give a real-time, 360° view of acoustic properties and defects in tissue.

It helps to identify abnormalities in sphincters, rectal wall, anal masses, and fistulas. Endoanal ultrasonography is performed in the left lateral or lithotomy position. The lithotomy position in females allows for the evaluation of other pelvic support defects.
- Anorectal manometry (ARM): ARM measures the tone in the anal sphincter and rectal muscles, the sensation in the rectum, and neural reflexes needed for normal bowel movements. It can also be used to evaluate rectal capacity and rectal compliance. Anal manometry measures how strong the sphincter muscles are and whether they relax as they should during defecation. This procedure can diagnose problems involving: resting, squeezing, releasing anal sphincter tone, muscle coordination, expulsion, and rectal sensation. During the procedure a small plastic tube with a small balloon at the end is inserted rectally. The balloon is inflated and measurements are taken, while muscles are squeezed and relaxed. Normal values for manometry vary among institutions as no uniformly accepted standard currently exists. An abnormally low sphincter pressure demonstrates that a sphincter defect is present. Decreased resting pressure suggests isolated IAS sphincter dysfunction, while decreased squeeze pressure suggests isolated EAS dysfunction. Patients with severe weakness of the EAS may have a prolapsed rectum. Maximum squeeze pressure has greatest sensitivity and specificity in FI. ARM is often done in conjunction with the balloon expulsion test.
- Balloon expulsion test: This test measures the time it takes to expel a balloon from the rectum. A small balloon is inserted into the rectum and then inflated with water. The patient goes to the bathroom and tries to expel the balloon. Prolonged balloon expulsion suggests a dysfunction in the anorectal area.
- Defecography: This is a radiologic test that uses barium to give important information on how the rectum empties, and if there are any structural abnormalities. It can also help in the diagnosis of:
  – Rectal intussusception
  – Rectal prolapse
  – Rectocele (bulging in the rectum)
  – Enterocele (falling of the bowels during evacuation)
  – Cystocele (bulging of the bladder)
  – Vaginal prolapse

Sitting in an upright position on a commode, the patient is asked to rest, squeeze, and strain certain muscles and then push the barium paste out, while X-rays are being taken.

- Pudendal nerve terminal motor latency (PNTML): The PNTML test measures the time from nerve stimulation to muscle contraction. PNTML evaluates the time required for an electrical stimulus to travel along the pudendal nerve from the ischial spine to the anus. Findings reflect myelin function of the peripheral nerve and pelvic floor neuromuscular integrity. The pudendal nerve is stimulated at the ischial spine transanally. The latency period between stimulation of the nerve and evoked response of the muscle is measured. Any damage to the neuromuscular unit results in the prolongation of the latency. Although prolonged PNTML indicates pudendal neuropathy, normal latency does not exclude nerve injury because only the fastest remaining conducting fibers are recorded. In addition, external sphincter innervation has been shown to have overlap. Another difficulty is with interpreting the findings, as the literature currently presents no uniformly accepted standards. Despite these factors, many investigators have suggested that PNTML is the most significant predictor of functional outcome of a sphincteroplasty.

Red Flags
- Bleeding
- Severe pain
- Sensory or motor deficits
- Decreased anal tone

Treatment

Goal
- To restore continence and improve the quality of life. A combination of strategies is most useful.
- Main approach is to stimulate a regular bowel program and treat underlying causes (e.g., fecal impaction, diarrhea, bowel disease, lactose intolerance).

Supportive therapies
- Education/counseling/habit-training
- Diet (e.g., increase fiber, avoid lactose/fructose)
- Reduce caffeine intake
- Anal hygiene/skin care

Specific therapies

Pharmacologic
- Constipation/incomplete evacuation: Rectal evacuants; glycerin suppository, bisacodyl suppository, and various enemas (e.g., saline, mineral oil, docusate, phosphate, tap water with/without digital stimulation).

- Antidiarrheals (overactive bowel) include
  - Loperamide: 2 to 4 mg 45 minutes before meal/social event to prevent evacuation.
  - Lomotil: 1 to 2 tablets twice to four times daily, as needed. Maximum: 8 tablets daily. Reduces stool frequency and urgency, and increases colonic transit time.
  - Anticholinergic: hyoscyamine (1–2 tablets every 4 hours, as needed. Maximum: 12 tablets daily).
  - Bile salt malabsorption: cholestyramine (2–4 g twice to four times daily before meals. Maximum: 16 g daily) and colestipol (2 g one to two times daily, increase 4 g every 1–2 months. Maximum: 16 g daily).
  - Estrogen replacement in postmenopausal women: estrogen increases resting anal and voluntary squeeze pressures.

  SCI—side effects of multiple medications should be assessed, particularly in older SCI individuals.
- Supraspinal lesion; reflex defecation intact: suppository or rectal stimulation.
- Cauda equina/lower motor neuron lesions; reflex defection impaired: laxatives, antidiarrheals, enemas, and digital stimulation.

Biofeedback therapy (neuromuscular conditioning)
- Manometry or skin-sensing electrodes are attached to visual or auditory feedback to tell the patient when the proper anal muscles are being used.

Anal sphincter muscle strengthening
- For sphincter weakness

Rectal sensory conditioning
- For impaired sensation

Rectoanal coordination training
- For dyssynergia

Others
- Anal plugs: temporarily occlude anal canal
- Sphincter bulking agents (collagen; glutaraldehyde cross-linked [GAX] silicone): augment surface area and seal of anal canal
- Electrical stimulation of sacral spinal nerves: stimulates anal contraction
- Pelvic floor muscle exercises (Kegel exercises): improves anal sphincter muscle tone/function. Contraction of perineal muscles as tightly as possible for 5 seconds followed by relaxation; repeated 30 times, three times daily

Surgery
- Sphincteroplasty (e.g., plastic reconstruction of sphincter)
- Muscle transposition; gluteus (buttock) or gracilis (inner thigh) used to encircle/strengthen anal canal
- Artificial bowel sphincter implantation
- Sacral nerve stimulation
- Colostomy—rare; if suitable techniques have failed, it is a safe option

Consults
- Gastroenterology
- Neurology
- Gynecology
- Oncology
- Physiatry
- Physical therapy

Prognosis
- Variable; better for functional incontinence, poor habits, and reversible causes; worse for neurologic or structural causes

Helpful Hints
- Determine the goals of bowel program (frequency, timing, location)
- Eating smaller and more frequent meals can reduce urgency and stool frequency.
- Minimize medications affecting bowel motility (e.g., anticholinergics, narcotics, tricyclic antidepressants, antacids)
- Caffeinated beverages, prune juice, and apricot nectar increase bowel evacuation.
- A high-fiber diet with fruits and vegetables normalizes stool consistency and reduces urgency.
- Minimize fatty foods and dairy products, which impair gut motility
- Toileting within 1 hour after breakfast and dinner helps to utilize the gastrocolic reflex.
- A foot stool to achieve a squatting position can aid in bowel motility.
- Avoid broad spectrum antibiotics, which alter the gut flora.
- Constipation prevention includes adequate daily fiber (25–35 g/day) and fluid intake (2500–3000 mL/day).
- For diarrhea symptoms, limit alcohol, caffeine, spicy foods, and leafy green vegetables. Add constipating foods such as cheese, yogurt, white rice, pasta, bananas, and applesauce, until resolution.
- Minimizing left lateral position allows gravity to assist with stool flow.
- Physical activity aids in regular and predictable bowel emptying.

Suggested Readings

Bellicini N, Molloy PJ, Caushaj P, et al. Fecal incontinence: A review. *Dig Dis Sci*. 2008;53(1):41.

Cheetham M, Brazzelli M, Norton C, et al. Drug treatment for fecal incontinence in adults. *Cochrane Database Syst Rev*. 2003;3:CD002116.

Landefeld CS, Bowers BJ, Feld AD, et al. National Institutes of Health state-of-the-science conference statement: Prevention of fecal and urinary incontinence in adults. *Ann Intern Med*. 2008;148:449.

Madoff RD, Parker SC, Varma MG, et al. Fecal incontinence in adults. *Lancet*. 2004;364:621.

Reilly WT, Talley NJ, Pemberton JH, et al. Validation of a questionnaire to access fecal incontinence and associated risk factors: Fecal Incontinence Questionnaire. *Dis Colon Rectum*. 2000;43:146–153.

Rockwood TH, Church JM, Fleshman JW, et al. Fecal Incontinence Quality of Life Scale: Quality of life instrument for patients with fecal incontinence. *Dis Colon Rectum*. 2000;43:9–16.

Sleisenger and Fordtran. *Gastrointestinal and Liver Disease*. 8th ed. Vol. 1. Philadelphia, PA: *Saunders; 2006*:199–213.

Whitehead WE, Bharucha AE. Diagnosis and treatment of pelvic floor disorders: What's new and what to do. *Gastroenterology*. 2010;138:1231–1235.

Whitehead WE, Borrud L, Goode PS, et al. Fecal incontinence in US adults: Epidemiology and risk factors. *Gastroenterology*. 2009;137:512–517.

Musculoskeletal: Arthritis of the Ankle and Hind Foot

Vivek S. Jagadale MD

Description
The most common disorder of the ankle and hindfoot is arthritis. There are often associated osteophytes or bone spurs. Arthritic joints are characterized by stiffness and pain. Patients often limp or turn their foot outward to reduce pain when walking. This chapter discusses ankle, subtalar, talonavicular, and calcaneocuboid arthritis.

Etiology/Types
- Degeneration
- Trauma
- Inflammation
- Infection
- Malalignment due to instability or muscle imbalance
- Congenital and developmental deformities
- Metabolic disorders: gout and pseudogout
- Hematological disorders
- Neoplasms
- Charcot neuroarthropathy

Epidemiology
- In all 50,000 new cases of hindfoot arthritis are reported each year.
- Post-traumatic cases make up approximately 70% of cases in the United States.
- Primary osteoarthritis of the ankle and hindfoot is less common than in the hips and knees.

Pathogenesis
- Joint trauma is a common cause of osteoarthritis.
- This can result from direct cartilage and chondrocyte damage or from abnormal weight-bearing stress due to articular incongruity and joint malalignment; can occur with an intra-articular fracture that is not, or cannot be, adequately reduced.
- Ligamentous instability can also lead to increased sheer stresses across a joint, predisposing to osteoarthritis.

Risk Factors
- In all 3 to 10 years after traumatic injury to the ankle or hindfoot, depending on the severity of cartilage injury or ligament instability
- Obesity

Clinical Features
- History of previous trauma or other risk factors
- Pain: Increased with activity, worse with uneven surfaces
- Stiffness
- Activity Limitations
- Gait alteration

Natural History
- Trauma to the hindfoot is the most common predisposing factor for arthritis.
- Pain and disability progress with time.

Diagnosis

Differential diagnosis
- Osteochondral lesions in joint
- Synovitis
- Intra-articular loose bodies
- Ankle instability or impingement
- Peripheral neuritis

History
- Patients present with complaints of pain that increases with activity. They may also complain of stiffness and difficulty walking. Often they will provide a history of previous trauma, inflammatory disease, infection, or deformity since childhood.

Examination
- Joint swelling
- Generalized joint tenderness
- Decreased range of motion
- Possibly palpable osteophytes
- Associated deformity
- Antalgic gait

Testing
- Diagnostic injections
- Standing radiographs
- Computerized tomography (CT) scan to rule out joint infection, Charcot's arthropathy, and so on
- Magnetic resonance imaging (MRI) to rule out additional tendon or ligament pathologies (more specific than CT)

Pitfalls
- As arthritis progresses, options for joint salvage surgery narrows. Early intervention may delay need for fusion or joint-replacement procedures.

Red flags
- Surgical complications increase in patients who smoke, who have diabetes or rheumatoid arthritis, or who are obese.
- Charcot joint: The cause should be identified.
- Unstable joint

Treatment

Medical
- Acetaminophen and nonsteroidal anti-inflammatory drugs (NSAIDs)
- Intra-articular or systemic corticosteroids (rarely indicated)
- Hyaluronic acid injection
- Ambulatory aids, such as canes or walkers
- Shoe modification, orthoses, or bracing

Exercise
- Range of motion
- Strengthening
- Functional exercises

Surgical
- Arthroscopy with joint debridement
- Realignment through ligament reconstruction and/or osteotomies
- Distraction arthroplasty with ring fixation for avascular necrosis of the talus and hindfoot collapse
- Arthrodesis (fusion) is still a gold standard for the majority of patients with arthritis of the ankle and subtalar joints.
- Total joint replacement (Scandinavian total ankle replacement, STAR) is one of the best emerging treatment modalities for ankle arthritis; only useful for selected patients with normal body mass index and less activity demand, as well as no gross ankle deformity, instability, infection, or osteopenia (Figures 1 and 2).
- Osteochondral allograft replacement for large osteochondral defects of the talus and early signs of arthritis in younger patients
- Amputation

Consults
- Orthopedic surgery
- Physical medicine and rehabilitation
- Prosthetics and orthotics

Complications of treatment
- Nonunion
- Malunion
- Wound complications
- Infection
- Hardware failure
- Arthrodesis of the ankle or subtalar joints can lead to later arthritis of the adjacent joints, minimal gait alterations, and interference with activities of daily living.

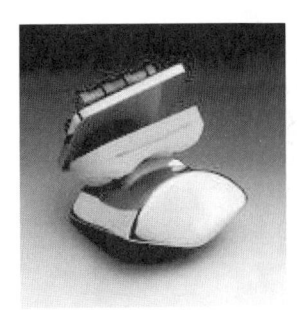

Figure 1 Scandinavian Total Ankle Replacement Prosthesis

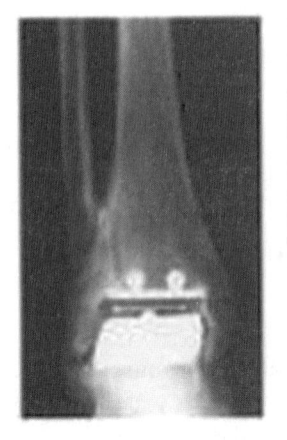

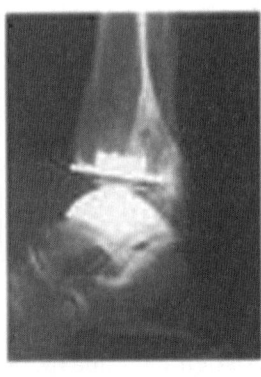

Figure 2 Radiographs of the Scandinavian Total Ankle Replacement Prosthesis

Prognosis
- Early diagnosis, identification of etiology, prompt intervention, good patient compliance, and a multidisciplinary approach (especially in patients with diabetes mellitus, peripheral vascular disease, etc.) favors good results.

Helpful Hints
- Hindfoot and ankle arthritis is a common and potentially debilitating problem.
- Arthrodesis remains the standard definitive surgical treatment in most patients.
- Based on improving results, ankle arthroplasty is becoming preferred for selected, low-demand patients.
- Realignment procedures and hyaluronic acid injections may play a role in optimizing pain relief and function for high-demand patients, who are not yet candidates for fusion or arthroplasty.

Suggested Readings
Hintermann B. *Total Ankle Arthroplasty*. 1st ed. New York: Springer; 2005.

Mann RA and Coughlin MJ. *Surgery of the Foot and Ankle*. 8th ed. St. Louis: Mosby; 1993.

Menz HB. *Foot Problems in Older People: Assessment and Management*. 1st ed. Churchill Livingston: Elsevier; 2008.

Musculoskeletal: Arthritis of the Thumb, Fingers, and Wrist

Christopher Parks MD ■ Theresa Wyrick MD

BASAL JOINT ARTHRITIS OF THE THUMB

Description
Debilitating and painful arthritis of the carpometacarpal (CMC) joint in the thumb.

Etiology/Types

Classification
- Stage I—mild joint widening
- Stage II—joint narrowing and sclerotic changes with small osteophytes (less than 2 mm)
- Stage III—joint narrowing with larger osteophytes (2 mm)
- Stage IV—pantrapezial involvement

Epidemiology
- The most commonly involved arthritic joint of the hand
- More common in women, especially postmenopausal
- Female-to-male ratio is 6:1
- No genetics or environmental link known

Pathophysiology
- Ability of the joint to move in three planes allows for significant axial loads during pinch and grip.
- Loss of ligament integrity allows for subluxation of the metacarpal on the trapezium.

Diagnosis

Differential diagnosis
- De Quervain's tenosynovitis
- Flexor carpi radialis tendonitis
- Stenosing flexor tenosynovitis of flexor pollicis longus
- Carpal tunnel syndrome

History
- Pain and weakness with pinch and gripping activities
- Night pain

Examination
- Painful grinding with axial compression and circumduction of metacarpal on trapezium
- Adduction deformity of thumb
- Localized tenderness over volar aspect of thumb at CMC joint
- Decreased radial and palmar thumb abduction

Treatment

Nonsurgical
- Nonsteroidal anti-inflammatory drugs (NSAIDs)
- Corticosteroid injections
- Thumb spica splinting
- Activity modifications

Surgery
- Ligament reconstruction and tendon interposition (LRTI)
- Trapezium excision
- CMC fusion
- Prosthetic replacement

FINGER ARTHRITIS

Description
Acute or chronic inflammation of the distal/proximal interphalangeal (DIP/PIP) joints, metacarpal joints, and the surrounding soft tissues.

Etiology/Types
- Osteoarthritis
  - Most common type of finger arthritis
  - Mostly affects the PIP and DIP joints
- Rheumatoid arthritis
  - Systemic disease that affects soft tissue (synovium) around joints
  - Begins in peripheral joints (hands, feet)
  - Often symmetric
  - Most commonly affects metacarpophalangeal joints

Epidemiology
- Females three times more likely to be affected
- Affects about 2.5% of the adult population

Pathophysiology
- Osteoarthritis
  - Matrix metalloproteinases (MMPs) and proinflammatory cytokines
  - Mediate cartilage destruction
  - Growth factors and inhibitors of MMPs and cytokines are inadequate to counteract
- Rheumatoid
  - Multiple theories exist
  - T-cells interact with an antigen to initiate and propagate the inflammatory process
  - Macrophages and fibroblasts create inflammation without T-cell involvement

Diagnosis

History
- Symptoms
  - Localized joint pain
  - Swelling, redness, and tenderness
  - Stiffness

Examination
- Signs
  - Decreased range of motion
  - Grinding of joint
  - Heberden's nodes (DIP)
  - Bouchard's nodes (PIP)
  - Swan-neck deformity
  - Boutonniere deformity

Treatment

Nonsurgical
- Change or reduction in activity levels
- NSAIDs
- Heat
- Finger splinting
- Physical therapy

Surgery
- Used as a last resort
- Arthrodesis
- Joint replacement

Suggested Readings
Barron OA, Glickel SZ, Eaton RG. Basal joint arthritis of thumb. *J Am Acad Orthop Surg*. 2000;8:314–323.

Laine VA, Sairanen E, Vainio K. Finger deformities caused by rheumatoid arthritis. *J Bone Joint Surg Am*. 1957;39:527–533.

Musculoskeletal: Dupuytren's Contractures and Trigger Finger

Christopher Parks MD ■ Theresa Wyrick MD

DUPUYTREN'S CONTRACTURE

Description
A thickening and tightening of the palmar fascia layer in the palm and fingers that causes flexion of fingers.

Etiology
- A cellular and fibroproliferative disorder that involves increased quantity of fibroblasts and myofibroblasts.
- Local microvascular ischemia can promote high cellularity and altered collagen profiles.

Epidemiology
- More common in men above the age of 40
- Ethnicity
  - Scandinavian
  - Irish
  - Eastern European
- Associations
  - Diabetes
  - Seizures
  - Alcohol abuse

Clinical Features
- Often a delayed presentation until joint motion is affected. It is usually painless, and begins as a nodule or cord.
- Nodule formation and skin-pitting near distal palmar crease are typical; bilateral involvement is common.
- Progression of disease is usually nodular to cords; unpredictable time course.
- "Dupuytren's diathesis"—severe form of disease with knuckle pads, plantar fibromatosis, and Peyronie's disease.

Treatment

Nonsurgical
- Effectiveness of creams and physical therapy inconclusive
- Heat
- Ultrasound
- Custom splint to stretch fingers
- Intralesional injection of steroids
- Educating about importance of early disease detection

Surgery
- Metacarpophalangeal (MCP) joint contractures of 30° and any proximal interphalangeal (PIP) contractures are indications for surgery.
- Selective fasciectomy is commonly used to resect diseased tissue in palm.
- Zigzag and transverse palmar incisions are used for exposure, and flaps for coverage.

Postoperative
- Reduce postoperative edema and scarring
- Early active flexion range of motion exercises
- Splinting

Complications
- Digital nerve injury, hematoma formation, poor wound-healing, stiffness in digits, and complex regional pain syndrome
- Progressive flexion contracture of digits
- Variable rate of recurrence

TRIGGER DIGITS

Description
Stenosing tenosynovitis is characterized by pain and/or the inability to flex or extend the thumb or fingers smoothly.

Etiology/Types
- Two types of tendon sheath pathology are
  - Nodular: confined swelling of tendon sheath
  - Diffuse: diffused inflammation
- Quinnell classification based on triggering in flexion or extension
  - 0: Mild crepitus or pain in a nontriggering digit
  - 1: Uneven movement of the digit
  - 2: Clicking without locking
  - 3: Correctable locking of digit
  - 4: Locked digit, irreducible

Diagnosis

History
- Initial painless triggering with mild click with progression to pain at MCP joint and finally triggering.

Examination
- Tenderness to palpation at palmar base of digit over metacarpal head
- Catching with extension of fingers from fist
- Locking of digit in flexion

Associated conditions
- Diabetes
- Gout
- Carpal tunnel syndrome
- Hypertension
- Rheumatoid arthritis
- Dupuytren's contracture
- Hypothyroidism

Treatment

Nonsurgical
- Early treatment with activity modification may be helpful.
- Nonsteroidal anti-inflammatory drugs (NSAIDs); massage can benefit types 1 to 3.

Injections
- Corticosteroid injections into tendon sheath from lateral or palmar approach, effective in 57% of patients

Surgery
- Surgical release of the A1 pulley can be achieved through open or percutaneous technique; considered curative

Complications
- Injection: permanent damage to digital nerve/artery; inject directly over tendon
- Surgery: tendon bowstringing, stiffness, and digital nerve transection

Suggested Readings

Benson LS, Williams CS, Kahle M. Duypuytren's contracture. *J Am Acad Orthop Surg.* 1998;6:24–35.

Saldana MJ. Trigger digits: Diagnosis and treatment. *J Am Acad Orthop Surg.* 2001;9(4):246–252.

Musculoskeletal: Hip Fracture

Patrick M. Kortebein MD

Description
The term "hip fracture" is applied to fractures involving the region from the femoral head to the proximal portion of the femoral shaft.

Etiology/Types
- Most common etiology—fall from a standing position: approximately 90%
- Hip fracture types/anatomic classification:
  - Intracapsular—femoral neck and head
  - Extracapsular—intertrochanteric and subtrochanteric

Epidemiology
- Incidence: World—1.6 million/year and United States—approximately 300,000/year
- Age (mean): women—77 years, and men—72 years
- Lifetime risk: women—17.5%, and men—6%
- Recurrent fracture: 5% to 10% within 1 year of initial fracture
- Mortality (1 year): 15% to 36%

Pathogenesis

Intracapsular fractures
- Higher rate of nonunion/malunion and avascular necrosis of the femoral head.

Subtrochanteric fractures
- Greater need for implant devices (e.g., intramedullary nail or rods)
- Higher rate of implant failure due to the higher stress on this part of the femur

Risk Factors
- White
- Female
- Osteoporosis
- Prior falls
- Dementia
- Premorbid living in a nursing home

Clinical Features
- Hip pain
- Inability to bear weight
- Present with shortened, externally rotated limb

Diagnosis

Differential diagnosis
- Arthritis
- Dislocation
- Pelvic fracture
- Other trauma

History
- Mechanism of injury: fall to the ground or twist with foot planted
- Hip or groin region pain, with immediate onset after injury
- Often unable to bear weight

Examination

Vital signs
- Elevated pulse and/or blood pressure (BP), if significant pain
- Alternatively, may be decreased BP due to blood loss/dehydration

Musculoskeletal/hip region
- Ecchymosis may be present about hip region
- Limb typically externally rotated and shortened; pain with range of motion

Neurologic
- Normal motor/sensory/reflex function, although motor impairment is possible due to pain.
- Ambulation: majority are unable to walk due to pain.

Skin
- Breakdown or wounds/abrasions

Vascular
- Dorsalis pedis/posterior tibial pulses, and capillary refill of both feet

Testing
- Radiographs: AP/lateral hip X-rays; infrequently, computerized tomography (CT) or magnetic resonance imaging (MRI)

- Laboratory: complete blood count (CBC), electrolytes, blood urea nitrogen/creatinine (BUN/Cr), and coagulation studies (prothrombin time [PT]/partial thromboplastin time [PTT])

Pitfalls
- Missing a fracture
- Significant blood loss
- Concomitant neurologic injury

Red flags
- Consider rhabdomyolysis if immobile for a prolonged period (hours) after fall/injury.
- Review medications, especially for anticoagulants and those with central nervous system effects.

Treatment

Surgical
- Surgical repair depends primarily on the type of fracture.
- Options include percutaneous pinning, intramedullary (IM) nail, open reduction/internal fixation (ORIF), or partial/total hemiarthroplasty

Higher risk surgical patients
- Age above 75 years
- Initial hemoglobin below 12 g/dL
- Peritrochanteric fracture
- Poor physical health (American Society of Anesthesiologists classification)
- Impaired premorbid cognition

Open reduction/internal fixation
- Lower morbidity (e.g., blood loss/need for transfusion)
- Typically, weight-bearing restrictions

Arthroplasty (total or partial)
- Lower reoperation rates and earlier recovery
- May reduce the risk of avascular necrosis and nonunion
- Typically, weight bearing as tolerated (WBAT)

Regardless of the type of surgical fixation, there is no difference in mortality or rate of regaining prior residential living status.

Potential complications of fracture treatment

Orthopedic
- Wound infection
- Nonunion/avascular necrosis (AVN)
- Dislocation/prosthesis loosening
- Nerve injury; peroneal (fibular) nerve most common
- Heterotopic ossification

Medical
- Adequate analgesia
- Deep vein thrombosis (40–60%)/pulmonary embolism (2–15%)
- Anemia; average ~3 gm/dL decrease
- Pressure/decubitus ulcer
- Genitourinary: urinary tract infection (e.g., prolonged Foley catheter), urinary retention, and renal failure
- Gastrointestinal: stress ulcers and constipation
- Delirium
- Myocardial infarction/pneumonia
- Depression
- Falls

Postacute rehabilitation

Settings/locations (see Chapter 91)
- Inpatient rehabilitation
- Nursing home/subacute rehabilitation
- Home health
- Outpatient
    Goals: Safe, independent mobility and performance of basic activities of daily living (ADLs).

Rehabilitation program

Key elements
- Weight-bearing precautions
- Mobility: transfers/ambulation (with or without a gait aid)
- Hip fracture/falls precaution/osteoporosis education
- Activities of daily living (ADLs) training with adaptive equipment

Medical management
- Pain management/analgesics
- Deep venous thrombosis prophylaxis
- Wound healing/pressure sore prevention
- Genitourinary: discontinuation of catheter (if not done) and monitoring for infection
- Gastrointestinal: ulcer prophylaxis
- Anemia: monitoring and transfusion as needed

Adjuvant treatment considerations
- Anabolic steroids; limited evidence of improved strength/functional recovery when used postoperatively
- Resistance exercise training; improved function and quality of life when initiated 4 months after hip fracture

Prognosis
- Independence: Only 50% of hip fracture patients return to independent living.

- Of patients living in the community prior to their fracture, 45% are institutionalized afterwards.
- Of the patients independent prior to their hip fracture, 45% can walk one block and only 10% can climb five stairs 1 year after fracture.

Inpatient rehabilitation
- Greater functional improvement
- Mobility generally improves with rehabilitation, but optimal method of rehabilitation is unclear.
- Lower rates of death and institutionalization/nursing home admission

Helpful Hints
- Evaluate for reversible risk factors to prevent recurrence or further falls
- Postoperative rehabilitation improves function
- Aggressively prevent complications and comorbidities

Suggested Readings
1. Halm EA, Wang JJ, Boockvar K, et al. The effect of perioperative anemia on clinical and functional outcomes in patients with hip fracture. *J Orthop Trauma.* 2004;18:369–374.
2. Magaziner J, Hawkes W, Hebel JR, et al. Recovery from hip fracture in eight areas of function. *J Gerontol A Biol Sci Med Sci* 2000;55A:M498–M507.
3. Binder Ef, Brown M, Sinacore DR, et al. Effects of extended outpatient rehabilitation after hip fracture: a randomized controlled trial. *JAMA* 2004;292:837–846.
4. Handoll HHG, Cameron ID, Mak JCS, et al. Multidisciplinary rehabilitation for older people with hip fractures. *Cochrane Database Syst Rev.* 2009;4:CD007125.
5. Handoll HHG, Sherrington C, Mak JCS. Interventions for improving mobility after hip fracture surgery in adults. *Cochrane Database Syst Rev.* 2011;3:CD001704.

Musculoskeletal: Joint Replacement

Danielle K. Powell MD

Description
Total joint replacement, or arthroplasty, is an orthopedic procedure, which involves resection of the diseased articular surfaces of a joint and replacing them with a prosthesis. It can be performed on any joint in the body, including the hip, knee, ankle, foot, shoulder, elbow, wrist, and fingers. The ultimate goal of arthroplasty is to relieve pain, improve function, and enhance quality of life.

Etiology/Types
- Osteoarthritis is the most common condition causing joint destruction.
- Other causes of joint destruction include rheumatoid arthritis, seronegative arthritides, crystal deposition diseases, avascular necrosis, and rare bone dysplasias.

Epidemiology
- It is estimated that 713,000 arthroplasty surgeries are performed annually in the United States.
- Hip and knee total joint arthroplasty are the most common, and it is estimated that 362,000 knee and 295,000 hip arthroplasties are performed each year in the United States.

Pathogenesis
- Primary osteoarthritis is an idiopathic phenomenon, occurring in previously intact joints, with no apparent initiating factor.
- The most common secondary causes of osteoarthritis are mechanical derangements, pyogenic infection, ligamentous instability, and fracture into a joint.

Risk Factors
- Any cause of osteoarthritis predisposes the person to needing a joint replacement.
- Obesity
- History of joint trauma, especially with cartilage damage
- Erosive arthritides
- Biomechanical abnormalities

Clinical Features
- Significant disabling pain, deformity, inability to perform activities of daily living (ADLs), and reduced quality of life are the primary indications for evaluation for arthroplasty.
- Stiffness, swelling, locking of the joint, pain with weight-bearing activities, constant pain unrelieved by rest, and night pain are the major symptoms that patients report.
- Morning stiffness

Natural History
- Osteoarthritis is a slowly progressive condition.
- Pain does not necessarily correlate with disease severity, but severely affected joints can be expected to hurt.
- With time, cartilage is lost, and there may be "bone-on-bone" joint changes. This can lead to loss of a range of motion and function, and severe pain.

Diagnosis

Differential diagnosis
- Peripheral vascular disease
- Radiculopathy
- Infection

History
- Onset, location, severity, functional effects, and previous treatments
- Quantification of the level of pain (e.g., mild, moderate, severe; numerical scale of 1–10)
- Assessment of how the patient's ADLs are affected

Examination
- A thorough musculoskeletal examination should be performed, including manual muscle testing, sensory testing, muscle stretch reflexes, range of motion, and arterial pulses.
- Gait assessment
- Special tests: leg length discrepancy, Trendelenburg sign, and straight leg raise

Testing
- Laboratory studies—complete blood count (CBC), basic blood chemistries, coagulation studies, and urinalysis
- Imaging—plain radiographs of the affected joint and chest X-ray
- Other tests—electrocardiogram (ECG)
  - Magnetic resonance imaging (MRI) may be necessary to evaluate certain disorders such as osteonecrosis.

Pitfalls
- Skin viability and blood supply must to be assessed prior to the procedure to ensure wound healing in the postoperative period.
- Aspirin and nonsteroidal anti-inflammatory drugs should be discontinued at least 1 week prior to surgery.
- Warfarin should be discontinued 3 to 5 days prior to surgery.

Red flags
- Arthroplasty is contraindicated in patients with active infection, skeletal immaturity, irreversible muscle weakness in the absence of pain, severe vascular disease, and preexisting significant medical problems such as recent myocardial infarction, unstable angina, heart failure, or severe anemia.
- Relative contraindications include medical conditions that preclude safe anesthesia and the demands of surgery and rehabilitation.
- Other relative contraindications include skin conditions within the field of surgery, a past history of osteomyelitis around the joint, a neuropathic joint, and morbid obesity.

Treatment

Medical
- Initial management of patients with osteoarthritis should be conservative.
- Conservative treatment includes medications, physical therapy, bracing, intra-articular steroid injection, viscosupplementation injection, weight reduction, and ambulatory aids.
- Once a patient has failed conservative treatment, arthroplasty should be performed.
- Pain control, bowel and bladder management, nutrition and hydration, thromboembolism prophylaxis should be a priority postoperatively.

Exercises
- Postoperative Day 1—initiation of bedside exercises, bed mobility, and transfer training; review of precautions and weight-bearing status
- Postoperative Day 2—initiation of gait training with the use of assistive devices, such as crutches and a walker, and continuation of functional transfer training
- Postoperative Days 3 to 5 (or on discharge to the rehabilitation unit)—range of motion and strengthening exercises to the patient's tolerance, progression of ambulation on level surfaces and stairs with the least restrictive device, and ADL training
- Postoperative Day 5, up to 4 weeks—strengthening exercises, stretching exercises to increase the flexibility of affected muscles, and progression to independence with ADLs

Consults
- Orthopedic surgery
- Cardiology
- Pulmonology

Complications of treatment
- Intraoperative complications include: fracture, nerve injury, vascular injury, and cement-related hypotension.
- Postoperative complications include: infection, dislocation, osteolysis and wear, aseptic loosening, periprosthetic fracture, implant failure/fracture, leg length discrepancy, heterotopic ossification, and thromboembolic disease.
- Arthroplasty does not always produce successful results, especially in patients with rheumatoid arthritis, because that condition may continue to narrow the joint space and accelerate the formation of scar tissue.
- As with any major surgery, there is always a risk of an allergic reaction to anesthesia, loss of blood, postoperative infection, or the formation of deep vein thrombosis.
- A joint that has undergone surgery is less stable than a healthy joint and dislocation or loosening of the joint may require revision.

Prognosis
- Death is more likely to occur in elderly patients and in those with other serious medical conditions.
- The 30-day mortality rate for a total hip arthroplasty is 0.7%; for knee arthroplasty it is 0.6%.

- Mortality rates are higher for patients who have a total hip arthroplasty for a hip fracture compared to those who have elective surgery for other indications.
- Prosthetic joints are generally well tolerated; however, they can wear out with time, especially in very active individuals. This may occur in a 15- to 20-year time frame, and may require revision surgery; revision surgery is more difficult and may have a worse prognosis.

Helpful Hints
- Low-impact activities are acceptable after arthroplasty (stationary bicycling, swimming, golf, and bowling). However, high-impact activities, such as racquet sports, jogging, and horseback riding, are not advised because they may lead to excessive wear or loosening of the prosthetic components.

Suggested Readings
Brotzman BS, Wilk KE, eds. *Clinical Orthopeadic Rehabilitation*. St. Louis: Mosby; 1996.

Canale ST, Beaty JH, eds. *Campbell's Operative Orthopedics*. St. Louis: Mosby; 2007.

Clagett GP, Anderson FA Jr, Levine MN, et al. Prevention of venous thromboembolism. *Chest*. 1992;102(Suppl. 4):391S–407S.

Kauffman TL, ed. *Geriatric Rehabilitation Manual*. New York: Churchill Livingston; 1999.

Musculoskeletal: Low Back Pain

Shahla M. Hosseini MD PhD ■ Gary P. Chimes MD PhD

Description
Low back pain (LBP) is a symptom with a broad range of causes, and it requires a thorough neurologic and musculoskeletal examination.

Clinical Features
- Pain localized to the axial spine
- May also have radiating lower limb pain
- May also have focal neurologic deficits to lower limb myotomes, reflexes, and dermatomes
- Usually has a directional plane of movement that characteristically worsens symptoms

Risk Factors
- Older age
- Trauma
- Smoking
- Obesity
- Poor general health
- Core muscle weakness
- Sedentary work
- Physically strenuous work
- Job dissatisfaction
- Anxiety and depression
- Poor stress-mediation skills
- Congenital spine abnormality

Etiology
Bone disorders
- Vertebral body compression fracture
- Central and neuroforaminal spinal stenosis
- Spondylolisthesis
- Spondylolysis (less common in the elderly)
- Degenerative scoliosis
- Functional leg length discrepancy

Joint disorders
- Lumbar facet abnormality
- Sacroiliac joint dysfunction

Soft tissue disorders
- Pelvic floor dysfunction
- Sarcopenia
- Muscle strain or ligament sprain
- Myofascial pain/trigger points
- Fibromyalgia

Endocrine disorders
- Metabolic bone disease
- Low vitamin D
- Low testosterone
- Referred visceral pain from abdominal (including abdominal aortic aneurysms, AAA), pelvic, or retroperitoneal organs
- Psychological, neoplastic, infectious, rheumatologic, and hematologic disorders

Disc disorders (less common in the elderly)

Epidemiology
- Prevalence estimates of LBP in people varies by setting for people of 65 years of age.
- About 13% to 49% in the community (rural and urban)
- About 23% to 51% in primary practice
- About 40% to 75% in long-term care facilities

Natural History
- Some back pain in the elderly is acute and self-limited, while in others it becomes chronic.
- Chronic LBP typically causes significant disability and risk of falling; it commonly occurs with depression.

Pathogenesis of Spondylosis and Spinal Stenosis
Intervertebral disc degenerative cascade
- Circumferential and radial tears
- Internal disruption of disc
- Disc height loss and bulging
- Vertebral body osteophyte formation and bulging of ligamentum flava

Zygapophyseal (facet) joint degenerative cascade
- Synovial reaction and cartilage destruction
- Osteophyte formation and enlargement of articular processes
- Capsular laxity and subluxation

Combined effects of degeneration
- Degeneration of the disc and Z-joints leads to instability of the Z-joints, lateral stenosis (encroachment on exiting nerve roots), and/or central stenosis (encroachment of cauda equina).
- The effect of recurrent strains at levels above and below the original lesion leads to multilevel spondylosis and spinal stenosis.

Diagnosis

History
- Age of patient, duration and description of symptoms (inciting event, recent acute change, radiation of pain, changes with valsalva), and impact of symptoms on activity
- Frequency and circumstances of falls
- Establish the direction of preference:
  - Worse with flexion (e.g., bending over to put on shoes)? Suggests anterior element pain, particularly discogenic low back pain, and vertebral body compression fracture in older adults or those at risk for metabolic bone disease
  - Worse with extension (e.g., standing and arching back or walking downhill)? Suggests posterior elements; most commonly, facet joint disease, spondylolisthesis, sacroiliac joint arthropathy, or spinal stenosis
  - Worse with transitional movements (e.g., getting up out of a chair)? Suggests spondylolisthesis or degenerative disk disease
- History of trauma (consider even heavy lifting as potential trauma in osteoporotic patient)
- History of cancer
- Pelvic floor weakness in both females and males
- Response to prior therapies (e.g., If a patient did not respond to oral steroids, what dose of steroids was prescribed? If physical therapy did not help, what types of exercises (if any) was he or she doing?)
- Consider the role of common comorbidities: depression, arthritis of peripheral joints, osteoporosis, vitamin D deficiency, and hypogonadism in males

Red flags
- Bowel or bladder incontinence
- Saddle anesthesia
- New onset of weakness in legs or gait disturbance
- Pain at night that is much worse than baseline pain
- Unexplained fevers, weight loss, or anorexia

Physical examination
- Observe posture and gait
- Inspect spine for scoliosis, assess for leg length discrepancy, pelvic obliquity, and examine muscle bulk for wasting
- Assess whether patient is able to stand from sitting in standard chair without using arms for assistance
- Palpate for concordant pain in the following regions: sacral sulcus, piriformis, lumbar facets, greater trochanter, quadratus lumborum, insertion of gluteus medius, and lower axial spine in midline
- Range of motion (ROM) of spine and quality of ROM
- ROM of surrounding joints (hip, knee, and shoulder)
- Manual muscle testing of hip flexors, hip extensors, knee extensors, ankle dorsiflexors, long toe extensors, and ankle plantar flexors. Hip abduction strength should be tested in the side-lying position with the hip placed at 10° of extension.
- Sensation in L1–S2 dermatomes (also include S3–S5 if indicated). In patients with a history of falls, check Romberg and lower extremity proprioception/vibration sense.
- Muscle stretch reflexes at the knee, medial hamstring, and ankle (Note that absent Achilles reflex is a common finding in the elderly.) Remember to check Babinski reflex.
- Slump sit test: With the patient in seated position, assist patient to full flexion of cervical, thoracic, and lumbar spine accompanied by full extension of one knee to cause maximal dural tension and reproduce radicular symptoms; assess for improvement with cervical extension.
- Modified stork test: With the patient in standing position, assist patient to shift weight onto one leg while using the other leg for balance, assist the patient to extend spine posterolaterally over the weight-bearing leg in order to load the posterior elements including the lumbar facets, pars interarticularis and the sacroiliac joint.
- For those patients able to tolerate these tests, remain close to the patient or support them by their hands while having them perform the following:
  - Single-leg stand: Assess balance and watch for drop of contralateral hip
  - Single-leg squat: Watch for medial knee deviation or "cork-screwing" (rotational instability)
- Posterior pelvic pain provocation test: With the patient in supine position, passively flex one hip and knee, and posteriorly load the hip using your own weight.
- Active straight leg raise: With the patient in supine position, assess patient's pain and ease of movement

with active unilateral hip flexion to 30°; then repeat the test to assess for any change in these parameters with the addition of manual pelvic stabilization.

Testing
- Electromyography (EMG): useful for evaluating radiculopathy and to determine which lesions on imaging are neurologically significant
- Plain radiograph
  - Indications: suspicion of fracture due to trauma or bony lesions due to tumor
  - Types of views: AP and lateral views are standard; oblique view for spondylolysis to visualize pars interarticularis; and lateral flexion-extension views to check for dynamic instability (e.g., spondylolisthesis)
- Magnetic resonance imaging (MRI)
  - Indications: suspicion of radiculopathy after acute injury; infection; tumor; progressive neurologic loss; and presurgical
  - Add gadolinium contrast if tumor or infection is suspected and in postsurgical patients.
- Computerized tomography (CT) indications: suspicion of bony lesions; sometimes indicated in postsurgical patients; used for those for whom MRI is contraindicated

Treatment

Therapeutic exercises
- Flexion-based exercises are used in older patients with evidence of lumbar spinal stenosis and a directional preference for flexion.
- Extension-based exercises are used in patients with symptoms distal to the buttock that centralizes with lumbar extension.
- Lateral shift exercises are used in patients with visible frontal plane deviation of the shoulders relative to the pelvis and in those who have a directional preference for lateral translation movements of the pelvis.
- Stabilization/motor control is recommended for some patients with aberrant movements during lumbar flexion/extension, who have decreased pain with spinal/core musculature activation.

Modalities
- Ice, superficial heat, ultrasound, and *transcutaneous electrical nerve stimulation* (TENS)

Medical
- Acetaminophen: first-line medication for arthritic back pain
- Nonsteroidal anti-inflammatory drugs (NSAIDs): for muscle strain or arthritic back pain; used when patients do not adequately respond to acetaminophen; consider alternatives for those with renal failure and those at risk of gastrointestinal bleed
- Consider topical NSAIDs (e.g., diclofenac) or other topical compounds (e.g., lidocaine, capsaicin) for those with contraindications to oral medications
- Anticonvulsants and tricyclic antidepressants (TCAs): for neuropathic pain; TCAs for fibromyalgia
- Short course of high-dose oral steroids: for suspected radiculopathy or inflammatory pathology
- Spinal injections with anesthetic and/or steroid for diagnostic and therapeutic purposes (e.g., transforaminal epidural; sacroiliac; and facet, lateral, and medial branch blocks)
- Opioids only for cases of moderate-to-severe chronic pain, which adversely impacts function or quality of life, and for those with medical contraindications to the above-listed medications

Other interventions
- May include acupuncture, movement re-education, soft-tissue manual techniques, cognitive–behavioral therapy, and progressive relaxation

Consults
- Nonsurgical: physical medicine and rehabilitation; spinal interventionists
- Surgical: orthopedic surgery and neurosurgery

Helpful Hints
- Keep in mind during the history and examination that determining the patient's direction of preference will help to narrow the differential diagnosis.
- Encourage patients with LBP to stay active. However, they may require movement re-education for improper body mechanics.

Suggested Reading
Dreyfuss P, Dreyer S, Cole A, et al. Sacroiliac joint pain. *J Am Acad Orthop Surg*. 2004;12(4):255–265.
Kirkaldy-Willis WH. The relationship of structural pathology to the nerve root. *Spine*. 1984;9(1):49–52.
Kirkaldy-Willis WH, Wedge JH, Yong-Hing K, et al. Pathology and pathogenesis of lumbar spondylosis and stenosis. *Spine*. 1978;3(4):319–328.
VanWye WR. Nonspecific low back pain: Evaluation and treatment tips. *J Fam Pract*. 2010;59(8):445–448.

Musculoskeletal: Neck Pain

Jonathan M. Stuart DO

Description
Pain perceived as arising in a region bounded superiorly by the superior nuchal line, laterally by lateral margins of the neck, and inferiorly by an imaginary transverse line through the T1 spinous process.
- This definition does not imply that the source of pain lies within this region, but only describes where the pain is felt.

Etiology/Types

Axial neck pain
- Pain localized to the neck and its surrounding tissues. This may be caused by any of the innervated zygapophyseal joints, cervical discs, vertebral periosteum, atlanto-occipital joints, cervical muscles, cervical dura mater, and vertebral arteries.

Cervical radiculopathy
- A phenomenon caused by damage to one of the cervical nerve roots. This can be due to compression or irritation and can come from the intervertebral disc, vertebral body, or zygapophyseal joints. Pain can be located both in the neck and in the area innervated by the affected nerve root.

Cervical myelopathy
- Damage to the spinal cord in the cervical area. This can be due to
  - Narrowing of the vertebral foramen at one or more levels, with compression of the spinal cord. Typically, an insidious onset of gait disturbance, upper/lower extremity sensory loss, lower extremity stiffness and jerking, upper/lower extremity weakness, urinary/bowel incontinence, Lhermitte sign, and neck and upper extremity pain are hallmarks of this condition.

Cervical spondylosis
- Age-related degenerative changes in the cervical spine affecting the vertebrae, intervertebral discs, ligamentum flavae, and zygapophyseal joints

Epidemiology
- Lifetime prevalence of neck pain: 67% of population
- Incidence is highest in middle age.
- Women are affected more than men.
- Point prevalence: 10% of the population
- One study of asymptomatic men and women above age 60 found that 86% of men and 89% of women had evidence of degenerative changes in the C2–7 intervertebral discs.
- For cervical spondylotic myelopathy, the onset is usually after age 40, typically between 50 and 70.

Natural History
- The majority of neck pain is axial in nature and is due to poor posture, poor ergonomics, stress, and/or chronic muscle fatigue; this pain usually resolves on its own.
- Pain due to cervical radiculopathy normally requires treatment of some kind. Whether this treatment will be conservative or surgical is dependent on the patient's history and physical presentation.
- Pain due to cervical myelopathy will require intervention. This intervention may be conservative or surgical, but surgical consultation is recommended. In these cases, the risk of long-term consequences from cord compression is significant.
- Cervical spondylosis is of particular concern in the elderly population. This is due to the increased incidence of osteophyte formation on the vertebral bodies and zygapophyseal joints. Formation of osteophytes occurs as the intervertebral discs age and deteriorate. The condition progresses with age.

Diagnosis

Differential diagnosis

Mechanical
- Cervical strain
- Cervical sprain
- Osteoarthritis

- Herniated nucleus pulposus
- Cervical spondylosis
- Cervical stenosis

Rheumatologic
- Rheumatoid arthritis
- Diffuse idiopathic skeletal hyperostosis (DISH)
- Polymyalgia rheumatica
- Fibromyalgia
- Reiter's syndrome
- Psoriatic arthritis
- Enteropathic arthritis

Infectious
- Vertebral osteomyelitis
- Diskitis
- Herpes zoster
- Infective endocarditis
- Granulomatous process
- Epidural, intradural, and subdural abscess
- Retropharyngeal abscess

Endocrine or metabolic
- Osteoporosis
- Osteomalacia
- Parathyroid disease
- Paget's disease
- Pituitary disease

Tumors
- Benign or malignant

Vascular
- Vertebral artery dissection
- Carotid artery dissection

Other
- Syringomyelia

History
- Location, quality, severity, duration of symptoms, frequency, inciting event, exacerbating activities, and alleviating activities
- Associated symptoms
- Prior episodes of pain
- Previous treatments and response to those treatments
- Past medical history
- Past surgical history

Examination
- Observation
- Active range of motion (AROM) and passive range of motion (PROM)
- Palpation; particularly of the posterior cervical musculature and muscles of the upper back
- Sensory and motor examination of all four extremities
- Reflexes in all four extremities
- Lhermitte's sign (electrical sensation in the spine with neck flexion)
- Spurling's maneuver (extending neck, rotating head, and applying downward pressure on head); fairly specific, but not overly sensitive for cervical radiculopathy
- Axial compression test (neck in neutral with downward pressure on head); this can cause local pain in the facet joints
- Shoulder examination; often shoulder problems overlap with cervical problems

Testing
- Cervical spine X-rays with posteroanterior (PA), lateral, and oblique views
- Cervical computerized tomography (CT) scan, if investigating bony anatomy not seen on plain X-ray
- Cervical magnetic resonance imaging (MRI) to evaluate soft tissues, especially the discs
- Electrodiagnosis to evaluate nerve root involvement versus peripheral neuropathy
- Ultrasound to evaluate the vascular structures of the neck

Red Flags
- Gait disturbance or jerky lower extremity movement
- Bowel/bladder incontinence
- Upper/lower extremity sensory loss
- Upper/lower extremity weakness

Treatment

Medical
- Ice for acute neck pain and heat for muscular pain lasting longer than 48 hours
- Nonsteroidal anti-inflammatory drugs
- Acetaminophen
- Opioids for severe pain
- Topical agents as adjunct treatment; topical lidocaine or diclofenac

Exercises
- Range of motion

- Strengthening exercise; flexion-based exercises for increasing neck flexor strength
- Posture and biomechanics; chin tuck

Injections
- Trans-foraminal epidural steroid injection
- Facet joint steroid injection

Surgery/procedures
- Radiofrequency ablation of medial branch may be considered when steroid injections provide good but temporary pain relief
- Laminectomy, discectomy, and cervical fusion

Complications of treatment
- Medication side effects
- Injection side effects
- Surgery side effects/chronic pain

Prognosis
- Generally, patients recover fully from sprains/strains with appropriate conservative care.
- Facet joint mediated pain has a more variable outcome; if radiofrequency ablation is performed, this may need to be repeated periodically.
- Degenerative problems generally progress, though symptoms often stabilize.
- Older patients with advanced degenerative pathology have a potential to develop a long-term waxing and waning course.

Helpful Hints
- Avoid overinterpretation of imaging studies.
- A long-term exercise and posture program can help manage pain.
- Patients may need to learn to "manage" their pain, rather than expecting a complete resolution.

Suggested Readings
1. Aprill C, Dwyer A, Bogduk N. Cervical zygapophyseal joint pain patterns. II: A clinical evaluation. *Spine*. 1990;14:458–461.
2. Bogduk N, Aprill C. On the nature of neck pain, discography and cervical zygapophysial joint blocks. *Pain*. 1993;54:213–217.
3. Jackson R. Cervical trauma: Not just another pain in the neck. *Geriatrics*. 1982;37:123.
4. Schellhas KP, Smith MD, Gundry CR, et al. Cervical discogenic pain: Prospective correlation of magnetic resonance imaging and discography in asymptomatic subjects and pain sufferers. *Spine*. 1996;21(3):300–312.
5. Wolff MW, Levine LA. Cervical radiculopathies: Conservative approaches to management. *Phys Med Rehabil Clin N Am*. 2002;13:589–608.

Musculoskeletal: Osteoarthritis

Kevin M. Means MD

Description
Osteoarthritis (OA) is a chronic disease that can change the lifestyle of the affected person by producing pain and decreasing function; OA can result in loss of mobility, pain, disability, and dependence.

Etiology/Types
- Primary
  - Related to age and cartilage changes
  - Related to genetic factors
  - Due to collagen disease
- Secondary
  - Related to joint trauma or surgery
  - Related to or exacerbated by obesity
  - Due to congenital joint problems
  - Metabolic: ex-gout and endocrine abnormalities

Epidemiology
- OA is the most common joint disease.
- OA is very common in older patients but can occur in younger patients, either through a genetic mechanism or, more commonly, because of previous joint trauma.
- OA affects over 20 million persons in the United States.
- Native Americans have a higher incidence of OA compared to the general population.
- Overall, OA is more common among Caucasians than in African Americans, although black women have a higher incidence of knee OA than other groups.
- The prevalence of OA is over 80% by age 65 (based on radiographic imaging).
- 28% of elderly persons have symptomatic OA of the knee and 23% have symptomatic OA of the hip.
- In individuals aged above 55, the prevalence of OA is higher among women than men; women are especially susceptible to OA in the distal interphalangeal (DIP) joints of the fingers and in the knee, compared to men (1.7:1 ratio).

Pathogenesis
- Excessive wear and tear changes on joints contribute to OA development; secondary nonspecific inflammatory changes in the joints also may contribute, so the former term "degenerative joint disease" is no longer used for OA.
- Biomechanical, immunologic, and biochemical factors are involved in cartilage destruction, which is at the core of OA; growth factors may play a role in the body's attempts to repair cartilage through cartilage synthesis.
- In early OA, increased chondrocyte metabolism leads to increased proteolytic breakdown of the cartilage matrix.
- Fibrillation and erosion of the cartilage surface ensues and proteoglycan and collagen fragments are released into the synovial fluid, stimulating a chronic inflammatory response in the synovium; metalloproteinases and cytokines produced by synovial macrophages can diffuse back into the cartilage and directly or indirectly destroy tissue.
- Other proinflammatory molecules may also be a factor.
- In addition to breakdown of the articular cartilage, OA involves the entire joint complex, including synovium and subchondral bone.
- Grossly, cartilage fissuring, pitting, and erosion are seen and can progress to the point that large areas of the joint surface are denuded of cartilage; bone underlying denuded cartilage becomes sclerotic.
- Simultaneously, cartilage and bone proliferate (a self-repair attempt), especially at the joint margin, leading to marginal osteophytosis.
- Genetic factors, obesity, and decreased bone density may make OA more likely to occur.

Risk Factors
- Age (due to reduced cartilage volume and perfusion; decreased proteoglycan content)
- Disorders of bone (e.g., Paget disease, avascular necrosis)
- Female gender
- Genetic factors
- Obesity (increases mechanical stress)
- Hemoglobinopathies (sickle cell disease, thalassemia)
- Infection
- Muscle weakness

- Neuropathic disorder leading to a Charcot joint (syringomyelia, tabes dorsalis, diabetes)
- Previous rheumatoid arthritis (RA)
- Repetitive use (i.e., jobs requiring heavy labor and bending)
- Trauma (injury-induced abnormal biomechanics)
- Underlying musculoskeletal disorders (congenital hip dislocation, slipped femoral capital epiphysis)

Clinical Features (See Table 1)
- OA generally has no significant inflammatory component, except in advanced disease; erythema, warmth, and marked joint swelling suggest another process (RA, joint sepsis, crystal arthropathy)
- OA affects the synovial joints, particularly the large weight-bearing synovial joints, including the hips, knees, and the cervical and lumbar–sacral spine
- The smaller joints of the hands (DIP and proximal interphalangeal, PIP) and feet are also commonly affected

Table 1 Clinical Features of Osteoarthritis

Pattern of (typical) joint involvement[a]: Axial: cervical and lumbar spine. Peripheral: distal interphalangeal joint, proximal interphalangeal joint, first carpometacarpal joints, knees, and hips

Symptoms: Joint pain. Morning stiffness lasting less than 30 minutes. Joint instability or buckling. Loss of function

Signs: Bony enlargement at affected joints. Decreased range of motion. Crepitus on motion. Pain with motion. Malalignment and/or joint deformity

[a]There is a less common OA subtype with multiple joint involvement; most commonly, OA affects the hands, hips, knees, and/or spine.

Natural History
- Early in OA, pain and stiffness is seen in and around the affected joint. This is worsened by joint use and is relieved by rest. This stage may last for years or decades.
- Later, as the disease progresses, pain onset can occur with minimal joint motion. Night pain is possible but is usually associated with severe or advanced OA; morning stiffness is not a prominent symptom and if present, it is typically brief.
- In large weight-bearing joints, advanced OA with progressive loss of joint space and subchondral bone erosion can result in joint deformity and progressive loss of joint function.

Diagnosis
Differential diagnosis
- OA should be differentiated from other arthritides, and other conditions that produce pain in and around the affected joints. Depending on the joint/joints involved, the following may be considered:
  - Crystal deposition disease
  - Pseudogout
  - Inflammatory arthritis
  - Seronegative spondyloarthropathies
  - Joint infection
  - Bursitis
  - Reactive arthritis
  - Fracture

History
- The typical OA symptoms: pain in the knee, hip, hand, or spine; onset usually insidious
- OA typically does not affect the wrists, elbows, or shoulders.
- Pain varies by site and nature; back, hip, or knee OA pain may be felt in the buttock, groin, thigh, or knee, and it can vary in character from a dull ache to a sharp, stabbing pain.
- Hip stiffness is common and can impair function (abnormal gait, difficult lower extremity dressing).
- Pain during grasp or other manual dexterity tasks, especially if the first carpometacarpal joint is involved.
- Neck pain/stiffness, difficulty looking to the side or rear (cervical facet joint OA)
- Occasionally, swallowing difficulties develop due to anterior cervical spine osteophytes.
- Low back pain (lumbar spine OA); vertebral osteophytes can narrow the foraminae and compress nerve roots; patients may have cervical or lumbosacral radicular symptoms, sphincter dysfunction or cord compression, pain, weakness, and numbness of the upper or lower limbs depending on the level of involvement.
- Localized signs and symptoms are typical; widespread joint involvement suggests other systemic disorders.

Examination
- Physical examination should include careful assessment of the affected joints, surrounding soft tissue, and bursae.
- Physical signs of OA include
  - Painful and decreased range of motion (ROM), joint deformity, and malalignment
  - Joint instability (excessive motion) or buckling, especially during stair descent (knee)

– Crepitus, on passive ROM (indicates cartilage surface irregularity)
– Periarticular tenderness may indicate bursitis, which should be differentiated from OA.
- Hand examination may reveal DIP enlargement (Heberden's nodes).
- PIP joints may develop Bouchard's nodes, which should be differentiated from RA; RA usually involves the metacarpal joints and rarely involves the DIP joints.
- The base of the thumb and the first interphalangeal joint are commonly affected.

Testing
- OA is likely to be present in older patients; superimposed abnormalities (RA, crystal arthropathy, spondyloarthropathy) are possible and should be ruled out.
- Laboratory findings in OA are usually within normal limits and confirm the absence of inflammatory arthritis; abnormalities raise suspicion for other diseases.
- Synovial fluid analysis is usually benign in OA with a good mucin clot formation, few mononuclear leukocytes, and no crystals.
- Radiologic studies usually show asymmetric joint involvement, bony sclerosis, marginal osteophytosis, and occasional bony cysts.

Pitfalls
- Missing connective tissue disease, infections, or treatable biomechanical problems

Red flags
- Fever, signs of infection
- Unstable joint
- Systemic symptoms

Treatment
Goals: reduce pain and improve function.

Nonpharmacologic treatment
- Braces and appropriate footwear may be helpful (for example, a medial unloading knee orthosis for OA with predominantly medial knee compartment narrowing)
- A cane may be used in the contralateral hand for hip osteoarthritis, or in the preferred hand of comfort for knee osteoarthritis
- Patient education: Instruction in joint-protection techniques to avoid stress on the affected joint/joints; activity modification to promote low-impact activities; and weight reduction (diet and exercise)
- Exercises: Muscle strengthening to assist in joint protection (for example, quadriceps and hamstring strengthening for knee OA); stretching exercises to maintain/increase ROM; low-impact aerobic exercise such as swimming, water aerobics, and aquatic walking programs have all been reported to be beneficial in OA; emerging nontraditional exercises such as tai chi also show potential; exercise adherence should be monitored and encouraged
- Thermal agents and therapeutic modalities may help to reduce pain and facilitate stretching
- Occupational therapy intervention: Education in joint-protection techniques, modification of activities of daily living (ADLs), provision of adaptive equipment, thermal agents (paraffin), and hand splinting may be useful, especially for advanced osteoarthritis with hand involvement

Pharmacologic treatments
- Early disease: acetaminophen (4 g/day maximum) for mild or moderate pain without apparent inflammation; patient education and lifestyle modification
- If response to acetaminophen is unsatisfactory or if the clinical presentation is inflammatory, consideration should be given to nonsteroidal anti-inflammatory drugs (etodolac, meloxicam, naproxen).
- Topical anti-inflammatory medications or capsaicin can be used for knee OA.

Injections
- Later, in the chronic phase of OA, where pain is progressive, intra-articular injection therapy with corticosteroids and viscosupplementation may be tried.
- Intra-articular corticosteroid injections (methylprednisolone, betamethasone, triamcinolone) reduce signs of inflammation (pain, increased warmth, erythema, effusion); pain relief onset is usually seen within days and lasts for several weeks; reduces pain by suppressing inflammatory responses.
- Viscosupplementation or intra-articular injection of sodium hyaluronate (Hyalgan, Synvisc) has been shown to be safe and effective for pain relief in knee OA, including repeat treatment; Hyaluronate is derived from rooster combs and poultry product, so an allergic reaction is possible; effects can last for months, possibly due to the viscosity of the material and other little understood mechanisms.

Surgery
- If conservative interventions are ineffective, or if the patient cannot perform ADLs despite maximal

therapy, an orthopedic surgical consultation should be considered.
- Orthopedic surgical procedures:
  - Arthroscopic joint lavage
  - Joint realignment osteotomy
  - Joint fusion (arthrodesis)—to eliminate motion
  - Joint replacement (arthroplasty)
- Depending on the orthopedic surgical procedure performed, postoperative patients may require rehabilitative intervention that can vary from crutch or cane ambulation, orthosis support, and outpatient exercise therapy after arthroscopy to possibly acute rehabilitation admission and/or several weeks of partial weight-bearing activities with an assistive device and extensive exercise therapy.

Complications of surgery
- Sciatic or other nerve damage
- Pain
- Loosening of hardware
- Wear of the prosthesis

Prognosis
- Depends on the joints involved and the severity of the condition
- For knee OA, in older patients and in those with a higher body mass index, varus deformity and multiple joint involvement are more likely to have disease progression.

Helpful Hints
- Appropriate medical management of OA requires early diagnosis and recognition of current factors that may influence prognosis or complicate the disease.
- The growing elderly population and the prevalence of OA present a substantial challenge to society and the health care system.

Suggested Readings
American College of Rheumatology Subcommittee on Osteoarthritis Guidelines. Recommendations for the medical management of osteoarthritis of the hip and knee: 2000 update. *Arthritis Rheum.* 2000;43:1905–1915.

Hinton R, Moody RL, Davis AW, et al. Osteoarthritis: Diagnosis and therapeutic considerations. *Am Fam Physician.* 2002;65:841–848.

Zhang W, Moskowitz RW, Nuki G, et al. OARSI recommendations for the management of hip and knee osteoarthritis, Part II: OARSI evidence-based, expert consensus guidelines. *Osteoarthritis Cartilage.* 2008;16:137–162.

Musculoskeletal: Osteoporosis and Vertebral Fractures

Mehrsheed Sinaki MD ■ Elizabeth Huntoon MD

Description
Osteoporosis consists of a heterogenous group of syndromes in which bone mass per unit volume is reduced in otherwise healthy bone, resulting in fragile bone. The increased bone porosity results in architectural instability and fracture.
- The World Health Organization has defined osteoporosis as a bone mineral density (BMD) of 2.5 standard deviations below the peak mean bone mass of young healthy adults. The *T* score shows the amount of one's bone density compared with a young adult (at the age of 35) of the same gender with peak bone mass. The *Z* score is adjusted for an individual's age.

Etiology/Types

Hereditary, congenital
- Osteogenesis imperfecta

Acquired
- Generalized
  - Idiopathic
    - Premenopausal women
    - Middle-aged men
    - Juvenile osteoporosis
  - Postmenopausal
  - Age related
  - Endocrine disorders
    - Estrogen deficiency
  - Sedentary lifestyle/immobility
  - Smoking
  - Nutritional
    - Malabsorption
  - Nephropathies
  - Chronic obstructive pulmonary disease
  - Malignancy
  - Medications
    - Glucocorticoids
    - Anticonvulsants
      - Phenytoin
    - Barbiturates
    - Cholestyramine
    - Heparin
- Localized
  - Inflammatory arthritis
  - Fractures
  - Limb immobilization
  - Limb dystrophies/paralysis

Epidemiology
- Osteoporosis is estimated to affect 200 million women worldwide.
  - About 20% of women aged 70
  - About 40% of women aged 80
  - About 66% of women aged 90
- Lifetime risk of an osteoporotic vertebral fracture in men aged above 50 is 30% and women is 50%.
  - About 30% of all hip fractures occur in men.
  - About 20% of all vertebral fractures occur in men.

Pathogenesis
- Bone remodeling is a process that allows removal of old bone and replacement with new bone tissue.
- Bone remodeling has five phases.
  - *Activation*: Osteoclastic activity is recruited.
  - *Resorption*: Osteoclasts erode bone and form a cavity.
  - *Reversal*: Osteoblasts are recruited.
  - *Formation*: Osteoblasts replace the cavity with new bone.
  - *Quiescence*: Bone tissue remains dormant until the next cycle starts.
- Peak adult bone mass is achieved between ages 30 and 35.
- High-turnover osteoporosis occurs due to an increased rate of bone remodeling and bone loss; examples include
  - *Hyperparathyroidism*
  - *Thyrotoxicosis*
- Secondary causes of osteoporosis are associated with an increased rate of activation of the remodeling cycle in the setting of decreased osteoblastic activity.

Risk Factors
- Age
- Female gender
- White
- Postmenopausal/surgical or otherwise
- Anorexia/low body mass index
- Physical inactivity
- Low calcium/vitamin D intake
- Cigarette smoking
- Excessive alcohol intake
- Long-term glucocorticoids
- Family history of osteoporosis
- Hypogonadism in men

Clinical Features
Asymptomatic, unless fractures have occurred. Most common fractures include:
- Distal forearm/wrist
- Thoracic vertebra; compression
- Hip/proximal femur
- Sacral insufficiency fractures may occur with no significant trauma or injury

Diagnosis
History
Risk factors include (see Risk Factors listed above):
- Weight/low body mass index
- Low physical activity level
- Calcium/vitamin D intake
- Cigarette smoking
- Alcohol intake
- Family history of osteoporosis
- Medications

Physical examination
- Normal or with back pain
- Kyphoscoliosis, if prior thoracic vertebral compression fracture

Testing/diagnostic studies
- Radiographs of chest and spine
- Dual-energy X-ray absorptiometry (DXA) for bone mineral density
- Complete blood cell count
- Metabolic profile
  - Calcium
  - Phosphorus
- Vitamin D
  - 25-hydroxyvitamin D
  - 1,25-dihydroxyvitamin D3
- Parathyroid hormone
- Bone-specific alkaline phosphatase
- Osteocalcin
- Erythrocyte sedimentation rate
- Serum protein electrophoresis
- Total thyroxine
- Urinalysis/24-hour urine

X-ray findings
- X-rays of the spine
- Increased lucency of the vertebral bodies
- Anterior wedging of vertebral bodies
- Biconcavity of vertebral bodies and compression fractures
- Kyphosis

Optional
- Bone scan
- Iliac crest biopsy
- Biochemical markers of bone turnover

Treatment
Management of acute vertebral fractures
- Analgesic medications
- Bracing/positioning
- Posture control
- Physical therapy
  - Modalities
    - Heat/ice
    - Transcutaneous electrical nerve stimulation (TENS) unit trial may help in some cases
  - Safe, pain-free transfers/ambulation
  - Gait aid, if necessary
  - Isometric back extension exercises
- Vertebral augmentation—Injection of polymethylmethacrylate into active/acute vertebral compression fracture.

Indications
- Persistent pain
- Magnetic resonance imaging (MRI) with acute edema/fracture
- Vertebroplasty—Stabilizes compression fracture
- Kyphoplasty—Injection of polymethylmethacrylate into vertebral compression fracture after restoring vertebral height

Management of chronic pain in patients with osteoporotic vertebral fracture
- Improve faulty/abnormal posture
- Analgesic medications; avoid codeine derivatives

- Avoid strenuous physical activities, particularly spine flexion.
- Patient-specific therapeutic exercise program
  - Isometric back extensor strengthening
    - In sitting or prone, unloaded
    - Leads to a decreased risk of vertebral fractures
    - Improves horizontal trabecular connections
    - Reduces recurrent fractures in persons with prior vertebroplasty

Sacral/pelvic insufficiency fractures
- Management
  - Analgesics
  - Orthopedic evaluation, generally for weight-bearing precautions

Orthoses
- Posture training program, including weighted kypho-orthosis: beneficial for reducing kyphosis

Medications (Food and Drug Administration–approved for postmenopausal osteoporosis)
- Estrogen
- Alendronate (Fosamax)
- Risedronate (Actonel)
- Ibandronate sodium (Boniva)
- Zoledronic acid
- Raloxifene (Evista)
- Calcitonin (Miacalcin)
- Teriparatide (Forteo; bone-forming agent)

Nutrition/dietary recommendations
- Calcium—1,200 mg per day; combined diet and supplements
- Vitamin D—800 IU per day; combined diet and supplements

Suggested Readings

Bonner FJ, Sinaki M, Grabois M, et al. Health professional's guide to rehabilitation of the patient with osteoporosis. *Osteoporos Int.* 2003;14(Suppl. 2):S1–S22.

Huntoon EA, Schmidt CK, Sinaki M. Significantly fewer refractures after vertebroplasty in patients who engage in back-extensor strengthening exercises. *Mayo Clin Proc.* 2008;83:54–57.

Kaplan RS, Sinaki M, Hameister MD. Effect of back supports on back strength in patients with osteoporosis: A pilot study. *Mayo Clin Proc.* 1996;71(3):235–241.

Khosla S. Increasing options for the treatment of osteoporosis. *N Engl J Med.* 2009;361(8):818–820.

National Osteoporosis Foundation. Osteoporosis disease statistics: "Fast Facts." http://www.Nof.Org/Osteoporosis/Diseasefacts.htm. Accessed March 21, 2006.

Sinaki M. Critical appraisal of physical rehabilitation measures after osteoporotic vertebral fracture. *Osteoporos Int.* 2003;8:774–779.

Sinaki M. Falls, fractures, and hip pads. *Curr Osteoporos Rep.* 2004;2(4):131–137.

Sinaki M. Nonpharmacologic interventions: Exercise, fall prevention, and role of physical medicine. *Osteoporos Clin Geriatr Med.* 2003;19:337–359.

Sinaki M. Prevention and treatment of osteoporosis. In: Braddom R, ed. *Physical Medicine and Rehabilitation*. Philadelphia, PA: Elsevier; 2011:913–934.

Sinaki M. The role of physical activity in bone health: A new hypothesis to reduce risk of vertebral fracture. *Phys Med Rehabil Clin N Am.* 2007;18:593–608.

Sinaki M, Brey RH, Hughes CA, et al. Significant reduction in risk of falls and back pain in osteoporotic-kyphotic women through a Spinal Proprioceptive Extension Exercise Dynamic (SPEED) program. *Mayo Clin Proc.* 2005;80:849–855.

Sinaki M, Itoi E, Wahner HW, et al. Stronger back muscles reduce the incidence of vertebral fractures: A prospective 10 year follow-up of postmenopausal women. *Bone.* 2002;30:836–841.

Sinaki M, Pfeifer M, Preisinger E, et al. The role of exercise in the treatment of osteoporosis. *Curr Osteoporos Rep.* 2010;8:138–144.

WHO Study Group. Assessment of fracture risk and its application to screening for postmenopausal osteoporosis. *World Health Organ Tech Rep Ser.* 1994;843:1–29.

Musculoskeletal: Posterior Tibial Tendon Dysfunction

Ruth L. Thomas MD

Description
Although progressive flatfoot deformity in adults has multiple possible etiologies, by far the most common cause is posterior tibial tendon dysfunction (PTTD). The severity of the tendon failure can be mild, with only tenosynovitis, or severe, with marked deformity of the hindfoot.

Etiology/Types
- Stage I—mild tenosynovitis without deformity
- Stage II—moderate tendon degeneration with flexible, correctable, hindfoot collapse and increasing forefoot abduction
- Stage III—severe PTTD with fixed hindfoot deformity
- Stage IV—severe PTTD associated with failure of the medial deltoid ligament and valgus opening of the ankle joint

Epidemiology
- PTTD is more common in females (75%).
- Average age at diagnosis is 57 years.

Pathogenesis
- PTTD results from degenerative changes in the posterior tibial tendon, leading to a painful hindfoot deformity, including loss of arch height, increasing heel valgus, and forefoot abduction.
- Probably due to attritional overuse of the tibialis posterior tendon
- As the tendon fails, the underlying medial ligaments stretch, and arch support is diminished.
- The Achilles tendon, which is lateral to the midline, increases valgus hindfoot position.
- Unopposed pull of peroneus brevis allows the foot to progressively abduct, uncovering the navicular.
- The forefoot supinates to accommodate the valgus hindfoot to the floor.
- With time, this deformity becomes increasingly rigid.

Risk Factors
- Female
- Accessory navicular
- Ligamentous laxity
- History of steroid exposure or major surgery around the tibialis posterior tendon
- Seronegative inflammatory disease
- Obesity

Clinical Features
- Swelling notable below the medial malleolus, best observed from behind
- "Too many toes" sign may be noted when the patient is examined from behind with both knees facing forward (i.e., more toes visible on one foot than the other, demonstrating abduction of the forefoot)
- Pain along the course of the tibialis posterior tendon with attempted single heel rise.
- Lack of heel inversion on heel rise, or inability to perform single heel rise.

Natural History
- Pain is initially seen medially along the course of the tibialis posterior tendon.
- Stage I tenosynovitis will occasionally resolve without progression to deformity.
- As PTTD progresses to Stage II, arch sag is observable. Heel valgus increases over time and the forefoot turns outward (abduction).
- Stage II deformity is manually correctable by placing the heel in a neutral position and rotating the forefoot out of supination.
- Eventually, the deformity becomes fixed (Stage III) and the medial pain often subsides. Frequently, lateral hindfoot pain will develop due to impingement between the fibula and calcaneus.

Diagnosis

Differential diagnosis
- Degenerative, traumatic, or inflammatory arthrosis

- Charcot neuroarthropathy
- Neurologic foot disease
- Tumors of the foot
- Loss of soft-tissue stabilizers (spring ligament or midfoot ligaments)

History
- Complaint of medial ankle pain along the course of the tendon
- 50% of patients recall sustaining an ankle sprain.
- Difficulty walking, especially up and down the stairs
- Patients often report that they are rolling their shoewear inward.

Examination
- Tenderness, warmth, and swelling along course of tibialis posterior tendon
- Hindfoot valgus
- "Too many toes" sign due to abduction of the forefoot in relation to the hindfoot
- Pain with attempt to go up onto the toes of the affected foot (single heel rise)
- Absence of heel varus with single heel rise
- Inability to perform a single heel rise

Testing
- Standing X-rays of both feet; to evaluate for pes planus on the lateral view and forefoot abduction on anterior–posterior view
- Magnetic resonance imaging (MRI); to evaluate for fluid in the tendon sheath, degenerative changes within the tendon, longitudinal splitting, and complete rupture

Pitfalls
- Untreated PTTD can lead to rigid valgus hindfoot deformity, chronic pain, and decreased mobility.

Red flags
- Steroid injection in and around a diseased tendon can lead to tendon rupture and should be avoided.

Treatment

Medical
- Anti-inflammatory medication
- Cast or boot immobilization for 6 to 8 weeks
- Exercise program for early disease after inflammation subsides
- For long-term management, custom orthosis for early disease with minimal arch collapse, or ankle bracing for advanced disease

Surgical
- Flexible deformities can be corrected with flexor digitorum tendon transfer to the navicular, combined with a calcaneal osteotomy
- Rigid deformities require hindfoot arthrodesis (fusion)
- Both realignment procedures and fusion often require lengthening of the Achilles mechanism.

Consults
- Orthopedic foot and ankle surgery
- Prosthetics and orthotics
- Physical therapy

Complications of treatment
- Inadequate correction or pain relief
- Painful scar
- Prolonged calf weakness is seen with gastrocnemius lengthening
- With fusion, there is a loss of motion

Prognosis
- Exercise is useful only in early disease without deformity.
- Orthoses are indicated for mild foot collapse, but do not support the ankle when deformity progresses.
- Bracing can slow the progression of arch collapse and abduction.
- Early surgical treatment can prevent the need for fusion.
- Surgical results are generally good for pain relief and correction of deformity.

Helpful Hints
- PTTD is the most common cause of acquired adult flatfoot deformity.
- PTTD should be suspected in older females with chronic medial ankle pain and progressive flatfoot deformity.
- Single heel rise is the best screening tool.

Suggested Reading
Deland JT. Adult-acquired flatfoot deformity. *JAAOS.* 2008;16(7):399–406.

Musculoskeletal: Shoulder

Jonathan Swenson MD

Introduction
- Shoulder pain is a common complaint in older adults and may be related to intrinsic pathology of the anatomic structures of the shoulder or referred pain.

Etiology/Types
- Intrinsic shoulder pain is typically due to acute or chronic pathology of the anatomic structures (e.g., muscles, tendons, ligaments, and bones) associated with the four articulations in this region:
  - Glenohumeral (GH)
  - Acromioclavicular (AC)
  - Sternoclavicular
  - Scapulothoracic

  The most common causes of shoulder pain in older adults include the following.

Impingement syndrome
- Compression of the rotator cuff tendons and subacromial bursa between the humeral greater tuberosity and coracoacromial arch

Rotator cuff tendinopathy/tears
- Supraspinatus and infraspinatus tendons are most frequently affected.
- Tendinopathy is a chronic process due to repetitive overhead activities with tendon microtrauma in regions with poor vascular supply.
- Tears are felt to occur due to chronic impingement and, less frequently, acute trauma.

GH joint osteoarthritis
- Characterized by destruction of joint cartilage with loss of joint space

Adhesive capsulitis ("frozen shoulder")
- GH capsule thickening with reduced active and passive range of motion (ROM)
- Etiology often idiopathic
- Risk factors include
  - Immobility due to injury/trauma
  - Hemiparetic side in stroke
  - Diabetes
  - Hypothyroidism

Biceps tendinopathy
- Similar to rotator cuff tendinopathy

AC joint osteoarthritis
- Prior AC sprain/trauma

  Causes of referred pain may include
- Cervical radiculopathy/radiculitis
- Neuralgic amyotrophy
- Cardiovascular disease
  - Angina
  - Myocardial infarction
- Pulmonary disease
  - Apical lung tumor (i.e., Pancoast tumor)
- Abdominal disease
  - Cholecystitis
- Dermatologic
  - Herpes zoster/postherpetic neuralgia

Epidemiology
- The prevalence of shoulder pain is 12% to 16% in the general adult population but is not specifically known in the older adult population.

Clinical Features

Impingement syndrome
- Gradual onset of anterior and lateral shoulder pain
- Exacerbated by the following:
  - Overhead activity
  - Sleeping on the affected side
- Night pain common

Rotator cuff tendinopathy/tear
- Anterolateral shoulder pain
- Night pain common
- Exacerbated by the following:
  - Overhead activity
  - Sleeping on the affected side
- Weakness and/or crepitus with overhead motion

GH joint osteoarthritis
- Gradual development of anterior shoulder pain and stiffness
- Exacerbated by activity
- Relieved by rest

Adhesive capsulitis
- Gradual onset stiffness
- Decreased ROM
- Diffused shoulder pain may be present
- Usually, a self-limiting course

Biceps tendinopathy
- Anterior shoulder pain
- Exacerbated by active shoulder and/or elbow flexion

AC joint osteoarthritis
- Anterior shoulder pain
- Exacerbated with cross-body adduction

Diagnosis
- Perform shoulder and upper extremity neurologic examination in all patients
- Shoulder examination is usually normal and does not alter pain in referred pain disorders.

Impingement Syndrome

Examination
- Tenderness of lateral shoulder/subacromial region
- Painful arc sign:
  - Pain between 120° and 60°, as the patient slowly adducts the shoulder
- Positive Neer sign:
  - Pain with maximal passive abduction in the scapular plane with internal rotation
- Positive Hawkins sign:
  - Pain when shoulder is forward flexed to 90° and elbow flexed to 90°. The shoulder is then internally rotated.

Tests
- Radiographs: narrowing of subacromial space on plain radiographs (normal greater than 7 mm)
- Diagnostic subacromial anesthetic injection
  - Repeat impingement testing with complete pain relief supports diagnosis.

Rotator Cuff Tendinopathy/Tear

Examination
- Tenderness in lateral shoulder/subacromial region
- Painful arc sign
- Drop arm sign
- Positive Neer and Hawkins signs
- Rotator cuff tear
  - Motor testing: weakness with rotator cuff muscle testing (e.g., external rotation)

Tests
- Magnetic resonance imaging (MRI)
- Musculoskeletal ultrasound

GH Joint Osteoarthritis

Examination
- Glenohumeral joint line tenderness
- Loss of ROM of external rotation and abduction
- Crepitus

Tests
- Radiographs
  - GH joint space narrowing
  - Flattening of the humeral head
  - Osteophytes
  - Subchondral sclerosis

Adhesive Capsulitis

Examination
- Decreased active *and* passive ROM, especially external rotation and abduction
- Positive Apley's scratch test:
  - Limited ROM when patient reaches behind neck and back to touch the opposite scapula.

Tests
- Clinical diagnosis; imaging not generally required
- Radiographs
  - Nonspecific; usually normal
- MRI with contrast
  - Thickening of the capsule and synovium may be noted

Biceps Tendinopathy

Examination
- Tenderness in bicipital groove
- Positive Speeds test:
  - Pain when patient's elbow is extended, forearm supinated, and shoulder elevated to 60°. Examiner then resists forward flexion.

Tests
- Radiographs normal
- MRI: tendinopathy

AC Joint Osteoarthritis

Examination
- Point tenderness at AC joint
- Positive scarf sign:
  - Pain when arm of the affected side is forcibly adducted across the chest/crossed body adduction test positive

Tests
- Radiographs
  - AC joint narrowing and osteophytosis

TREATMENT

Impingement Syndrome
- Relative rest; avoid overhead activities
- Trial of nonsteroidal, anti-inflammatory drugs (NSAIDs)/analgesics
- Physical therapy
  - ROM exercises
  - Stretching of capsular structures
  - Strengthening scapular stabilizers followed by rotator cuff muscles
- Corticosteroid injection; subacromial
  - Increased compliance with therapy

Rotator Cuff Tendinopathy/Tear
- Trial of NSAIDs/analgesics
- Physical therapy
  - Shoulder mobility and ROM
  - Stretching anterior and posterior joint capsule
  - Strengthening scapular stabilizers followed by rotator cuff muscles
- Eccentric strengthening for tendinopathy
- Corticosteroid injection; subacromial
- Surgical management
  - If conservative treatment fails
  - Acute traumatic full thickness tears

GH Joint Osteoarthritis
- Trial of NSAIDs/analgesics
- Physical therapy
  - Moist heat followed by gentle stretching/ROM exercises
  - Rotator cuff/scapular stabilizer-strengthening exercises
- Corticosteroid injection; intra-articular
- Sodium hyaluronate injection; intra-articular
- Total shoulder replacement or hemiarthroplasty
  - Advanced arthritis
  - Failure of conservative treatment

Adhesive Capsulitis
- Trial of NSAIDs/analgesics
- Physical therapy
  - Moist heat/ultrasound followed by ROM exercises
- Corticosteroid injections; intra-articular
  - May hasten recovery when combined with physical therapy
- Refractory cases
  - Capsule adhesiolysis
  - Manipulation under anesthesia

Biceps Tendinopathy
- Trial of NSAIDs/analgesics
- Physical therapy
  - Shoulder mobility and ROM
  - Stretching biceps tendons
  - Strengthening biceps muscles
    - Emphasizes eccentric strengthening with chronic tendinopathy
- Corticosteroid injection; subacromial

AC Joint Osteoarthritis
- Trial of NSAIDs/analgesics
- Corticosteroid injection
  - Ultrasound or fluoroscopic guidance helpful

Prognosis
- Most shoulder disorders can be treated conservatively
- More prompt surgical evaluation should be initiated for
  - Acute rotator cuff tears
  - Severe GH osteoarthritis
- Full recovery of adhesive capsulitis may take 6 to 18 months.

Suggested Readings
Anderson BC, Anderson RJ, Fields KB, et al. Evaluation of the patient with shoulder complaints. UpToDate.com 18.3. September 2010.

Griffin LY, Andrews JR, Davies M, et al. Section Two: Shoulder. In: Griffin LY, ed. *Essentials of Musculoskeletal Care*. 3rd ed. Rosemont, IL: American Academy of Orthopaedic Surgeons; 2005:145-233.

Schultz JS. Clinical evaluation of the shoulder. *Phys Med Rehabil Clin N Am*. 2004;15:351-371.

Warren RF, O'Brien SJ. Approaches to senior care #6. Shoulder pain in the geriatric patient. Part I. Evaluation and pathophysiology. *Orthopedic Rev*. 1989;18(1):129-135.

Warren RF, O'Brien SJ. Approaches to senior care #7. Shoulder pain in the geriatric patient. Part II. Treatment options. *Orthopedic Rev*. 1989;18(2):248-253,256-263.

Musculoskeletal: Spinal Stenosis

Ted A. Lennard MD

Description
Spinal stenosis is the narrowing of the central canal, neural foramen, or extraforaminal zones within the spinal column. This narrowing may result in compression of the neural elements and/or vascular structures and can exist concurrently in any or all of these zones.

Etiology/Types
- Traditionally, stenosis is categorized as either congenital or acquired.
- In the elderly, stenosis is identified by its location: central canal, foraminal, or extraforaminal.
  - Central: the area of the spinal column that contains the spinal cord from C1 to L2 and the cauda equina from L2-sacrum
  - Foraminal: the canal that contains the spinal nerve root posterior to the lateral disc and facet (i.e., zygapophyseal) joint
  - Extraforaminal: the area lateral to the neural foramen

Epidemiology
- About 3% to 4% of low back pain patients who see a general physician
- About 13% to 14% of patients seen by a spine specialist
- About 3% to 5% of the adult population have asymptomatic central stenosis.
- About 7% to 16% of adults have neuroforaminal stenosis.
- The proportion of stenotic, asymptomatic individuals is larger in older age groups (21% of adults above the age of 60 vs. less than 1% of adults under 60).
- An estimated 400,000 Americans, most above the age of 60, may have symptoms of lumbar spinal stenosis.
- Males are more affected than females.

Pathogenesis
- Degenerative: spondylosis, spondylolisthesis; thickening of adjacent ligaments (e.g., ligamentum flavum), hypertrophy of bony prominences or facet joints, disc bulges, or protrusions; and synovial cysts
  - Progressive disc degeneration with bulging and narrowing. This causes stress to be transferred to the adjacent facet joints, which then begin to degenerate and develop hypertrophy. Osteophytes form and the ligamentum flavum thickens. Neural structures are compressed.
- Traumatic: vertebral fractures and subluxations, herniated discs, and postsurgical changes, including fibrosis.
- Skeletal: metastatic cancer of the spine, Paget's disease, diffuse idiopathic skeletal hyperostosis (DISH), ankylosing spondylitis, and rheumatoid arthritis
- Metabolic: hypoparathyroidism, renal osteodystrophy, acromegaly, and pseudogout

Risk Factors
- Age above 50
- Congenital stenosis; short pedicles
- History of spinal surgery, such as discectomy or fusion

Clinical Features

Central stenosis from C1 to L2 (myelopathic signs)
- Upper and/or lower extremity and/or trunk weakness and/or numbness
- Spasticity/hypertonicity
- Gait disturbances
- Bowel or bladder dysfunction

Central stenosis from L2-sacrum (cauda equina or multilevel nerve root compression)
- Lower extremity weakness and/or numbness
- Bowel or bladder dysfunction
- Foraminal or extraforaminal stenosis
- Symptoms depend on the spinal nerve root compressed

Natural History
- Degenerative changes within the spinal column are a natural part of the aging process.
- As discs degenerate and bulge, abnormal stress is placed on the adjacent ligaments and joints causing hypertrophy of these structures.
- The result is progressive narrowing of the spinal nerve foramen or of the central canal.

- As the canals narrow, the neural structures become compressed, resulting in symptoms.

Diagnosis

Differential diagnosis
- Peripheral neuropathy
- Peripheral vascular disease/vascular claudication
- Bilateral hip and/or knee joint osteoarthritis
- Spinal cord tumor
- Large central single-level disc herniation
- Diabetes

History
- Cervical central stenosis: Patients can have diffuse numbness, pain, or weakness in the upper and/or lower extremities and/or trunk; patients may or may not have neck pain. As the stenosis worsens, gait disturbances, spasticity, or bowel and bladder problems may occur.
- Thoracic or lumbar central stenosis: Patients can have diffuse pain, numbness, or weakness in the lower extremities, typically worse with standing/ambulation and better with sitting/flexed lumbar posture (neurogenic claudication); patients may or may not have trunk/back pain. If the central stenosis is located in the thoracic spine or in the upper lumbar spine (to L2), spasticity or changes in gait may be present, when severe.
- Foraminal stenosis: Patients may experience numbness, tingling, weakness, or pain in the extremity controlled by the specific spinal nerve root affected.

Examination
- Range of motion of the spine and peripheral joints
- Neurological examination, including
  - Deep tendon reflexes
  - Sensory examination
  - Manual muscle testing
  - Assessment of atrophy
  - Evaluation for pathological reflexes (e.g., Hoffmann's, Babinski's)
  - Gait evaluation
  - Lhermitte's sign (cervical conditions; paresthesias/dysesthesias of thoracic region with flexed neck)
- Vascular examination: distal pulses

Testing
- Computerized tomography (CT) scan (with or without myelography)
- Magnetic resonance imaging (MRI) scan
- Electrodiagnostic studies

Pittfalls
- Missing a single or multilevel radiculopathy
- Missing myelopathy
- Missing spinal instability
- Missing diffuse neuropathic processes
- Missing peripheral vascular disease
- Missing compression from tumor

Red Flags
- Progressive motor and/or sensory deficits in the extremities
- Bowel or bladder dysfunction
- Myelopathic signs (hyper-reflexia/clonus, spasticity, Babinski and/or Hoffmann reflex, abnormal gait)
- Cauda equina syndrome (progressive loss of sensation and strength in the lower extremities; bowel, bladder, and/or sexual dysfunction)

Treatment

Medical
- Medications: neuropathic analgesics (e.g., amtriptyline/nortriptyline, gabapentin, pregabalin, duloxetine) and analgesics (e.g., nonsteroidal anti-inflammatories, tramadol)
- Orthoses: cervical soft collar, lumbar corset/thoracolumbar sacral orthosis (TLSO), and antiextension lumbar brace

Exercise
- Exercise: neutral/flexion biased cervical/lumbar stabilization, range of motion, and ambulation with gait aid with a flexed posture

Injections
- Interlaminar epidural steroid injections (above or below the level of stenosis)

Surgery
- Decompressive laminectomy with or without foraminal decompression and fusion

Prognosis
- Lumbar spinal stenosis may have a relatively slow progression; one study of nonsurgical patients noted 70% unchanged, 15% worse, and 15% better at 4-year follow-up.
- After surgical decompression, most patients should be able to return to most of their normal activities.
- If the diagnosis is delayed, permanent nerve damage or paralysis may occur.

Helpful Hints

- Maintain a high level of suspicion for stenosis in older patients who present with bilateral extremity complaints.
- Always perform a thorough neurologic examination on older patients with neck and low back pain.

Suggested Readings

Jakola AS, Sørlie A, Gulati S, et al. Clinical outcomes and safety assessment in elderly patients undergoing decompressive laminectomy for lumbar spinal stenosis; a prospective study. *BMC Surg.* 2010;10:34.

Pollintine P, et al. Time-dependent compressive deformation of the ageing spine. *Spine.* 2010;35(4):386–394.

Szpalski M, Gunzburg R. Lumbar spinal stenosis in the elderly: An overview. *Eur Spine J.* 2003;12(Suppl. 2): S170–S175.

Neurologic: Alzheimer Disease and Other Neurodegenerative Disorders

Jamil R. Dibu MD ■ Salah G. Keyrouz MD

Description
Neurodegenerative diseases are a group of conditions, also known as dementia syndromes, characterized by memory and cognitive decline, leading to functional impairment in daily living activities.

Etiology/Types
- Alzheimer disease (AD)
- Vascular dementia (multi-infarct, Binswanger's disease)
- Mixed dementia (AD and vascular)
- Frontotemporal dementia (FTD)
- Parkinson's disease dementia (PD)
- Dementia with Lewy bodies (DLB)
- Creutzfeldt–Jacob disease
- Multiple system atrophy (MSA)
- Progressive supranuclear palsy (PSP)
- Huntington disease
- Corticobasal degeneration (CBD)

Epidemiology
- 5% of the population between ages of 65 and 70 have dementia. The prevalence rises to more than 45% above the age of 85.

Alzheimer disease
- Accounts for 50% to 70% of dementia cases
- More than 35 million people worldwide are affected
- Incidence is age related, doubling every 5 years after the age of 65
- Prevalence is 30% or higher in populations with age ≥85

Pathogenesis
Despite uncertainties, the pathophysiology of Alzheimer disease revolves around the accumulation of neurofibrillary tangles (intracytoplasmic hyperphosphorylated tau protein), and amyloid protein aggregates surrounded by degenerating nerve terminals (neuritic "senile" plaques) that scattered throughout the cerebral cortex. At the molecular level, there is depletion of cortical acetylcholine.

Risk Factors

Alzheimer disease
- Age (strongest)
- Family history
- Genetic factors (ApoE e4 gene)
- Baseline mild cognitive impairment
- Mental and social exercises slows cognitive decline by enhancing neurogenesis.

Vascular dementia
- Hypertension, diabetes mellitus, smoking, and hypercholesterolemia
- Physical activity has an inverse relationship with the incidence of dementia by reducing cardiovascular risk factors and stroke incidence, improving physical functioning.

Clinical Features
- Memory impairment
- Cognitive dysfunction: language, visuospatial ability, calculation, judgment, and problem solving
- Neuropsychiatric: depression, withdrawal, hallucinations, delusions, agitation, insomnia, and disinhibition
- Specific features: rigidity, bradykinesia, and tremors at rest (parkinsonism), downward gaze palsy (PSP), hemiballismus (Huntington's disease), visual hallucinations (DLB), and rapid progressive behavioral changes (FTD)

Natural History
- Insidious episodic memory impairment (misplacing objects, repetitive questioning, forgetting names of familiar individuals, and difficulty with tasks that were otherwise automatic prior to disease onset)
- Visuospatial dysfunction
- Language deterioration
- Other cognitive dysfunction (i.e., executive dysfunction, agnosia, apraxia)
- Neuropsychiatric symptoms: depression, apathy, disinhibition, and agitation

- Late stage: individuals become bed-bound, and are dependent on others for basic activities of daily living such as toileting and feeding.
- Death

Diagnosis

A definitive diagnosis of neurodegenerative diseases can be only made postmortem. In clinical practice, the diagnosis of these conditions relies on history, neurologic examination, and the exclusion of many reversible causes of memory disturbance and cognitive impairment (listed below in "Differential diagnosis").

Differential diagnosis
- Hypothyroidism
- Vitamin B_{12} deficiency
- Drug intoxication (anticholinergics, antihistamines, benzodiazepines)
- Normal pressure hydrocephalus (NPH)
- Alcoholism
- Chronic subdural hematoma
- Chronic meningitides
- Brain tumor
- Wilson's disease
- HIV-associated dementia
- Conversion reaction
- Severe depression

History
- Short-term memory loss
- Functional impairment
- Fluctuating level of attention or alertness
- Motor symptoms associated with parkinsonism
- Vascular risk factors
- Visual hallucinations
- Sleep schedule and behavior
- Nutritional status
- Autonomic function (bladder, bowel)
- List of current and recently used medications and supplements

Examination
- Mental status (minimental status examination)
- Cranial nerves (ocular motor dysfunction)
- Sensory (peripheral neuropathy in metabolic and infectious causes of neurodegenerative diseases, unilateral sensory loss in stroke, cortical sensory dysfunction with CBD)
- Motor (upper and lower motor neuron signs, extrapyramidal signs)
- Cerebellar (cerebellar dysfunction is prominent in the cerebellar form of MSA)
- Gait (magnetic-difficulty getting feet off the ground in NPH, shuffling, short-stride in parkinsonism, spastic/hemiparetic in stroke)
- Signs of systemic diseases

Testing
- Screen for depression
- Complete blood count (CBC), chemistry panel, vitamin B_{12}, thyroid stimulating hormone, urine analysis, and urine and blood drug screen
- Liver function tests and ammonia
- Basic rheumatologic screen (erythrocyte sedimentation rate, C-reactive protein, antinuclear antibody)
- Computerized tomography (CT), magnetic resonance imaging (MRI; neuronal loss leading to diffuse cortical atrophy, sulcal widening, and compensatory ventricular dilatation [later stages]).
- Screen for Lyme, syphilis, HIV, and paraneoplastic syndrome if clinical suspicion arises.
- Electroencephalogram (EEG), cerebrospinal fluid studies if indicated

Pitfalls

Frequent seizures, especially of the complex-partial type, could present with memory and cognitive impairment mimicking certain neurodegenerative conditions, namely Alzheimer disease. This is a reversible illness, and an erroneous or delayed diagnosis could lead to unduly investigations, treatments, and prognostication.

Red flags

Neurodegenerative diseases have an unrelenting progression and an inexorable course, therefore, all reversible causes that mimic neurodegenerative diseases need to be excluded, or if present, corrected before diagnosing a primary condition for which there is no cure.

Treatment

Treatment is supportive in most cases, and what is currently available in our pharmacologic armamentarium merely delays progression.

Pharmacologic
- Cholinesterase inhibitors: donepezil, galantamine, and rivastigmine (oral, transdermal)
- N-methyl-D-aspartic acid receptor antagonist: memantine
- Atypical neuroleptics (treatment of hallucinations and delusions)
- Antidepressants (serotonin selective reuptake inhibitor)

Nonpharmacologic
- Physical and occupational therapies; randomized studies showing 30 minutes of daily exercises and individualized therapy sessions to compensate for functional deficits (i.e., training patients in the use of aids and coping behavior) showed less severe decline in activity of daily living performance.
- Behavioral interventions
- Family education regarding home safety and behavioral interventions
- Education regarding caregiver support resources
- In late stages, skilled nursing care, most typically in long-term facilities becomes necessary.
- Nutrition: provide oral supplements, tube feedings if needed (percutaneous endoscopic gastrostomy/jejunostomy, PEG/PEJ).

Consults
- Psychiatry
- Neurology
- Physical medicine and rehabilitation
- Nutrition

Complications of treatment
- Cholinesterase inhibitors: gastrointestinal symptoms, insomnia, vivid dreams, and bradycardia
- Antipsychotic drugs: sedation, extrapyramidal symptoms, and QT interval prolongation

Prognosis
- Cognitive decline in neurodegenerative diseases progresses inexorably to death.
- In the late stages of the disease, patients will be totally dependent on others for their daily activities; they will become bedridden, mute, and require tube feedings for their nutrition.

Helpful Hints
The pre-mortem diagnosis of most neurodegenerative conditions can be ascertained by exclusion of other treatable diseases, and routine follow-up to establish classical progression of symptoms.

Suggested Readings
American Academy of Neurology. *Continuum*, Dementia. Vol.16(2); 2010.

Querfurth HW, LaFerla FM. Alzheimer's disease. *N Engl J Med.* 2010;362:329–344.

Ropper AH, Samuels MA. *Adams & Victor's Principles of Neurology.* 9th ed. New York, NY: Mc-Graw Hill; 2009.

Neurologic: Amyotrophic Lateral Sclerosis and Other Neuromuscular Disorders

Ozun Bayindir MD ■ Nathan Prahlow MD ■ Ralph M. Buschbacher MD

Description
- Amyotrophic lateral sclerosis (ALS), or Lou Gehrig's disease, is a progressive and lethal neurodegenerative disease with combined upper motor neuron (UMN) and lower motor neuron (LMN) degeneration.

Etiology/Types
- The main cause of the disease is unknown; however, it is believed to be due to a multifactorial process.
- Sporadic cases: 90% to 95%
- Hereditary cases: 5% to 10%
  - Mutant SOD 1 gene (Cr 21): mutation in gene coding zinc–copper superoxide dismutase (20% of familial ALS and 3% of sporadic ALS)
  - ALS2, SETX, and VAPB gene mutations are also seen.
- The most common form of ALS is classical ALS (Charcot's); other types include
  - Pseudobulbar palsy
  - Progressive bulbar palsy: only bulbar muscles affected
  - Flail arm syndrome (brachial amyotrophic diplegia): LMN symptoms with proximal upper extremity weakness
  - Flail leg syndrome (pseudopolyneuritic form): LMN symptoms with weakness in the lower extremities and foot drop
  - ALS with multisystem involvement

Epidemiology
- Approximately, 1 to 2 cases per 100,000 people.
- Incidence of ALS rises with advancing age.
- Usually diagnosed at age 50 to 70.
- Affects men more than women (ratio 1.3:1).

Pathogenesis
- The most widely accepted hypothesis is a combination of genetic susceptibility and environmental factors. It is known that motor neuron death is an apoptotic process and apoptosis may result from the following:
  - Oxidative toxicity: Decreased intracellular enzyme (superoxide dismutase, SOD) activation causes free radical damage, leading to ischemia.
  - Excitotoxicity (glutamate-induced neuronal toxicity): An increase in intracellular glutamate (or increased glutaminergic activity) causes N-methyl-D-aspartate (NMDA) receptor activation and a subsequent increase in intracellular calcium, resulting in apoptosis.
  - Mitocondrial dysfunction (aging mitocondria)
  - Exogenous factors, such as lead, mercury, or viral agents may contribute.

Risk Factors
- Advancing age
- Male gender
- Genetic susceptibility

Clinical Features
- Painless, asymmetric, progressive muscle weakness and atrophy
- Cramps and fasciculations may be seen.
- LMN signs and symptoms: weakness, atrophy, and fasciculations
- UMN signs and symptoms: brisk reflexes, spasticity, and pathologic reflexes
- Pseudobulbar effect, due to imbalance of the UMNs and loss of control
- Dementia: Approximately, 5% of people with ALS have a form of dementia (the most common form is frontotemporal).
- Sensation is spared.
- Sphincters are spared.
- Extraocular muscles are spared.

Natural History
- Progression of weakness leads to impaired mobility and inability to perform activities of daily living (ADLs)
- Death occurs on average 3 to 5 years after the onset of symptoms.

- Respiratory failure and dysphagia are the most frequent causes of death.
- Only 10% of patients with ALS live more than 10 years.

Diagnosis

Differential diagnosis
- Cervical myelomalacia
- Primary lateral sclerosis
  - Symmetric UMN findings, usually with initial symptoms of spasticity instead of weakness
- Inclusion body myositis
  - Inflammatory myositis, with weakness and atrophy, but none of the UMN findings
- Multifocal motor neuropathy
  - Only LMN findings seen
- Kennedy disease: X-linked bulbospinal atrophy
  - Symmetric proximal extremity and bulbar weakness with atrophy, cramps, and fasciculations, but without UMN findings

History
- Family history
- Weakness in the bulbar region, upper extremities, and/or lower extremities
- Difficulty performing ADLs
- History of foot drop or falling

Examination
- Motor strength
- Reflexes
- Observation of ambulation
- Bedside respiratory function testing

Testing
- Other possibilities in the differential diagnosis must be ruled out
- MRI of the brain and spine
- Genetic testing
- Depending on the symptoms, the following should be considered: muscle biopsy, complete blood count and chemistries, B_{12}, folate, protein electrophoresis, antiganglioside IgGM1 antibody (monofocal motor neuropathy), tumor markers, heavy metals (Pb, Mn), HIV, human T-cell lymphotropic virus (HTLV), and/or Lyme serology.
- Electromyography
  - Sensory responses should be normal.
  - Motor responses may be affected, with slowed conduction velocity, decreased motor amplitude, and/or mildly prolonged distal latency.
  - Needle examination generally detects fibrillations, positive sharp waves, and fasciculations at rest; motor unit potentials are polyphasic, with increased amplitude, prolonged duration, and decreased recruitment.
  - El Escorial criteria include
    - Definite ALS; LMN and UMN findings in three regions (including bulbar)
    - Probable ALS; LMN and UMN findings in two regions
    - Probable ALS—laboratory supported; LMN and UMN findings in one region or UMN signs in ≥1 region and with acute denervation in ≥2 limbs
    - Possible ALS; LMN and UMN findings in one region
    - Suspected ALS; LMN signs only in ≥1 region, or UMN signs only in ≥1 region

Pitfalls
- Misdiagnosis is not uncommon, often leading to surgical procedures such as discectomy, cervical foraminotomy, or carpal tunnel release.

Red flags
- Fasciculations in atrophic muscles
- Tongue fasciculations

Treatment

Medical
- Currently, there is no effective treatment or known cure for ALS.
- Medications
  - Only riluzole is approved by the Food and Drug Administration (FDA) to treat ALS; may help slow disease progression and extend life by 2 to 3 months.
  - Other treatment options include glutamate antagonists (lamotrigine), gabapentin, topiramate, insulin-like growth factor 1 (IGF-1), and antioxidants such as vitamin E and CoQ10.
  - There are many medication trials in progress, including for memantine, arimoclomol, ceftriaxone, and lithium.
  - Pain control medications may be necessary for cramping, trauma due to falls, underlying degenerative changes, and wounds.
- Management of associated symptoms:
  - For dyspnea, bilevel positive airway pressure may be considered. Some patients elect ventilatory support, in which case tracheostomy may be considered.

- Alternative speech options include letter boards, dry-erase boards, and text-to-speech programs and devices.
- For dysphagia, tube feeding may be necessary. Nasogastric (short term) or percutaneous endoscopic gastrostomy (PEG) tube placement are options. PEG placement is generally recommended before forced vital capacity drops below 50%.
- For sialorrhea; sublingual atropine, amitriptyline, or scopolamine patch may be considered. Botulinum toxin injection to the salivary glands may be necessary in some cases.
- For symptoms of depression, various antidepressants may be used. It may be advantageous to use certain agents for "helpful" side effects (such as amitriptyline).
- Constipation is often an issue due to low liquid intake, immobilization, and opioid usage. Increased fluid intake, stool softeners, and dietary fiber may help to reduce symptoms.

Exercise
- The goals of treatment are to relieve symptoms and to maintain quality of life.
- Energy conservation is extremely important.
  - Strengthening exercises at best worsen fatigue, and at worst, may cause further weakness.
  - Submaximal and low-intensity exercises are used to avoid/minimize disuse atrophy and muscle deconditioning.
- A home stretching program should be instituted to promote maintenance of range of motion.

Adaptive equipment
- Ankle-foot orthoses are helpful in cases of foot drop.
- Depending on leg strength, patients may benefit from the use of a cane, walker, or wheelchair.
  - Powered wheelchairs may be configured to optimize patient care, including tilt-in-space, power recline, elevating leg rests, and alternative control interface features.
- ADLs should be assessed, and assistive devices prescribed as indicated.
- Splinting of the wrists may be necessary.
- Cervical collars may be considered; for wheelchairs, head rests may be useful.

Modalities
- As indicated for symptomatic relief

Injections
- None specifically indicated, but can be of benefit for concomitant degenerative joint disease symptoms or other associated problems.

Surgery
- PEG tube placement

Consults
- Neurology
- Physical medicine and rehabilitation
- Medical genetics
- Pulmonology
- General surgery
- Hospice

Complications of treatment
- Side effects of medications
  - Hepatotoxicity for riluzole
- Fatigue

Prognosis
- Life expectancy is generally between 2 to 5 years after the onset of symptoms, but some 10% of patients may live beyond 10 years.

Helpful Hints
- The intrinsic hand muscles and tibialis anterior are often among the earliest affected muscles in ALS.
- ALS should be considered in the patient with UMN and LMN signs.

Suggested Readings
Kiernan MC, Vucic S, Cheah BC, et al. Amyotrophic lateral sclerosis. *Lancet.* 2011;377:942–955.

Phukan J, Hardiman O. The management of amyotrophic lateral sclerosis. *J Neurol.* 2009;256:176–186.

Neurologic: Balance Disorders

Kevin M. Means MD

Description
- Balance—The ability to successfully maintain the body's center of mass (COM) over the available base of support.
- Maintenance of balance relies on the harmonious integration and coordination of
  - Input from visual, vestibular, proprioceptive, tactile, and kinesthetic sensation
  - Central nervous system (CNS) processing
  - Execution of appropriate (head, eye, trunk, and limb) motor output via the musculoskeletal system
- Balance control is a dynamic process achieved by the complex integration of several neurophysiologic mechanisms and biomechanical factors. This requires ongoing provision of perceptual information of the body's position and rapid correction for inadvertent displacement of the COM outside certain limits.
- Maintenance of balance may be either
  - Static (at rest) or
  - Dynamic (during motion)

Epidemiology
- A recent longitudinal study showed impaired balance in 21.5% (619) of the 2,925 participants.
- Prevalence of poor balance was higher in women than men and rates rose with increasing age.

Risk Factors
- Age
- Diabetes
- Arthritis
- Visual impairment
- Poor grip strength
- Lower income

Pathogenesis
- With advancing age, normal aging changes and pathologic changes associated with diseases or their treatments can affect the integrity and function of the visual, vestibular, musculoskeletal, central, and peripheral nervous systems.
- These effects are further compounded by a reduced capacity for plasticity and repair in the elderly, can result in balance control failure.

Differential Diagnosis (Etiology)

Visual
- Age-related changes in visual acuity, fields, depth perception, contrast and glare sensitivity, and dark adaptation affect quality or quantity of visual input.
- Conditions such as diabetic retinopathy, cataracts, or stroke can impair vision.

Sensation
- Conditions including atherosclerosis, radiculopathy, or myelopathy from spinal stenosis, peripheral neuropathy can impair somatosensory function and proprioception

Vestibular
- Age-related inner ear hair cell and vestibular nuclei neuronal loss; increased vestibulo-ocular reflex latency
- Vestibular failure seen in vestibular neuronitis, cerebellar, or brainstem ischemia

Musculoskeletal system
- Age-related increases in postural response latency, reduced muscle mass (sarcopenia)
- Reduced muscle strength and flexibility decrease response to balance perturbations
- Abnormalities such as myopathy impair muscle function; decreased joint mobility from arthritis, restrict postural adjustments; kyphosis, scoliosis, and leg length discrepancy can alter the center of gravity

Cardiovascular/autonomic nervous system
- Age-related impairment in the baroreflex may lead to postural hypotension, which affects balance.
- Many diseases (congestive heart failure, CHF, diabetes, Parkinson's disease) and drugs are associated with postural hypotension.

CNS
- Age-related decline in reaction time; influence of medications, polypharmacy, alcohol, and decreased attention impair CNS activity.

Balance and falls
- Regardless of the etiology, a failure of the body's physiologic balance control mechanism to successfully function will usually result in a fall.

DIAGNOSIS

History and Examination
See chapter Neurologic: Falls.

Tests of Balance Function
See chapter Evaluation of Balance and Mobility.

Natural History
Untreated balance disorders can result in falls and fall-related injuries (see chapter Neurologic: Falls).

Treatment
Treatment for balance disorders is aimed at treatment, correction, compensation, and/or substitution to the extent possible, for the various contributing etiologies mentioned above. This includes identifying and addressing the multiple pathologic and age-related changes in the visual, vestibular, musculoskeletal, CNS, and peripheral nervous system. Additional treatment could include the following:

Assistive devices
- Canes crutches, and walkers can improve balance of patients with balance impairments by widening the base of support and improving somatosensory feedback.
- Assistive devices are available without prescription and are often obtained informally; the appropriate device should be tried and properly fitted; instruct patients in safe use or risk no benefit and potential harm.

Balance rehabilitation therapy: therapeutic exercise
- Numerous studies have shown that well-prescribed exercise can improve physical abilities in older people.
- Interventions involving gait, balance, co-ordination and functional exercises, muscle strengthening, and multiple exercise types appear to have the greatest impact on indirect measures of balance.
- Evidence-based reviews on the efficacy of exercise on balance are inconclusive, due to methodological variability in the types of exercises and the outcome measures to determine balance ability.
- There is now strong evidence to support exercise interventions in the prevention of falls in older people, especially balance training.

Postural correction
- Although not studied extensively, postural malalignment can affect COM and the ability to control the COM if displaced (examples: hypolordosis, anterior pelvic tilt, thoracic kyphosis, forward head posture, shoulder protraction).
- A combination of stretching and strengthening of postural muscles (hip flexors, erector spinae, abdominals, hamstrings, gluteus maximus, cervical and thoracic paraspinals, middle trapezius, rhomboids) helps to improve balance by correcting and maintaining standing posture.

Nontraditional therapy

Tai Chi
- A form of martial arts has been used successfully to improve balance performance in the elderly and decrease falls.
- Mechanism is unclear, but thought to improve postural stability, attentional control, and emotional state.

Computerized devices and electronic games
- Although its efficacy has not been widely studied, the use of videogame systems like the Wii Balance Board and related game software is gaining popularity in the clinical physical therapy setting.

Prognosis
- Prognosis depends on the cause of pathology, level of impairment, and other factors, such as comorbidity.
- Some CNS disorders (Parkinson's disease) are progressive, and while rehabilitation intervention can slow the decline of function, the overall prognosis is fair at best.
- Depending upon the extent of the damage, cerebellar lesions or stroke may allow for slight to significant functional improvement.
- For nonneurological etiologies (arthritis, sarcopenia, etc.), recovery may be less complicated.

Helpful Hints
- Etiology of balance problems is typically multifactored. Factors should be identified and correctable conditions should be corrected.

Suggested Reading
Howe TE, Rochester L, Jackson A, et al. Exercise for improving balance in older people. *Cochrane Database Syst Rev.* 2007;4:CD004963. Doi: 10.1002/14651858.CD004963.pub2

Matsumura BA, Ambrose AF. Balance in the elderly. *Clin Geriatr Med.* 2006;22:395–412.

Sturnieks DL, St. George R, Lord SR. Balance disorders in the elderly. *Clin Neurophysiol.* 2008;38:467–478.

Neurologic: Carpal Tunnel Syndrome

Christopher Parks MD ■ Theresa O. Wyrick MD

Description
Carpal tunnel syndrome (CTS) is a compression neuropathy of the median nerve at the wrist.

Etiology/Types
Acute CTS—sudden onset of symptoms (may require urgent surgical decompression). Causes include
- Trauma
- Infection
- Hemorrhage

CTS—more common; includes idiopathic, anatomic, systemic, and exertional causes.
- Idiopathic:
  - Most common cause of CTS
  - More common in women
  - Incidence increases with age
- Anatomic:
  - Compression of median nerve within carpal canal by edema
  - Scar
  - Infection
  - Fluid
  - Mass
- Systemic: related to body conditions
  - Pregnancy
  - Diabetes
  - Obesity
  - Hypothyroidism
- Exertional: caused by repetitive use of wrist and/or digits

Epidemiology

Frequency
- Incidence of 3.5 cases per 1,000 subjects
- Prevalence of 3.7%

Race
- More common in whites
- Very rare in some ethnic groups (nonwhite South Africans)

Sex
- Female to male ratio is 3:1 to 10:1

Age
- Peak age range of 45 to 60 years
- Rare in a younger population

Pathogenesis
- The carpal tunnel borders in the wrist consist of a concave arch of carpal bones and the transverse carpal ligament.
- Tunnel contents include nine flexor tendons and the median nerve.
- Sustained increase in pressure in the canal can cause damage to the nerve.

Risk Factors
- Obesity
- Pregnancy
- Rheumatoid arthritis
- Diabetes
- Hypothyroidism

Clinical Features
- Paresthesias in median nerve innervated fingers
- Complaints of swelling
- Numbness in median nerve distribution
- Weakness of median nerve innervated hand muscles
- Increased symptoms at night
- Patients report relief of symptoms by shaking the hand.

Natural History
- Variable course
- During pregnancy, the symptoms generally resolve after delivery.

Diagnosis

Differential diagnosis
- Radiculopathy
- Tendonitis
- Other median nerve injury
- Brachial plexopathy
- Arthritis
- Multiple sclerosis

History
- Paresthesias with prolonged wrist flexion or extension; numbness/tingling in thumb, index, long, and ring fingers.
- Dropping things
- Night-time symptoms
- Subjective swelling

Examination
Examination findings are often of limited and questionable usefulness. Signs are not sensitive but fairly specific.
- Square-shaped wrist
- Median nerve hypesthesia
  - Sensitivity 51%; specificity 85%
- Phalen's sign (putting the backs of the hands together in a forced wrist flexion position for up to 1 minute)
  - Sensitivity 51%; specificity 76%
- Median nerve compression test
  - Sensitivity 28%
- Tinel's sign (tapping of the nerve reproduces symptoms)
  - Sensitivity 23%

Testing
- Plain radiographs can rule out anomalous bony anatomy.
- Electromyography/nerve conduction velocity (EMG/NCV); physiologic test: probably the gold standard.
- Ultrasound and magnetic resonance imaging (MRI) shows median nerve swelling or flattening, but cannot determine abnormal nerve function.

Pitfalls
- Missing a cervical radiculopathy or other median neuropathy as the cause of symptoms.
- Anomalous innervation

Red flags
- If there is evidence of atrophy, or denervation/conduction block on EMG, surgery might be considered sooner.

Treatment

Medical
- Immobilization: splinting of wrist at night/intermittently during day has been proven to give lasting benefit.
- Medications: nonsteroidal anti-inflammatory drugs, diuretics, and oral steroids can decrease tunnel interstitial fluid pressures: not usually a long-term solution, but can be considered if CTS is expected to resolve.

Injections
- Corticosteroid injections are most effective in the case of mild symptoms.
- They tend to give only temporary relief, but a good response to the injection is indicative of a good surgical outcome.

Surgery
- Release of the transverse carpal ligament via open incision, endoscopy, or limited incision provides definitive treatment.
- Open and endoscopic procedures have shown similar efficacies at 3 month follow-up.
- Endoscopic cases recover slightly faster.
- Drawback of endoscopic surgery is its dependence on surgeon expertise.

Consults
- Physical medicine and rehabilitation
- Neurology for EMG
- Orthopedic hand or plastic surgery and neurosurgery

Complications
- Pillar pain
- Surgical injury of the palmar cutaneous branch of the median nerve
- Incisional pain

Prognosis
- In all 75% success rate with surgery
- In all 8% worse with surgery
- Lower surgical success rate if EMG is normal
- Worse surgical outcome in older persons and in worker's compensation cases

Helpful Hints
- Splinting can give lasting relief of symptoms.
- Surgery in the face of a normal EMG gives less optimal outcomes.
- EMG should be done, both to confirm the diagnosis and to exclude other pathology.

Suggested Readings
Brown LG, Wright JG. Endoscopic compared with open carpal tunnel release. *J Bone Joint Surg Am.* 2003;85:964–964.

Cranford CS, Ho JY, Kalainov DM, et al. Carpal tunnel syndrome. *J Am Acad Orthop Surg.* 2007;15:537–548.

Neurologic: Charcot Foot

Ralph M. Buschbacher MD ■ Ruth L. Thomas MD

Description
A condition of joint deformity and destruction, usually in the feet/ankles, seen in persons with significant peripheral neuropathy.

Etiology/Types

Theories
- Neurotraumatic theory: loss of pain perception and proprioception leads to repetitive mechanical trauma that results in fractures and bone destruction.
- Neurovascular theory: inappropriate control of blood flow to the foot and ankle bones by the autonomic nervous system leads to osteopenia and fracture with minimal trauma.

Causes of charcot joints
- Diabetes—the most common cause
- Leprosy
- Syringomyelia
- Toxic exposure
- Multiple sclerosis
- Congenital neuropathy
- Trauma
- Tertiary syphilis
- Congenital insensitivity to pain
- Myelomeningocele

Epidemiology
- 0.08% of the general diabetic population
- 13% of high-risk diabetic patients
- Up to 35% have bilateral involvement
- Most commonly presents in the age range of the 50s and 60s, as opposed to most diabetic complications, which become problematic at a later age.

Pathogenesis
- Peripheral neuropathy causes an insensitivity to pain.
- Stress injuries are unrecognized and begin the deterioration of the joint:
  - Stage 0 (inflammation): erythema, edema, and warmth; X-rays normal
  - Stage 1 (development): bone resorption/osteopenia, periarticular fragmentation, fracture, joint subluxation/dislocation, and bony debris; X-rays show damage
  - Stage 3 (coalescence): bony consolidation, osteosclerosis, and fusion after bone destruction; X-rays show absorption of bone fragments/debris, fusion of joints, and sclerosis.
  - Stage 3 (remodeling): joint arthrosis, osteophyte formation, subchondral sclerosis, and progressive fusion; deformity is permanent

Risk factors
- Any cause of significant peripheral neuropathy
- Trauma, often minor, superimposed on the neuropathy can initiate the onset of symptoms

Clinical features
- Feet and ankles are most commonly affected.
- Early on there is marked swelling, warmth, and erythema of the involved area of the foot or ankle.
- Erythema improves with simple elevation of the limb.
- Continued weight-bearing leads to bone destruction and increasing deformity of the foot.
- Often confused with infection, but usually not associated with significantly elevated white blood cell (WBC) count, erythrocyte sedimentation rate, fever, or hyperglycemia.
- Patients with Charcot neuroarthropathy usually have bounding peripheral pulses.
- Midfoot involvement is common.
- The condition is often painless, due to the peripheral neuropathy.

Natural History
- Begins with marked swelling, warmth, and erythema, which is usually painless.
- Foot and ankle deformity develops due to bone destruction and ligament laxity. The deformity will usually become worse with continued unprotected weight-bearing.
- Swelling, warmth, and erythema gradually resolve; the length of time required depends on the location of the Charcot process; midfoot manifestation can resolve within weeks or months, but the hindfoot may take up to 2 years.

- Ulceration can occur due to pressure points.
- Long-term ulcerations may lead to amputation.

Diagnosis

Differential diagnosis
- Cellulitis
- Abscess
- Osteomyelitis
- Osteoarthritis
- Acute gout
- Neuropathic fracture
- Deep venous thrombosis
- Tumor
- Reflex sympathetic dystrophy/complex regional pain syndrome

History
- There is often a history of minor trauma.
- Usually, the initial presentation is unilateral.
- Early presentation is suggestive of infection.
- History should investigate other possible diagnoses.
- Diabetic history should be investigated.

Examination
- Sensory testing (Semmes–Weinstein monofilament test) reveals neuropathy.
- Raising the leg will decrease redness, distinguishing this condition from cellulitis.
- Deep venous thrombosis evaluation
- Temperature measurement: significant side-to-side difference (over 2°C) is suggestive of Charcot neuroarthropathy.
- Volumetric measurement—water displacement compared to opposite extremity as active Charcot process is associated with marked swelling.
- Pulses are easily palpated, due to widened pulse pressure.

Testing
- X-rays: to assess for fracture, bone deformity, and/or dislocation; weight-bearing films may be more sensitive.
  - X-rays will be normal early in the disease process.
- Nuclear medicine studies: may be helpful in differentiating between soft-tissue infection, osteomyelitis, and Charcot arthropathy.
  - Bone scan alone can be misleading; a technetium scan combined with an indium WBC study improves accuracy; in Charcot arthropathy there is an increased uptake on technetium scanning, but not on the indium scan.
- Magnetic resonance imaging (MRI) may not be able to differentiate between Charcot arthropathy and infection.
  - Shows early Charcot changes: ligament disruption and joint deformity
  - Can be misleading because of bone destruction
- Single-photon emission computed tomography (SPECT)/computerized tomography (CT)—combination of indium WBC study and colloid study performed together offers a very sensitive alternative study to determine if osteomyelitis is present when other studies are inadequate.
- Positron emission tomography-computed tomography (PET-CT): excellent sensitivity and specificity
- Dual energy X-ray absorptiometry (DEXA) scan shows lower bone mineral density.
- Labwork
  - No test specific for Charcot arthropathy, but tests can be helpful in ruling out other causes, such as infection.

Pitfalls
- Treating for a different condition, especially infection
- X-rays are normal early in the process
- Diabetes is the most common cause, but not the only one.

Red flags
- Missing a deep infection can be limb or life threatening

Treatment

Medical
- As soon as Charcot neuroarthropathy is diagnosed, weight-bearing on the affected limb should cease. The goal is to maintain the structural stability of the joint and to prevent skin ulceration.
  - A total contact cast can effectively manage swelling, equalize plantar pressures, and support the affected limb.
  - Casts are changed every 2 weeks until erythema, swelling, and warmth resolve; and X-rays show stabilization of the deformity.
- Long-term management requires protective shoewear and possible bracing.
  - Bracing options include double upright braces, polypropylene ankle foot orthoses, and leather corset braces; the choice of brace will depend on the nature of the deformity.
  - Custom extra-depth shoes with a custom insert may be needed.

- Bisphosphonates have been shown to be effective in treatment; however, optimal dosing/administration has not been determined; calcitonin nasal spray has also been studied and advocated.

Surgical
- Surgical management is only indicated after the inflammatory phase has resolved; it may be necessary to correct deformity associated with resultant instability or chronic ulceration.

Consults
- Orthopaedic foot and ankle surgery
- Wound management clinic
- Prosthetics and orthotics vendor

Complications/side effects
- Risk of further joint deterioration
- Skin breakdown with bracing
- Risk of amputation

Prognosis
- The goal of treatment is a stable, plantigrade foot that will fit in a shoe without recurrent ulcerations. With appropriate management, this goal can usually be achieved.
- Severe cases, especially those leading to ulceration, may require amputation.

Helpful Hints
- Charcot neuroarthropathy presents at a somewhat younger age than seen with other diabetic complications.
- Other emergency conditions need to be ruled out, especially infection.
- Early aggressive nonweight-bearing is needed to treat the condition.

Suggested Readings
Botek G, Anderson MA, Taylor R. Charcot neuroarthropathy: An often overlooked complication of diabetes. *Cleveland Clinic J Med.* 77;2010:593–599.

Wukich DK, Sung W. Charcot arthropathy of the foot and ankle: Modern concepts and management review. *J Diabetes Complicat.* 23;2009:409–426.

Neurologic: Delirium

Melissa Sinkiewicz DO ■ Dale C. Strasser MD

Description
- Delirium is an acute state marked by altered consciousness, fluctuating symptoms, and inattention.
- It is commonly unrecognized, potentially preventable, and is associated with functional loss, along with increased morbidity and mortality.

Etiology/Types
- Etiology is not fully understood, but can be related to excessive stimuli, alcohol/drug withdrawal, and various medications, medical problems, and metabolic abnormalities.
  - Hypoactive delirium is characterized by lethargy and apathy (most common).
  - Hyperactive delirium is characterized by agitation and restlessness.

Epidemiology
- Delirium occurs in up to 56% of all acute care hospital admissions.
- Up to 20% of hospitalized patients above the age of 65 develop complications due to delirium.
- Delirium occurs during an estimated 60% of nursing home admissions.

Pathogenesis
- Not entirely understood
- Multifactorial
- Disturbances occur in higher cortical functions
  - Prefrontal cortex, thalamus, and basal ganglia
  - Electroencephalogram (EEG) shows diffuse slowing, correlating with severity of disease

Risk Factors
- Age 65 or above
- More common in males than females
- History of delirium
- Recent trauma and/or recent surgery
- Medical comorbidities
  - Dementia
  - Depression
  - Renal failure
  - Hepatic disease
- Vision and hearing loss
- Specific medications
  - Anticholinergics
  - Narcotics
  - Benzodiazepines
  - Hypnotics
  - Anti-inflammatories
  - Beta-blockers
  - Diuretics
  - Antidepressants
- Polypharmacy
- Excessive environmental stimuli and sleep deprivation
- Alcohol or drug withdrawal
- Metabolic abnormalities (e.g., electrolyte abnormalities, blood glucose level)
- Acute infections (e.g., urinary tract infection, UTI, pneumonia)
- Inadequate pain control

Clinical Features
- Acute onset
- Fluctuating course
- Inattention
- Altered mental status and cognition
- Perceptual deficits
- Psychiatric disturbances
- Altered sleep–wake cycle

Natural History
- Interventions directed at metabolic disturbances and acute medical conditions along with discontinuing inappropriate medications and reducing environmental stimulation can reduce the incidence and diminish the symptoms.
- When left undiagnosed and untreated, serious medical decompensation and even death can occur.

Diagnosis

Differential diagnosis
- Dementia
- Depression
- Encephalopathy

- Postictal confusion
- Dissociative disorder
- Stroke

History
- History of current condition, including neurocognitive symptoms
- Medication assessment
- History of alcohol use, illicit drug use, and smoking

Examination
- Vital signs, including orthostatic blood pressure, pulse rate, and oxygen saturation
- Complete physical examination, including mental status

Testing
Laboratory studies and imaging were carried out when appropriate.
- Evaluation may include
  - Blood glucose level
  - Complete blood count (CBC)
  - Metabolic panel
  - Ammonia level
  - Arterial blood gas
  - Electrocardiogram (ECG)
  - Chest X-ray
  - Neuroimaging studies
  - Others tests based on clinical presentation
- The confusion assessment method (CAM) is a tool to evaluate and diagnose delirium.
  - CAM states that a patient must display inattention and the acute onset of fluctuating symptoms, in addition to either altered level of consciousness or disorganized thinking for diagnosis.

Pitfalls
- Missing other conditions, such as seizure disorder
- Missing alcohol or drug withdrawal

Red flags
- Abnormal vital signs
- New changes on physical examination—focal weakness, pulmonary rales, lower extremity edema, and abdominal distention
- Metabolic abnormalities
- Positive findings on computerized tomography (CT) scan or magnetic resonance imaging (MRI) suggestive of new stroke or intracranial hemorrhage

Treatment

Medical/environmental
- All causative medical conditions (e.g., dehydration, infection, pulmonary embolus) must be addressed.
- Potentially offending medications should be removed, weaned, or reduced.
- Excessive environmental stimulation should be reduced.
- Reorientation and reassurance of the patient
  - Extra supervision, including sitters, as needed
  - Glasses and hearing aids, as needed
- To assist with orientation, the physical and social environment should be optimized.
  - Allow access to clocks, calendars, and familiar objects such as photographs
  - Provide appropriate lighting, including access to natural sunlight
  - Limit use of catheters, lines, and restraints
  - Allow patient to move around unrestrained, as appropriate
  - Reduce sleep interruptions
- Chemical restraints (e.g., medications) should be used only when the above management steps have been initiated and the behavior poses a danger to self or others.
- Physical restraints are used only to ensure patient safety.
- Neither chemical or physical restraints should be used simply for the convenience of the staff.

Medications for agitation
- Risperidone (Risperdal)
  - Dosing—0.5mg orally, twice daily
  - Adverse effects
    - Extrapyramidal symptoms
    - QT prolongation
    - Hyperglycemia
    - Orthostatic hypotension
  - Should be avoided in elderly patients with dementia
- Olanzapine (Zyprexa)
  - Dosing—2.5 to 5 mg orally, daily
  - Adverse effects
- Anticholinergic effects such as the following should be avoided in elderly patients with dementia:
  - Hypotension
  - Extrapyramidal symptoms
  - QT prolongation
  - Orthostatic hypotension
  - Elevation in liver enzymes
  - Lowering of seizure threshold
- Quetiapine (Seroquel) should be avoided in elderly patients with dementia:
  - Dosing—25 mg orally, twice daily
  - Adverse effects
    - Extrapyramidal symptoms

- QT prolongation
    - Orthostatic hypotension
    - Lowering of seizure threshold
- Haloperidol (Haldol)
  - Dosing—0.5 to 1 mg orally or intramuscularly (IM), twice daily, can repeat oral dosing every 4 hours or IM dose every hour, up to 3 mg/day
  - Contraindications—hepatic disease, history of neuroleptic malignant syndrome
  - Adverse effects
    - Extrapyramidal symptoms
    - QT prolongation
    - Increased mortality in patients with dementia-related psychosis
- Lorazepam (Ativan)
  - Dosing—0.5 to 1 mg orally, repeated every 4 hours as needed.
  - Used when withdrawal from alcohol or benzodiazepines is the suspected cause of delirium
  - Adverse effects
    - Paradoxical agitation
    - Sedation
    - Respiratory depression

Consults
- Neurology
- Psychiatry
- Internal medicine

Prognosis
- With prompt diagnosis and treatment, acute delirium can resolve within hours.
- An episode of delirium, even if treated, increases the risk of mortality.
- Mortality rate is 22% to 76% in hospitalized patients with delirium.
- One-year mortality rate is 35% to 40%.

Helpful Hints
- Physical restraints should only be used when needed to ensure patient safety.
- Engage family members, friends, and caregivers in reorienting the patient.

Suggested Readings

Cole MG. Delirium in elderly patients. *Am J Geriatr Psychiatry*. 2004;12:7–21.

Fong TG, Tulebaev SR, Inouye SK. Delirium in elderly adults: Diagnosis, prevention and treatment. *Nat Rev Neurol*. 2009;5:210–220.

Inouye S. Delirium in older persons. *N Engl J Med*. 2006;354:1157–1165.

Inouye S, Studenski S, Tinetti ME, et al. Geriatric syndromes: Clinical, research, and policy implications of a core geriatric concept. *J Am Geriatr Soc*. 2007;55:780–791.

Inouye SK, van Dyck CH, Alessi CA, et al. Clarifying confusion: The confusion assessment method. A new method for detection of delirium. *Ann Intern Med*. 1990;113:941–948.

Shaughnessy M, Rudolph J. Advancing delirium science: Systems, mechanisms and management. *J Am Geriatr Soc*. 2011;59:S233–S304.

Young J, Inouye SK. Delirium in older people. *Br Med J*. 2007;334:842–846.

Neurologic: Dizziness and Vertigo

Kevin M. Means MD

Description

Dizziness is among the most common presenting symptoms in patients 75 years and above seen in an office practice. Vertigo is less common, but is a subtype of dizziness.

Dizziness
- A nonspecific term
  - Could be vertigo, unsteadiness, or disequilibrium
  - Half of all dizziness is associated with vertigo

Vertigo
- A type of dizziness
- Associated with a perception of movement (usually spinning)
- Can be associated with nausea, emesis, and diaphoresis
- Should be distinguished from other types of dizziness

Unsteadiness
- Nonvestibular dizziness and not in above categories (anxiety, giddiness, etc.)

Disequilibrium
- Feeling of imbalance or sensation of "falling," while standing or walking

Etiology/Types
- Medication side effect is a common cause of dizziness.
- Vertigo has a central or peripheral etiology.
- Disequilibrium usually has a locomotor etiology.
- Central vertigo is caused by hemorrhagic or ischemic insults to the cerebellum, vestibular nuclei, or their brainstem connections; central nervous system (CNS) tumors; infection; trauma; and multiple sclerosis.
  - Central vertigo is much less common than peripheral vertigo.
- Peripheral vertigo (three main types):
  - Benign paroxysmal positional vertigo (BPPV)—most common; BPPV is a clinical diagnosis; caused by displacement of otoconia within the semicircular canals
  - Labyrinthitis (acute suppurative, serous, chronic, or toxic)
  - Ménière's disease

Epidemiology
- In all 5% to 30% of elderly persons have dizziness.
- In all 5% to 10% of all initial physician visits are for dizziness.
- Dizziness is more common than low back pain by age 75.

Pathogenesis

Vestibular neuronitis
- Results from herpes simplex virus reactivation or other viral infection affecting the vestibular ganglion and vestibular nerves

Benign paroxysmal positioning vertigo
- Occurs with canalithiasis (otoconia floating in the endolymph) or cupulolithiasis (otoconia adherent to cupula) due to
  - Post-traumatic injury to peripheral vestibular structures
  - Vestibular neuronitis
  - Ménière's disease
  - Endolymphatic hydrops

Ménière's Disease
- Disordered inner ear fluid homeostasis, with endolymphatic hydrops, due to hereditary, autoimmune, infectious, or idiopathic causes.

Central dizziness and vertigo
- Hemorrhagic or ischemic insults to the cerebellum, the vestibular nuclei, and their connections in the brain stem with impairment of axonal activity in the affected area or areas.
- Structural or physiologic changes due to other diseases affecting the CNS and cranial nerve VIII (tumors, infection, trauma, and multiple sclerosis) result in impairment of neuronal activity.

Clinical Features

Vertigo symptom patterns
- Labyrinthitis, acute onset, constant vertigo for days, resolves in 1 to 2 weeks

- BPPV—episodic vertigo when turning in bed lasting seconds; single position usually elicits vertigo; no hearing loss or tinnitus
- Meniere's disease: also episodic but lasts hours and recurs over months to years

Diagnosis

Differential diagnosis
- Peripheral vertigo labyrinthine disorders
  - BPPV
  - Labyrinthitis
  - Ménière's disease
  - Vestibular neuronitis
  - Acoustic neuroma
- Central vertigo
  - Vertebrobasilar or cerebellar disease
  - Atherosclerotic disease of the vertebral or basilar arteries
  - Compression of the vertebral arteries
  - Thromboembolism
  - Brain stem lesion
  - Cerebellar hemorrhage
  - Multiple sclerosis
  - Traumatic brain and neck injury

History
The clinical history can help determine the type of dizziness (unsteadiness, disequilibrium, vertigo). Additional questions about dizziness and vertigo characteristics can further narrow the diagnostic possibilities.

Several dizziness questionnaires have been developed for use in the clinical setting.
- Sensation of movement
- Onset and duration
- Auditory or neurologic disturbances
- Unusual eye movements
- History of head or neck trauma
- Past medical history
- Medications and alcohol intake

Peripheral vertigo labyrinthine disorders (most common cause of true vertigo)

Benign paroxysmal positional vertigo
- Horizontal rotary nystagmus with crescendo–decrescendo pattern after a short latency period
- Less pronounced with repeated stimuli
- Typically can be reproduced at bedside with positioning maneuvers

Labyrinthitis
- Associated hearing loss and tinnitus
- Involves the cochlear and vestibular systems
- Abrupt onset, usually continuous
- Four types of labyrinthitis:
  - Serous labyrinthitis
    - Due to infection/inflammation of adjacent tissues or meninges
    - Causes mild to severe vertigo with nausea and vomiting, with some permanent impairment possible
  - Acute suppurative labyrinthitis
    - Due to acute bacterial infection in middle ear or meningitis
    - Causes severe hearing loss and vertigo
    - Treated with intravenous (IV) antibiotics
  - Toxic labyrinthitis
    - Toxic effects of medications (vancomycin, erythromycin, phenytoin, furosemide, salicylates, alcohol)
    - Causes vertigo in acute phase; then mild tinnitus and high-frequency hearing loss; ataxia in the chronic phase
- Chronic labyrinthitis
  - Localized inner ear inflammatory process due to middle-to-inner ear fistula
  - Most occur in horizontal semicircular canal
  - Due to destruction by a cholesteatoma

Ménière's disease
- Triad of vertigo, tinnitus, and hearing loss
- Due to cochlea "hydrops" (excess of endolymphatic fluid in the inner ear that overflows from its normal channels in the ear into other areas causing damage)
- Unknown etiology
- Possibly autoimmune
- Ménière symptoms are variable; abrupt, episodic, recurrent episodes of severe rotational vertigo usually lasting from minutes to several hours; may occur in clusters with long episode-free remissions.
- Unilateral or bilateral, usually low-pitched tinnitus that can increase in volume
- Fluctuating, progressive, unilateral or bilateral low-frequency hearing loss that can improve after an attack
- Some Ménière patients experience "drop attacks"—sudden, severe dizziness or vertigo resulting in a fall without warning.

Vestibular neuronitis—(vestibular neuropathy)—an idiopathic condition (possibly viral etiology)
- With sudden loss of afferent neuronal input from one or both vestibular apparatuses; results in acute onset of vertigo that increases in intensity over several hours

before gradually subsiding over several days; or mild vertigo lasting several weeks; may be associated with nystagmus, nausea, and vomiting; usually no auditory symptoms.

Acoustic neuroma
- Intracranial Schwann cell tumors surrounding the vestibular or cochlear nerve (CN VIII)
- Can cause vertigo with hearing loss and tinnitus, but vertigo is less common in early disease

Central vertigo syndromes
- Vertebrobasilar or cerebellar insufficiency/occlusion/infarction
- Atherosclerotic disease of the vertebral and basilar arteries and compression of the vertebral arteries by the cervical vertebrae cause transient posterior fossa hypoperfusion during head turning and neck extension, resulting in vertigo.
- Thromboembolism (during infarction)
  - Other common symptoms include: dysarthria, ataxia, facial numbness, hemiparesis, diplopia, and headache.
  - Tinnitus or hearing loss is unlikely.
- Vertical nystagmus is characteristic of a (superior colliculus) brain stem lesion.
- Cerebellar hemorrhage
  - A life-threatening cause of vertigo; neurosurgical emergency
  - Causes: hypertensive vascular disease; anticoagulation
  - Sudden onset headache, vertigo, vomiting, and ataxia
- Multiple sclerosis (vertigo is presenting symptom in 5% to 10%)
- Traumatic brain and neck injury
  - Vertigo and dizziness are common complications.
  - Caused by petechial hemorrhages in the brainstem vestibular nuclei from shearing forces

Examination
A neurologic and cardiovascular examination should be performed in all patients. Targeted components of the physical examination based on suspicion of the underlying diagnosis should be employed. Physical examination tests should attempt to reproduce the patient's symptoms.
- Orthostatic (supine to standing) vital signs
- Cranial nerve examination
- Presence of nystagmus
- Extraocular muscle function
- Hearing acuity
- Weber–Rinne test (*Weber test*: A vibrating tuning fork (256 Hz) is placed in the middle of the forehead. The patient is asked to report in which ear the sound is heard louder. A normal test: Sound is heard equally in both sides; *Rinne test*: A vibrating tuning fork (512 Hz) placed initially on the mastoid process behind each ear, until sound is no longer heard. Then, the fork is immediately placed just outside the ear with the patient asked to report when the sound caused by the vibration is no longer heard. A normal test is when the sound heard outside of the ear is louder than the initial sound.)
- External auditory canal examination
- Muscle strength
- Gait and cerebellar function
- Dix-Hallpike maneuver (used to diagnose BPPV):
  - Patient sits on the examination table facing forward, with eyes open
  - Turn patient's head 45° to the right; patient lies back quickly from sit to supine position with head hanging down 20° off the examination table; remains in position for 30 seconds
  - Sit the patient up and observe for 30 seconds
  - Repeat maneuver with patient's head turned to the left. Test is positive if any maneuvers produce vertigo with or without nystagmus.

Testing
Ancillary tests are only indicated when specific causes of dizziness and vertigo are suspected.
- Computerized tomography (CT) scan—if cerebellar mass, hemorrhage, or infarction suspected
- Caloric reflex testing (introduction of hot or cold water in the external auditory canal) can induce nystagmus and vertigo in patients with vestibular lesions.
- Angiography—for suspected vertebrobasilar insufficiency
- Magnetic resonance imaging (MRI; brain, neck)—to detect intracranial and/or spinal abnormalities
- Electronystagmography (ENG)—can detect vestibular abnormalities
- Audiometry—quantifies hearing loss; important in acoustic neuroma and Meniere disease
- Dynamic posturography—tests the vestibular system and the visual and somatosensory equilibrium
- Neuro-otologic examination—A neuro-ophthalmologist or an otolaryngologist puts the patient through specialized examination procedures.

Treatment
See treatment for selected conditions in Table 1.

Table 1 Treatment for Selected Causes of Dizziness and Vertigo

Condition	Treatment	Notes
Benign paroxysmal positional vertigo (BPPV)	Medications: Vertigo symptoms commonly treated with meclizine, but now increasingly less popular	• Evidence for meclizine effectiveness is lacking; meclizine has sedative side effects and vestibular suppression can prolong symptoms
	• Epley maneuver for otolith repositioning; • See a video demonstration of the procedure at: http://www.youtube.com/watch?v=59EIKztATiw&NR=1	• This is the main recommended treatment for BPPV; evidence supports the safety and efficacy of this procedure
	Brandt-Daroff repositioning exercises—One of the several exercises to facilitate compensation and reduce symptoms of vertigo. Brandt-Daroff exercise: Start in upright, seated position. • Move to the lying position on one side with nose pointed up at a 45° angle. • Remain in this position for about 30 seconds (or until the vertigo subsides, whichever is longer), then return to a seated position. Repeat on the other side. In all 20 repetitions, twice a day. See a video demonstration of Brandt-Daroff exercise at: http://www.youtube.com/watch?v=nIEguL0AaEw&NR=1&feature=fvwp	• Brandt-Daroff exercises are safe and effective in relieving BPPV vertigo symptoms, but also may exacerbate vertigo, nausea, and vomiting. This can possibly discourage people from continuing the exercise
	• Vestibular rehabilitation (VR)—A series of therapeutic head and neck exercises used in patients with balance disorders of vestibular origin. Proposed action is based on central mechanisms of neuroplasticity, known as adaptation, habituation, and substitution, aiming a vestibular compensation. • See a video demonstration of VR at: http://www.youtube.com/watch?v=hhinu_oU_hM	• Evidence supports the safe use of VR protocols for reduction or remission of dizziness and vertigo, improved postural instability, and improved static and dynamic balance, but further high-quality studies are needed
Vestibular neuritis	Medications: Methylprednisolone 100 mg orally, daily; then lower to 10 mg orally, daily, over 3 weeks	Vestibular neuronitis is usually self-limited and improves in 1 to 2 weeks. Demonstrated effectiveness in some trials
	Brandt-Daroff repositioning exercises	Demonstrated effectiveness in some trials
Labyrinthitis	Acute labyrinthitis—symptom treatment with meclizine 12.5 to 25 mg orally, every 6 to 8 hours, as needed; or diazepam 2 mg orally, daily Systemic steroids for 5 to 10 days can reduce the course of severe symptoms	
	Suppurative labyrinthitis—may require treatment with intravenous (IV) antibiotics Toxic labrynthitis—stop the offending agent if possible VR exercises	Referral to otolaryngologist or infectious disease consultant recommended
Ménière's disease	Medications: meclizine, droperidol, prochlorperizol, and diazepam are used to mask vertigo symptoms by suppressing inner ear signals. Diuretics (hydrochlorothiazide and triamterene, acetazolamide, methazolamide) decrease fluid pressure in the inner ear.	There is insufficient evidence to determine the efficacy of these treatments. Diuretics help prevent attacks, but do not help after the attack is triggered
	Dietary: salt restriction (1–2 g of sodium per day) used to decrease inner ear fluid pressure	There is insufficient evidence to determine the efficacy of these treatments
	Oral, intramuscular, or transtympanically administered steroids (dexamethasone) may reduce endolymphatic hydrops via their anti-inflammatory properties	Some studies report less than 80% reversal of vertigo, tinnitus, and hearing loss with steroids. Referral to an otolaryngologist required for transtympanic administration

(Continued)

Table 1 *(Continued)*

Condition	Treatment	Notes
	Intratympanic administration of aminoglycosides such as gentamicin are preferentially toxic to the vestibular (balance) end organ and reduce sensitivity to inner ear pressure fluctuations seen in Ménière disease	Not useful in bilateral Ménière's disease because bilateral treatment would result in complete loss of inner ear balance function
	Histamine agonist medications such as betahistine (Serc) are widely used in Europe and South America	Successful use in Ménière's disease reported, but insufficient evidence of efficacy; not approved by the U.S. Food and Drug Administration
	The Meniett device delivers pulses of pressure to the inner ear via a tympanostomy tube that is surgically inserted	Mechanism of action is unclear; long-term results not fully evaluated. Referral to an otolaryngologist required
	Surgical intervention: endolymphatic sac decompression or shunt, vestibular nerve section, labyrinthectomy, and transtympanic medication perfusion	Referral to an otolaryngologist required
Vertebrobasilar insufficiency	Treatment consists of controlling risk factors (diabetes, hypertension, hyperlipidemia) and using antiplatelet drugs (aspirin, clopidogrel)	
Disequilibrium	Treatment of underlying cause (e.g., peripheral neuropathy, Parkinson's disease), which is typically multifactored	Because disequilibrium is generally a symptom of an underlying condition, treatment of the condition improves symptoms of disequilibrium

- Treatment approach varies and is based on etiology.
- The main initial treatment of peripheral vertigo has been with anticholinergic antihistamines (meclizine, diphenhydramine, droperidol), but their long-term efficacy is unproven.
- The Epley maneuver works well for BPPV.
- Vestibular neuronitis:
  - Antiemetic and vestibular suppressants can improve acute symptoms, but can delay central vestibular compensation with prolonged use.
  - Corticosteroids may improve long-term outcomes.
  - Early vestibular rehabilitation is helpful.
  - Antiviral medications are not helpful.
  - One third of patients have chronic vestibular symptoms and develop BPPV.
- BPPV:
  - Canalith repositioning is usually effective after one or two treatments.
  - Medications are not effective for BPPV.
- Ménière's disease:
  - 80% of patients respond to conservative therapy with salt restriction and diuretics; corticosteroids (oral or intratympanic) can stabilize active disease.
  - Intratympanic gentamicin (chemical labyrinthectomy) is effective for treating vertigo.
  - Effectiveness of surgical therapy (shunting the endolymphatic sac) varies widely.
- Central dizziness and vertigo:
  - The course of patients with central vertigo is highly variable and depends on the etiology and severity of the underlying disease.
  - The prognosis for patients with basilar or vertebral artery infarction or spontaneous cerebellar hemorrhage is poor.
  - Neurosurgical advancements have improved the prognosis for many central dizziness patients.

Prognosis

- Older adults most likely to benefit from a vestibular rehabilitation program include those with unilateral or bilateral peripheral vestibular disorders.
- Other patients who can be helped by physical therapy include those with traumatic brain injury and neck trauma, cerebellar stroke or dysfunction, and multiple sclerosis.
- Patients with bilateral peripheral disorders may have slower and less complete improvement with physical therapy than unilateral patients.
- It is much more difficult to treat individuals with central disorders, anxiety disorders, and combined central/peripheral vestibular disorders

than patients presenting with peripheral vestibular dysfunction.

Helpful Hints
- Listen and understand what the patient means by "dizzy."
- Try to differentiate central from peripheral vertigo.
- Central causes are usually insidious and more severe, while peripheral causes are mostly abrupt and benign.
- Most patients will not need imaging or special tests.
- Meclizine is probably overprescribed.

Suggested Readings

Bhattacharyya N, Baugh RF, Orvidas L, et al. Clinical practice guideline: Benign paroxysmal positional vertigo. *Otolaryngol–Head Neck Surg.* 2008;139:S47–S81.

Furmana JM, Razb Y, Whitney SL. Geriatric vestibulopathy assessment and management. *Curr Opin Otolaryngol Head Neck Surg.* 2010;18:386–391.

Kerber KA, Fendrick AM. The evidence base for the evaluation and management of dizziness. *J Eval Clin Pract.* 2010;16:186–191.

Lang EE, Walsh RM. Vestibular function testing. *Ir J Med Sci.* 2010;179:173–178.

Matsumura BA, Ambrose AF. Balance in the elderly. *Clin Geriatr Med.* 2006;22:395–412.

Post RE, Dickerson LM. Dizziness: A diagnostic approach. *Am Fam Physician.* 2010;82:361–368.

Neurologic: Dysphagia

Martin B. Brodsky PhD ■ Jeffrey B. Palmer MD

Description
Dysphagia, or abnormal swallowing, is common in the elderly and can lead to serious sequelae including aspiration pneumonia, dehydration, malnutrition, and airway obstruction.

Etiology/Types

Physiological
- Stroke
- Neurodegenerative or neuromuscular disorders
- Esophageal motility disorders
- Medication-induced (anticholinergics, benzodiazepines, neuroleptics)
- Traumatic brain or spinal cord injury

Structural
- Diverticulae of the pharynx or esophagus (e.g., Zenker)
- Eosinophilic esophagitis
- Strictures, webs, or rings
- Head and neck cancer (oral cavity, pharynx, larynx, or esophagus)
- Surgical deletions
- Radiation fibrosis

Dysphagia is commonly classified by phase relative to bolus position:
- Oral phase: bolus acquisition, mastication, manipulation, and transport to the pharynx
- Pharyngeal phase: bolus movement from the oral cavity, through the pharynx, and into the esophagus through pressures by the tongue and pharyngeal constrictor muscles
- Esophageal phase: bolus movement via peristalsis from the pharynx to the stomach.

Epidemiology
- In the United States, the prevalence of dysphagia is 7% with an increasing incidence with age.
- Dysphagia occurs most commonly as a result of neurologic disorders (e.g., stroke, Parkinson's disease, PD), although esophageal (e.g., reflux, scleroderma) and mechanical (e.g., neoplasm) disorders may also cause dysphagia.
- There is limited data on the incidence of dysphagia, although up to 40% of stroke patients will experience this disorder.

Pathogenesis
- Variable, depends on the neurologic or mechanical process involved

Risk factors
- Stroke
- Traumatic brain injury
- Various medications
- Esophageal diverticuli/structural abnormalities/surgery
- Radiation
- Intubation/tracheostomy

Clinical Features

Symptoms
- Pain on swallowing (odynophagia)
- Weight loss
- Change in dietary habits
- Coughing and choking with swallowing suggest pharyngeal dysphagia.
- Complaint of food sticking in the chest suggests esophageal dysphagia.
- Complaint of food sticking in the neck is common in both pharyngeal and esophageal dysphagia.
- Dysphagia for solid foods is more common in structural conditions (e.g., strictures).
- Nasal regurgitation suggests pharyngeal dysphagia.
- Dysphagia can be asymptomatic in stroke and neurologic conditions.

Signs
- Dysarthria or dysphonia (abnormal speech or voice quality)
- Tongue weakness
- Drooling
- Difficulty initiating swallowing
- Unexplained weight loss

Natural History
- Most people have dysphagia after stroke; about 50% improve substantially within 2 weeks, 85% within 6 months.
- Most people have dysphagia after treatment for head and neck cancer; the dysphagia generally persists with limited improvement over time.
- Silent aspiration (without symptoms) is common in stroke, neurologic disorders, and head and neck cancer.

Diagnosis

Differential diagnosis
- Barrett's esophagus
- Gastroesophageal reflux disease
- Postnasal drip
- Reactive airway disease
- Visceral hypersensitivity
- Iron deficiency (Plummer–Vinson syndrome)
- Psychogenic disorder

History
- Neurologic disorders
- Cancer
- Problems with different foods and/or liquids
- Quality of speech
- Regurgitation
- Weight loss

Examination
- Palpation of hyoid bone, thyroid cartilage, and cricoid cartilage
- Inspection of oral cavity
- Neurologic examination, including cranial nerves and gag reflex

Instrumental examination
- Assessment of oral and pharyngeal anatomy and physiology can be done using a videofluoroscopic swallow study (VFSS) and/or a fiberoptic endoscopic evaluation of swallowing (FEES).
- VFSS permits evaluation of structures not seen on FEES (e.g., esophageal sphincters).
- FEES excels in observation of secretions and pharyngeal/laryngeal mucosa, and does not require radiation.
- The mechanism of swallowing impairment and compensatory maneuvers should be assessed to improve safety and efficiency (e.g., modifying food consistency, posture, or respiration).
- Finding aspiration on VFSS or FEES is an indication of increased risk of aspiration pneumonia.
- Esophageal swallowing can be assessed with esophagogastroduodenoscopy (EGD) or traditional barium swallow.

Pitfalls
- Bedside swallowing evaluation is not highly reliable for detecting dysphagia and aspiration.
- Swallow performance may differ with time of day or situation, so findings on VFSS or FEES may not generalize to other situations.

Red flags
- Aspiration pneumonia

Treatment
- Treatments are individualized; what helps one patient may exacerbate impairment in another patient (e.g., thickened liquids reduce aspiration in some patients, but increase it in others).
- Treatment may include any combination of
  - Exercise
  - Diet modifications (texture or consistency of foods or liquids)
  - Postures of the head, neck, and body (e.g., chin down, head turn)
  - Techniques to improve oral and pharyngeal sensation (e.g., thermal stimulation)
  - Surface electromyography (EMG) biofeedback
  - Respiratory maneuvers (e.g., supraglottic swallow)
- Electrical stimulation: frequently used, but data on safety and effectiveness are lacking.
- Dilatation for stricture or stenosis, especially of esophagus and its sphincters.
- Surgery (e.g., hyoid suspension or cricopharyngeal myotomy): infrequently used to treat dysphagia.
- Tube feedings: used for patients who cannot safely take sufficient alimentation or hydration by mouth.
- Gastrostomy/jejunostomy tube feedings: controversial with respect to safety and efficacy in the institutionalized elderly individual.

Consults
- Otolaryngology, head and neck surgery
- Speech therapy
- Neurology
- Physical medicine and rehabilitation

Prognosis
- Stroke: About 50% improve substantially within 2 weeks, 85% within 6 months.
- Stricture: Most patients will experience immediate improvement following dilatation, but recurrence is common.
- PD: Often asymptomatic initially, though swallowing is abnormal. Progresses gradually.

Helpful Hints
- The absence of a gag reflex does not necessarily indicate dysphagia, nor does the presence of a gag indicate normal swallowing function.
- Be sensitive to patient complaints of swallowing difficulties, including food refusal/avoidance.

Suggested Readings
Groher ME, Crary MA, eds. *Dysphagia: Clinical Management in Adults and Children.* Maryland Heights, MO: Mosby Elsevier; 2010.

Logemann JA. *Evaluation and Treatment of Swallowing Disorders.* 2nd ed. Austin, TX: Pro-Ed; 1998.

Palmer JB, ed. Dysphagia. *Phys Med Rehabil Clin N Am.* 2008;19(4).

Neurologic: Falls

Kevin M. Means MD

Description
- Fall: An involuntary change from standing, walking, bending, reaching, and so on to no longer being supported by both feet; accompanied by (partial or full) contact with the ground or floor.
- Syncopal fall: A fall associated with or resulting from a loss of full consciousness, such as from fainting or a seizure. Most falls are nonsyncopal.
- Injurious fall: A fall associated with any detectable residual adverse physical change persisting after the fall.

Etiology
- Multifactorial etiology theory:
  - Falls in older persons are usually due to an accumulation of multiple modest impairments, rather than any single deficit.

Epidemiology
- 33% of community-dwelling elderly persons fall annually (half of these persons fall multiple times).
- 40% to 60% of nursing home residents fall; this population has the highest injury percentage.
- Elderly hospital patients have intermediate (35–40%) fall incidence.
- Community-dwelling elderly persons report the lowest incidence of falls, but this (largest) group of elderly persons has the most total falls; community falls may be under-reported.
- Fall risk increases with age nonlinearly (an 80-year-old has eight times the risk of a 65-year-old).

Pathophysiology
- Multiple factors have been reported to contribute to an increased risk of falling (see Risk Factors below).

Risk Factors

Intrinsic
- Previous falls or multiple stumbles
- Poor health status
- Polypharmacy (≥4 medications)
- Specific drugs: tricyclics, diuretics, benzodiazepines, alcohol, and antihypertensives
- Syncope and dizziness
- Frequent nocturnal urination
- Vision or hearing impairment
- Dementia
- Muscle weakness
- Gait abnormalities
- Musculoskeletal problems
- Specific diagnoses: Parkinson's disease stroke and peripheral neuropathy
- Vestibular disorders
- Foot disorders
- Number of chronic disabilities

Environmental
- Stairs
- Poor lighting and unstable furniture
- Clutter and loose throw rugs
- Pets
- Ill-fitting clothing or shoes

Situational
- Inattention and divided attention
- Rushing and impulsivity
- Poor safety awareness
- Extreme or unusual activity
- Unfamiliar setting or hazards
- Risk-taking behavior

Natural History

Impact of falls
- Morbidity
  - Fractures in 5%
  - Other injuries in 10% to 20%
- Mortality
  - Hip fracture mortality is approximately 15% and is the seventh leading cause of death in older persons.
  - 75% of fall-related deaths are seen in the elderly.
- Disability
  - Falls result in an increased incidence of disability.
  - The presence of a disability increases fall risk.
- Early institutionalization
  - Persons hospitalized for falls are more likely to be discharged to nursing homes and to need more

in-home services; they are less likely to regain preinjury mobility status.
- Health care costs
  - Annual U.S. fall-related health care expenses are $20 billion.
  - Hip fracture generates $2 billion in health care system costs.
  - Cost to individuals with hip fracture is $16,000 to $18,000 within 1 year of the fracture.

Clinical Features
- Fear of falling—A lack of self-confidence in one's ability to avoid falls during everyday activities.
- "Ptophobia," extreme fear, hesitancy, or refusal to walk with or without assistance can lead to autorestriction in activities, immobility, and physical decline.
- Depression
  - Increased among fallers
- Low self-efficacy/self-esteem
  - Increased among fallers
- Social isolation
  - Results from activity of daily living (ADL) and mobility self-restriction

Diagnosis

History
- Medical history
- Falling history: when and how, during what activity, location; if multiple falls, is there a pattern?
- Fall-associated symptoms: syncope, dizziness, vertigo, generalized or lower limb weakness, pain, and foot or visual problems
- Medication inventory: including over-the-counter and herbal medications
- Alcohol use
- Activity history

Examination
- General physical examination
- Orthostatic blood pressure recording
- Visual screening (Snellen chart)
- Mental status
- Cranial nerve function; nystagmus
- Romberg test and sharpened Romberg (the Romberg test performed in tandem/heel-to-toe stance)
- Cerebellar function
- Observation of gait
- Focused musculoskeletal and foot examination

Functional balance and mobility testing
See Chapter 21, Evaluation of Balance and Mobility, for more information.

Treatment

Barriers to managing falls
- The etiology of the fall is not always obvious.
- Most falls are unobserved and under-recognized.
- Knowledge about specific intervention is still evolving.

Intervention approach
- Identification of possible contributing factors, especially in complex patients
- Management of contributing neuromuscular and musculoskeletal problems
- Formulation and monitoring of a specific rehabilitation plan
- Fix what is fixable, help compensate, substitute for, or avoid nonfixable conditions or factors

Falls rehabilitation team interventions
- Revise/reduce medications
- Assistive devices, as necessary
- Orthotics, footwear modifications
- Energy conservation instruction
- Home safety modifications, adaptive equipment; clutter removal
- Patient/caregiver education
- Emergency alarm systems
- Transfer and functional training
- Therapeutic exercise

Situational preventive measures
- Avoid fatigue; encourage rests
- Avoid distraction, increase attention and concentration
- Improve safety awareness
- Build confidence, self-esteem
- Arrange for support services

Evidence-based interventions
- One type of exercise as the sole intervention—not effective.
- Health education alone or one type of exercise plus health education—not effective.
- Comprehensive (physical, behavioral, environmental) interventions targeting multiple risk factors in high-risk individuals significantly reduce falls.
- Other effective measures (as part of a comprehensive fall-prevention program:
  - Calcium and vitamin D can reduce fall and fracture risk (type and dose are unclear).
  - Hip pads can help reduce fall-related hip fractures in the nursing home setting.
  - Reduction of psychotropic medications, early cataract surgery

- Professional home hazard evaluation and modification
- Exercise is an essential part of a comprehensive fall-prevention program
  - Most effective exercise programs have included multiple exercises such as strengthening and balance exercises or three-dimensional exercises (including Tai Chi, qi gong, dance, and yoga).
  - There is either no or insufficient evidence to support or refute the effectiveness of general physical activity, including walking or cycling.
  - Optimal exercise conditions (frequency, duration, setting, etc.) are unclear; but in a recent evidence-based review, the most effective programs ran three times a week for 3 months.

Prognosis
- Comprehensive programs reduce injury and non-injury fall rate by 15% to 50%.
- Higher intensity exercise programs have better outcomes.
- Higher risk people have lower rates of fall reductions.

Helpful Hints
- Falls prevention is possible and important.
- Rehabilitation depends on identifying contributing factors, correcting the correctable, and, otherwise, compensating.

Suggested Readings
Ganz DA, Bao Y, Shekelle PG, et al. Will my patient fall? *JAMA*. 2007;297:77–86.

Gillespie LD, Gillespie WJ, Robertson MC, et al. Interventions for preventing falls in elderly people. *Cochrane Database Syst Rev.* 2009; 2:CD000340. Doi: 10.1002/14651858.CD000340.pub2.

Howe TE, Rochester L, Neil F, et al. Exercise for improving balance in older people. *Cochrane Database Syst Rev.* 2011;11:CD004963. Doi: 10.1002/14651858.CD004963.pub3.9.

Panel on Prevention of Falls in Older Persons, American Geriatrics Society, British Geriatrics Society. Summary of the updated American Geriatrics Society/British Geriatrics Society clinical practice guideline for prevention of falls in older persons. *J Am Geriatr Soc*. 2011;59:148–157.

Tinetti ME. Preventing falls in elderly persons. *N Engl J Med*. 2003;348:42–49.

Neurologic: Gait Disorders

Kevin M. Means MD

Description
Gait disorders are deviations from the normal walking pattern (gait).
- Gait disorders are especially important in the elderly because they can compromise independence and increase the risk of falls and injury.
- Many older people limit their activity because of concerns about ambulation and fear of falling.

Etiology/Types
- Some changes in gait in the elderly are due to age-related changes.
- Gait disorders are also a common manifestation of neurologic, musculoskeletal, and cardiovascular disease, particularly in the elderly.
- Many common pathological conditions can influence gait and result in gait disorders.

Common pathologic gait disorders
- Weakness gaits
  - Trendelenburg
  - Waddling
  - Steppage or foot-drop
- Cautious gait (short hesitant steps)
- Stiffness gaits (limited movement of joint, trunk segment, or limb)
  - Skeletal and joint disorders (antalgic)
  - Spasticity and dystonia
  - Vestibular disorders (head/neck/trunk stiffness)
  - Festinating (short, jerky steps; accelerating, with difficulty stopping after starting); parkinsonism
  - Muscle hypertonicity
- Ataxic gait (wide-based; irregular cadence, steps, and trunk movements)
  - Sensory ataxia, cerebellar ataxia, and chorea
- Deviating gaits (veering off to side)
  - Unilateral vestibular disorders
  - Nondominant parietal stroke with neglect
- Freezing gait (motionless attempt to initiate gait; narrow base)
  - Parkinsonism
  - Progressive supranuclear palsy
  - Hydrocephalus, frontal lobe lesions

Epidemiology
- The prevalence of gait disorders is difficult to estimate due to the absence of standard diagnostic criteria.
- Studies have reported that 15% of volunteers above 60 years, 29% of those age 75 to 84, and 49% of the population 85 and above have an abnormal gait on neurologic examination.
- In a 2009 survey, 18% to 45% of elderly Americans reported difficulty in walking.

Pathogenesis

Gait changes with aging
- Decreased velocity (increased double limb support, decreased step length)
- Step length decreases 10% from age 25 to 75
- Increased stance time and decreased swing
- Decreased pelvic rotation
- Decreased cadence (number of steps per minute)
- Increased anterior pelvic tilt and thoracic kyphosis
- Decreased ankle plantar flexion (PF); decreased heel rise during terminal stance
- Decreased PF push off power
- Decreased vertical movement of the center of mass
- Increased sway path

Gait disorders and falls
- Gait disorders increase the risk of falling and injury.
- Sequelae from a fall-related injury can exacerbate gait disorders

Risk Factors
Risk factors are usually multifactorial.
- Degenerative joint disease
- Acquired musculoskeletal problems
- Cardiorespiratory diseases
- Intermittent claudication
- Impairments following orthopedic surgery
- Impairments following stroke
- Postural hypotension
- Neurologic diseases
- Cognitive dysfunction
- Affective disorders
- Fear of falling

Clinical Features
See the section on Etiology/Types.

Diagnosis

History
- History of known neuromuscular or musculoskeletal conditions
- Onset, chronicity, and progression of walking difficulty
- History of falls (temporal pattern, frequency, location, etc.)
- The presence and pattern of any of the following symptoms associated with walking:
  - Limping
  - Fatigue, generalized weakness
  - Poor balance
  - Dizziness and vertigo
  - Numbness and tingling
  - Sphincter dysfunction
  - Tremor
  - Lower limb muscle weakness
  - Stiffness (trunk or limb)
  - Pain
- Medications
- Alcohol use
- Functional status and activity history

Physical Examination
- Neurologic examination
  - Mental status, affect
  - Cranial nerve function
  - Romberg
  - Hoffmann's sign
  - Cerebellar function
  - Manual muscle testing and tone
  - Balance and posture
  - Sensory testing
  - Reflexes
  - Babinski sign
  - Musculoskeletal and foot examination
  - Range of motion and posture
  - Joint deformity and asymmetry

Observational gait analysis
- Approach systematically; observe movement from head to toe.
- View from front, side, and back.
- As appropriate, note the following:
  - Smoothness of movement
  - Arm swing
  - Trunk movement
  - Body rise
  - Speed
  - Cadence (steps per minute)
  - Step length and symmetry
  - Step width
  - Path
  - Stability
  - Specific deviations

Functional performance tests

Timed Up and Go test
- Equipment: chair with arms, tape measure, tape, and stop watch
- The patient begins sitting in a chair with the back resting on the back of the chair.
- The patient is asked to arise and walk at a normal pace to a line marked on the floor 3 m away from the chair, turn around, return to the chair, and sit down.
- The patient wears regular footwear and may use any gait aid that is normally used during ambulation, but may not be assisted by another person.
- The patient is timed but there is no time limit—may stop and rest if necessary; the patient should be given a nontimed practice trial before testing.
- Results correlate with gait speed, balance, functional level, ability to go out, and can change over time.
- Interpretation of results:
  - If less than 10 seconds—normal
  - If less than 20 seconds—good mobility without a gait aid; can go out alone
  - If less than 30 seconds—cannot go outside alone; requires a gait aid
  - If ≥14 seconds—high risk of falls

Tinetti gait evaluation
- A functional mobility skills test
- Gait subscale includes 10 characteristics as follows:
  - Initiation of gait
  - Step length and height
  - Right and left step length
  - Right and left foot clearance during swing
  - Step symmetry
  - Step continuity/discontinuity
  - Path
  - Use of walking aid
  - Trunk sway
  - Step width
- Test items are scored on a 0 to 1 or 2 scale (maximum gait score = 12).
- Results are interpreted when Tinetti gait and Tinetti balance subscales are combined (maximum

balance score = 16; maximum balance + gait score = 28)
- If less than 19—high risk of falling
- If 19 to 23—increased risk of falling
- If less than 24—low risk of falling

Timed 10-m walk test
- Used for higher level functioning patients
- Patient walks at preferred speed without assistance 10 m (32.8 ft) and the time is measured for the intermediate 6 m (19.7 ft—timing is started when the leading foot crosses the 2-m mark; it is stopped when the leading foot crosses the 8-m mark), allowing for acceleration and deceleration.
- Assistive devices can be used, but should be kept consistent and documented from test to test.
- If physical assistance is required to walk, this test should not be performed.
- Average time for three trials is used.
- Gait laboratory analysis (if available)—note that this approach requires special equipment and reimbursement is limited.

Testing
Testing can be done as needed for specific disorders:
- X-ray/computerized tomography (CT) scan/magnetic resonance imaging
- Electromyography (EMG) and nerve conduction studies
- Electronystagmogram

Treatment
- Treat (or refer for treatment) all treatable conditions.
- Treatments vary by condition and include pharmacologic and nonpharmacologic treatment of neurologic and musculoskeletal disorders.
  - Medications: analgesics, antispasticity agents, and anti-Parkinson's drugs
  - Therapeutic exercise
  - Gait training
  - Therapeutic modalities
  - Orthoses
  - Appropriate assistive devices
  - Shoe modifications

Helpful Hints
- Use all clinical information, including gait examination, to identify the gait disorder and underlying contributing factor/factors.

Suggested Readings
Axer H, Axer M, Sauer H, et al. Falls and gait disorders in geriatric neurology. *Clin Neurol Neurosurg.* 2010;112:265–274.

Sudarsky L. Neurologic disorders of gait. *Curr Neurol Neurosci Rep.* 2001;1:350–356.

Sudarsky L. Geriatrics: Gait disorders in the elderly. *N Engl J Med.* 1990;332:1441–1446.

Van Hook FW, Demonbreun D, Weiss BD. Ambulatory devices for chronic gait disorders in the elderly. *Am Fam Physician.* 2003;67:1717–1724.

Whittle MW. Clinical gait analysis: A review. *Hum Mov Sci.* 1996;15:369–387.

Yves J, Gschwind YJ, Bridenbaugh SA, et al. Gait disorders and falls. *GeroPsych.* 2010;23:21–32.

Neurologic: Homonymous Hemianopsia

Joseph G. Chacko MD

Description
Homonymous hemianopia is the loss of vision of the right or left visual field in both eyes, and respecting the vertical midline.

Etiology/Types
- The disease process is in the brain, not the eyes.
- Most common causes include
  - Stroke (over 70%)
  - Trauma
  - Brain tumor
  - Rare causes include posterior form of Alzheimer, multiple sclerosis, and infections.

Epidemiology
- Prevalence approaches 1% in the general population above age 49.

Pathogenesis
- Brain pathology is contralateral to the side of vision loss, and posterior to the optic chiasm.
- The optic tract may be involved, but more commonly the temporal, parietal, or occipital lobes of the brain are affected.

Risk Factors
- Primary risk factors include those associated with stroke (see chapter on Neurologic: Stroke), traumatic brain injury.

Clinical Features
- Patient bumping into objects, people, or doorways on one side of visual space.
- Patient in recent motor vehicle accident and did not see other car/object in blind hemifield.

Natural History
- Most recovery occurs in the first 3 months after onset.
- Up to 40% of patients may have spontaneous recovery.
- Less pronounced recovery typically occurs 6 months after onset.

Diagnosis

History
- Vision loss
- Accidents/bumping into things
- Some patients may experience visual hallucinations on the side of the blind hemifield (i.e., Charles Bonnet syndrome).
- Rarely, dementia patients may deny the blindness (i.e., Anton's syndrome).

Examination
- Visual acuity testing: Patient may fail to see letters toward the side of the chart corresponding to the hemianopia.
- Confrontational visual field testing, one eye at a time: One or two fingers are placed in each visual quadrant to test vision. The patient should look at the examiner's nose with the unoccluded eye during testing.
- Blood pressure: Untreated hypertensive stroke may be the etiology.

Testing
- Computerized tomography (CT) or magnetic resonance imaging (MRI) of the brain may be performed with referral to neurology depending on the results.
- If stroke is the cause, carotid Doppler studies and an echocardiogram should be performed.

Red Flags
- Changing neurologic status
- Patient should not drive; the patient/family should be counseled, but the physician is not compelled to contact the motor vehicle department. This should be documented in the chart.

Treatment
- Three main rehabilitation programs are currently used:
  - Optical therapy
  - Eye movement therapy
  - Visual field restitution
- Optical therapy most commonly involves prism lenses that may be used for one or both eyes, and over the

entire visual field or only the hemianopic field; these lenses are meant to replace part of the intact visual field with a portion of the impaired field.
- Eye movement therapy involves practicing finding objects in the blind hemifield by increased voluntary saccades to this area.
- Visual field restitution attempts to restore functional vision within the damaged visual field; this process entails "retraining" vision by practicing for detecting stimuli in the impaired area of vision. This remains a controversial program with conflicting research findings.
- All of these rehabilitation programs involve multiple hours devoted to the particular training regimen (e.g., 20–100 hours).

Consults
- Neurology
- Ophthalmologist or neuro-ophthalmologist can perform formal visual field testing and consider vision-based rehabilitation strategies (e.g., hemianopic mirrors/prisms).

Helpful Hints
- Teach patient to move the head left and right to improve recognition of objects in their environment.
- Use straight-edge while reading to avoid losing their line of text.

Suggested Readings
Gilhotra JS, Mitchell P, Healey PR, et al. Homonymous visual field defects and stroke in an older population. *Stroke*. 2002;33:2417–2420.

Schofield TM and Leff AP. Rehabilitation of hemianopia. *Curr Opin Neurol*. 2009;22:36–40.

Zhang X, Kedar S, Lynn MJ, et al. Homonymous hemianopias. Clinical-anatomic correlations in 904 cases. *Neurology*. 2006;66:906–910.

Neurologic: Parkinson's Disease

Kevin M. Means MD

Description
Parkinson's disease (PD) is a degenerative disorder of the basal ganglia that is typically characterized by the presence of a tremor. PD is progressive and can have debilitating effects on function by impairment of mobility, communication, activities of daily living, and swallowing.

Etiology/Types
- PD affects the central nervous system and results from the death of dopamine-containing cells in the substantia nigra region of the midbrain.
- The cause of cell death is unknown.
- The basal ganglia exert a constant inhibitory influence on several motor systems, preventing their activity at inappropriate times.
- Released dopamine reduces inhibition, allowing activation for motor movements.
- A high level of dopamine function promotes motor activity and dopamine depletion (as is seen in PD) producing hypokinesia—reduced motor output.

Epidemiology
- PD is one of the most common neurologic disorders, affecting 1% of individuals above 60 years of age and 4% of individuals above 80 years of age.
- Mean age of onset is approximately 60 years; onset in persons younger than 40 years is relatively uncommon.
- The incidence and prevalence of PD increase with age.
- The estimated incidence of PD is 4.5 to 21 cases per 100,000 population per year.
- Most studies report a prevalence of approximately 120 cases per 100,000 population.
- Some studies report that PD is less common (about 1.0:1.5) in women and in persons of African or Asian descent, but other studies report an equal prevalence.

Pathophysiology
- The specificity and sensitivity of neuropathologic diagnostic criteria are variable.
- Two major neuropathologic findings:
  - Loss of pigmented dopaminergic neurons in the substantia nigra
  - The presence of Lewy bodies (concentric, eosinophilic, cytoplasmic inclusions) within pigmented neurons of the substantia nigra and other areas
- PD affects five major pathways in the brain (motor, oculomotor, associative, limbic, and orbitofrontal circuits) that connect other brain areas with the basal ganglia.
- This explains the wide variety of symptoms seen in PD, including difficulty with movement, attention, and learning.

Risk Factors
- In most people, the disease is idiopathic and believed to be due to a combination of genetic and environmental factors.
- Less than 5% of cases are solely due to genetic factors.
- Genetic factors are important when PD onset is before the age of 50 years.
- Other risk factors have been associated with developing PD, but no causal relationship has been proven.
- Environmental risk factors for PD include
  - Use of pesticides
  - Rural living environment
  - Consumption of well water
  - Herbicide exposure
  - Proximity to industrial plants

Clinical Features
- Problems with movement
  - Tremor
  - Rigidity
  - Slow movement
  - Weakness
  - Postural difficulties
  - Clumsiness
  - Difficulty with walking
- Cognitive and emotional problems
  - Late onset of dementia
- Autonomic dysfunction

- Pain
- Sleep disorder

Natural History
- Without treatment, motor symptoms advance aggressively in the early stages of PD with a functional decline over 8 to 10 years from independent ambulation to nonambulatory status.

Diagnosis
PD is a clinical diagnosis based on the medical history and neurologic examination. No laboratory study is diagnostic of PD.

Differential diagnosis
In a patient with tremor, clinical signs and symptoms should be assessed to differentiate parkinsonian tremor from other types of tremor seen in the following conditions:
- Alzheimer disease
- Cardioembolic stroke
- Chorea in adults
- Cortical basal ganglionic degeneration
- Dementia with Lewy bodies
- Dopamine-responsive dystonia
- Essential tremor
- Hallervorden–Spatz disease
- Huntington disease
- Lacunar syndromes
- Multiple system atrophy
- Neuroacanthocytosis
- Normal pressure hydrocephalus
- Olivopontocerebellar atrophy
- Parkinson-plus syndromes
- Progressive supranuclear palsy
- Striatonigral degeneration
- Vascular dementia
- Wilson disease

History
- The most obvious symptoms are as follows:
  - Tremor
  - Rigidity
  - Slow movements
  - Difficulty with walking
  - Decrease in dexterity (20% of PD patients first experience clumsiness in one hand)
- Later developing symptoms include
  - Cognitive and behavioral problems
  - Dementia (usually occurs in advanced PD)
- Other symptoms
  - Sensory: regional pain and anosmia (decreased sense of smell)
  - Decreased swallowing (this may lead to excess saliva in the mouth and drooling)
  - Sleep disturbances
  - Emotional problems such as depression or anhedonia (inability to experience pleasure from activities usually found enjoyable)
  - Generalized weakness or malaise
  - Symptoms of autonomic dysfunction (constipation, sweating abnormalities, seborrheic dermatitis, urinary incontinence or retention, erectile dysfunction)

Examination
There are four cardinal signs of PD. Two of the first three below are required to make the clinical diagnosis. The fourth cardinal sign—postural instability—occurs late in PD (usually after 8 or more years).
- Resting tremor (can test while seated or standing with outstretched arms)
- Rigidity (increase in resistance to passive movement of a joint)
- Bradykinesia (paucity of spontaneous movements and slowed intentional movement)
- Postural instability (imbalance and loss of righting reflexes—tested by carefully assessing the reaction to an intentional postural perturbation while standing)

Testing
- Magnetic resonance imaging and computed tomography scans of the brain are unremarkable, but may be obtained to rule out other diagnoses.
- Positron emission tomography and single-photon emission computed tomography may show findings consistent with PD, but are usually not necessary in patients with a typical presentation.

Medication trial
- A trial of levodopa resulting in relief of motor symptoms can help to confirm the diagnosis.

Treatment
- There is no cure for PD.
- Medications, surgery, and multidisciplinary management can provide symptomatic relief.

Medical
- The main medications used for treatment of motor symptoms include
  - Levodopa (usually combined with a dopa decarboxylase inhibitor such as carbidopa or

benserazide, or a catechol-O-methyl transferase inhibitor like entacapone)
- Dopamine agonists (bromocriptine, pergolide, pramipexole, ropinirole, apomorphine)
- Monoamine oxidase B (MAO B) inhibitors (selegiline and rasagiline)

Surgical
- Surgical treatment for PD is increasing in popularity and includes surgical lesions and deep brain stimulation of the thalamus, the globus pallidus, or the subthalamic nucleus.

Injections
- Botulinum injections administered by specially trained physiatrists or neurologists for limb dystonia can be helpful.

Rehabilitation
- The physiatrist, through appropriate identification and management of problems associated with PD and coordination of rehabilitation team efforts, may be able to improve the patient's ability to perform activities of daily living, improve mobility, reduce pain, and avoid fractures and other injuries from falls.

Speech pathology
- Speech therapy is effective in treating the laryngeal manifestations of PD.
- A commonly utilized speech therapy technique used to treat speech problems by optimizing intelligibility in PD is the Lee Silverman voice treatment (LSVT).
- Unfortunately, a relatively small percentage (3–4%) of patients with PD are referred for speech therapy.
- In late-stage PD, the use of assistive technologies such as augmentative communication devices can aid communication.
- Assessment of dysphagia and management of swallowing problems may help to minimize the risk of aspiration.

Occupational therapy
- Evidence from randomized clinical trials on occupational therapy (OT) interventions in PD is limited. However, it is possible that OT can help with
  - Improvement and maintenance of transfers and mobility
  - Improvement of personal self-care activities of daily living
  - Environmental modifications to improve safety and maximize motor function
  - Cognitive assessment and appropriate intervention

Physical therapy
- Evidence-based reviews have found exercise, with or without formal physical therapy, to be beneficial to physical functioning, health-related quality of life, strength, balance, and gait speed for people with PD.
- The optimal content of exercise interventions (exact content, dosage, intensity, duration) at different stages of PD remains unknown.
- In one study, an exercise program supervised by a physical therapist demonstrated more improvements in motor symptoms, mental and emotional functions, daily living activities, and quality of life compared to a self-supervised home exercise program.
- Strengthening exercises may improve strength and motor function for PD patients with muscle weakness and generalized weakness and deconditioning.
- Flexibility and range of motion exercises may help reduce rigidity in PD.
- Relaxation techniques can help to decrease muscle tension.
- Physical therapists commonly use several strategies to improve functional mobility, safe ambulation, and to prevent falls, including use of assistive devices and gait training.
- Evidence to support or refute the value of exercise in reducing falls in PD patients is insufficient.

See the chapter titled Neurologic: Parkinson's Disease—Postural Instability, Freezing, and Falls.

Consults
- Neurology
- Physical medicine and rehabilitation
- Neurosurgery

Complications of treatment
- Dyskinesia, from medications

Prognosis
- PD progresses with time.
- It is difficult to predict the course of PD for a given individual.
- In people taking levodopa, the progression time of symptoms to a stage of high dependency from caregivers may be over 15 years.
- In advanced PD, disability is more related to
  - Motor symptoms that do not respond as well to medication (dysphagia, speech difficulties, and gait/balance problems)
  - Motor complications (primarily dyskinesia) from medication side effects, which appear in up to 50% of individuals after 5 years of levodopa usage.

- After 10 years, most people with PD have autonomic disturbances, sleep problems, mood alterations, and cognitive decline; these symptoms greatly increase disability.
- Mortality risk
- Life expectancy of people with PD is reduced, with mortality ratios that are two times greater than in persons without PD.
- Mortality risk factors:
  - The presence of cognitive decline
  - The presence of dementia
  - Age 70 years or above at diagnosis
  - Advanced disease state
  - Presence of swallowing problems
  - If tremor (instead of rigidity) is the main disease symptom, mortality is lower.

Helpful Hints
- The goal of medical management of PD is control of signs and symptoms for as long as possible and to minimize adverse effects.
- Medications usually provide good symptomatic control of motor signs for 4 to 6 years.
- The goal of rehabilitation is to restore and preserve function and to prevent and/or treat secondary complications.
- Quality of life deteriorates quickly, if treatment is delayed.

Suggested Readings
Davie CA. A review of Parkinson's disease. *Br Med Bull.* 2008;86:109–127.

Dereli EE, Yaliman A. Comparison of the effects of a physiotherapist-supervised exercise programme and a self-supervised exercise programme on quality of life in patients with Parkinson's disease. *Clin Rehabil.* 2010;24:352–362.

Gage H, Storey L. Rehabilitation for Parkinson's disease: A systematic review of available evidence. *Clin Rehabil.* 2004;18:463–482.

Goldenberg MM. Medical management of Parkinson's disease. *P T.* 2008;33:590–606.

Goodwin VA, Richards SH, Taylor RS, et al. The effectiveness of exercise interventions for people with Parkinson's disease: A systematic review and meta-analysis. *Mov Disord.* 2008;23:631–640.

Jankovic J. Parkinson's disease: Clinical features and diagnosis. *J Neurol Neurosurg Psychiatr.* 2008;79:368–376.

Rodriguez-Oroz MC, Jahanshahi M, Krack P, et al. Initial clinical manifestations of Parkinson's disease: Features and pathophysiological mechanisms. *Lancet Neurol.* 2009;8:1128–1139.

Neurologic: Parkinson's Disease—Postural Instability, Freezing, and Falls

Aparna Wagle Shukla MD

Description
Parkinson's disease is an incapacitating degenerative disorder that negatively affects quality of life; freezing of gait and falls constitute two of the most important contributing factors.

Freezing of Gait

Definition
- Freezing of gait is defined as a gait disorder in which parkinsonian patients are unable to initiate or continue locomotion.

Clinical presentation
- It manifests as transient arrests of ambulation, with the patient's feet appearing to be "stuck" to the ground.
- Freezing occurs usually when the patient initiates walking (start-hesitation), takes turns (turn-hesitation), passes through a doorway, or becomes distracted. Freezing episodes are generally transient, last for a few seconds to few minutes and may occur during either "on" or "off" the dopaminergic medications.

Risk factors
- Men affected greater than women
- Longer disease duration
- Increased disease severity

Treatment options

Cueing strategies
Auditory and visual stimuli helpful in the initiation of a movement in the midst of a freezing spell.
- Marching like a soldier
- Walking to music
- Walking sideways
- Walking briskly and taking long steps
- Stepping toward a target on the ground
- Stepping over a cane laid on the floor in front of the foot
- Use of a laser beam stick and modified inverted stick
- Clapping hands
- Counting out a rhythm or singing and then trying to walk in concert with the rhythm
- Performing rocking movements of the body

These cueing strategies when tested for control of freezing in various studies did not demonstrate as impressive results as anticipated. This suggests freezing of gait is a complex phenomenon with various motor control deficits at play and Parkinson's disease patients have a small capacity for compensation.

Medical and surgical therapies
Unfortunately, no definite treatment is available.
- Selegiline therapy, when followed long term, has been found to reduce freezing of gait.
- Bilateral subthalamic nucleus deep brain stimulation has shown some benefits for freezing, only when tested off medication.
- Pedunculopontine nucleus stimulation has been proposed as a promising treatment modality for postural instability and freezing of gait.

Falls in Parkinson's Disease

Risk factors
- Old age
- Longer duration of disease
- Advanced stage of disease
- Inability to rise from a chair
- Postural instability
- Levodopa-induced dyskinesia
- Mental status changes
- Vestibular dysfunction
- Depression
- Decreased proximal muscle strength
- Fear of falling

Predisposing conditions
- More likely in atypical parkinsonism such as multiple system atrophy and progressive supranuclear palsy, particularly early in the course of the illness.

Pathophysiological mechanisms
In one study, the following mechanisms were found:
- Unstable posture (29.0%)
- Freezing or festination (25.8%)
- Sudden loss of postural reflexes (toppling falls; 25.8%)
- Coexisting neurologic disorders (6.5%)
- Cardiologic disorders (6.5%)
- Symptomatic orthostatic hypotension (3.2%)

Treatment of falls
- Prevention is the best strategy.
- Underlying cause should be determined and corrected.
- Identify any relationship between falling and the timing of dopaminergic therapy and adjust treatment accordingly.

Physical aids for safety
- Knee pads, wrist guards, and helmets
- Mechanical aids such as a walker, a tripod cane, or a wheelchair
- A home visit by a trained physical or occupational therapist to evaluate areas for improvement in home safety (e.g., loose throw rugs, torn carpeting, slippery surfaces, small objects on the floor, poor lighting, unsafe stairways) is highly recommended.

Suggested Readings
Boonstra TA, van der Kooij H, Munneke M, et al. Gait disorders and balance disturbances in Parkinson's disease: Clinical update and pathophysiology. *Curr Opin Neurol.* 2008;21:461–471.

Brichetto G, Pelosin E, Marchese R, et al. Evaluation of physical therapy in parkinsonian patients with freezing of gait: A pilot study. *Clin Rehabil.* 2006;20:31–35.

Fahn S. The freezing phenomenon in parkinsonism. *Adv Neurol.* 1995;67:53–63.

Okuma Y, Yanagisawa N. The clinical spectrum of freezing of gait in Parkinson's disease. *Mov Disord.* 2008;23(Suppl. 2): S426–430.

Olanow CW, Stern MB, Sethi K. The scientific and clinical basis for the treatment of Parkinson's disease (2009). *Neurology.* 2009;72:S1–136.

Nieuwboer A. Cueing for freezing of gait in patients with Parkinson's disease: A rehabilitation perspective. *Mov Disord.* 2008;23(Suppl. 2):S475–481.

Neurologic: Spinal Cord Injury

Ralph M. Buschbacher MD ■ Lois Buschbacher MD

Description
Elderly persons can develop traumatic spinal cord injury (SCI), just as in the younger population. But, the elderly also have a greater propensity to developing SCI due to tumor and degenerative changes. They have a higher risk of SCI due to falls, which in the elderly are the more common cause of SCI as opposed to motor vehicle accidents, which predominate in the younger population.

Etiology/Types
- Traumatic: falls and motor vehicle accidents; a higher incidence of central cord syndrome
- Degenerative (cervical spinal stenosis); due to narrowing of the central canal
- Tumor
- Infectious (abscess)
- Herniated disc; usually superimposed on degenerative changes
- Vascular: abdominal aortic aneurism or perioperative ischemia causing spinal cord infarction
- Autoimmune: transverse myelitis
- Unstable spine: pathological fracture

Epidemiology
- Traumatic causes
  - Falls, 71.0%; 69% of falls occur on level ground
  - Motor vehicle accidents, 21.7%
  - Other, 6.8%
- Nontraumatic causes
  - Tumor, 28.0%
  - Vascular, 27.9%
  - Degenerative disease, 26.1%
  - Inflammation, 17.2%
- Incidence rises with age.
- Incidence and prevalence are increasing over time.
- In the younger population, males generally predominate; in the elderly, this trend is less pronounced.
- Nontraumatic causes are more common in the elderly.
- Most SCI in the elderly is in the cervical area.
- Elderly persons have a higher rate of incomplete injuries than do younger persons.
- Over 90% of elderly SCI patients have comorbid medical conditions.

Pathogenesis
- Trauma, causing a direct disruption of the cord tissue; this can lead to any of the levels and SCI syndromes seen in younger persons.
- Trauma that causes buckling of the ligamentum flavum in the cervical spine; this causes a higher incidence of central cord syndrome. The ligamentum flavum in the elderly is less elastic. During neck extension, the ligament in the elderly is more likely to "buckle" inward and compress the spinal cord. This tends to damage the central part of the cord causing a central cord syndrome.
- Lower energy injuries predominate in the elderly, which likely accounts for a higher proportion of incomplete injuries.
- Tumor
  - Direct invasion
  - Causing pathologic fractures in the spine
- Vascular; ischemic injury, often a perioperative complication
- Degenerative; gradual narrowing of the spinal canal can lead to myelomalacia. Narrowing also leads to a propensity to injury from trauma.

Risk Factors
- Male (less so than in the younger population)
- Risk of falls
  - Impaired balance and cognition
  - Medical reasons (orthostatic hypotension)
  - Environmental reasons (unsafe home environment)
- Spinal stenosis/degeneration
- Spondyloarthropathies (ankylosing spondylitis, diffuse idiopathic skeletal hyperostosis)

Clinical Features
- Complete or incomplete SCI
- Central cord syndrome
- Myelomalacia
- Vascular insult
- Pathologic fracture
- Tumor invasion
- Elderly with SCI have higher rates of complications and a slower and more incomplete progress of rehabilitation.

- Early on, there is spinal shock and areflexia.
- Sequelae of SCI
  - Orthostatic hypotension
  - Hypercalcemia
  - Spastic bladder if upper motor neurons are damaged
  - Lower motor neuron bladder if sacral micturition center, conus medullaris, and cauda equina are damaged
  - Urinary tract infection
  - Bowel dysfunction
  - Contracture
  - Spasticity
  - Heterotopic ossification (normal bone in an abnormal location)
  - Pressure ulcers
  - Neuropathic pain
  - Sexual dysfunction
  - Musculoskeletal overuse syndromes
  - Long-term increased risk of cardiovascular disease due to a sedentary lifestyle.
  - Late development of syringomyelia
  - Central cord syndrome: upper extremities more involved, bladder dysfunction, sensory loss, and sacral sparing

Natural History
- Elderly who sustain an SCI have higher rates of complications.
- Accelerated aging
- Aggravation of pre-existing medical conditions.
  - Impaired strength in muscles needed for transfers, propulsion, and self-care; leads to lower level of independence
  - Greater incidence of comorbidities, such as cardiovascular disease, emphysema, osteoporosis, cancer, and bowel/bladder issues; leads to greater rate of complications and a lower functional reserve
  - Impaired pre-existing posture, decreased range of motion, and prior musculoskeletal issues (rotator cuff tear) limit rehabilitation efforts
- Common complications/effects (early):
  - Skin breakdown
  - Hypercalcemia
  - Urinary tract infection
  - Pneumonia
  - Deep venous thrombosis/pulmonary embolism
- Common complications (intermediate):
  - Heterotopic ossification
  - Autonomic dysreflexia
  - Contractures/spasticity
  - Abnormal thermoregulation
- Common complications (late):
  - Tracheal stenosis (especially with long-term intubation)
  - Syrinx
  - Neuropathic pain
  - Musculoskeletal pain (Carpal tunnel syndrome, shoulder impingement, overuse)
  - Kidney/bladder stones
  - Osteoporosis

Diagnosis

Differential diagnosis
- Other central nervous system disorders
  - Tumor
  - Multiple sclerosis
  - Transverse myelitis
  - Infarction
- Peripheral neuropathy
- Peripheral arterial disease/claudication
- Intramedullary hematoma

History
- Trauma
- Prior degeneration
- Surgery
- Aortic aneurism
- Cancer
- Osteoporosis
- Signs of concomitant traumatic brain injury

Examination
- Complete general examination
- Complete neurological examination
- Assess comorbidities: skin, contractures, rotator cuff, neuropathies, and cardiopulmonary health

Tests
- X-ray: assess degenerative changes and stability
- Magnetic resonance imaging (MRI): assess myelomalacia, cord damage, and soft tissues
- Computerized tomography (CT): assess fractures and impingement into the central canal
- Lab tests:
  - Concomitant disease: diabetes
  - SCI complications: urinary tract infection, hypercalcemia, and alkaline phosphatase (heterotopic ossification)
- Triple-phase bone scan: heterotopic ossification

- Doppler studies/ventilation/perfusion scans for deep venous thrombosis/pulmonary embolism

Pitfalls
- Missing comorbidities
- Missing concomitant traumatic brain injury

Red flags
- Progressive neurologic decline
- Deep venous thrombosis/pulmonary embolism
- Hypercalcemia
- Cancer
- Unstable spine

Treatment

Acute
- Consideration of high dose of steroids
- Avoidance of the development of preventable complications: skin breakdown, contractures, and so on.
- Orthoses, as needed, for stability; halo vest (not used as frequently)
- Teaching self-catheterization, bowel and bladder care, transfers, pressure release, and so on.

Late
- Functional orthoses, as needed; wrist and ankle
- Wheelchair; power chair should be considered as a first-line option, even when the patient can use a manual chair. The power chair may prevent overuse and musculoskeletal complications.

Exercise
- Range of motion
- Strength
- Functional activities

Surgical
- Spinal stabilization, as needed
- Resection of mature heterotopic ossification, if it limits function
- Skin flaps for pressure ulcers
- Urinary diversion
- Tendon transfers for function

Complications
- Poor tolerance of halo vest: swallow, balance, coordination, and respiratory problems
- Osteoporosis—preinjury and postinjury may weaken surgical fixation
- More difficult to wean from ventilator than in younger persons

Consults
- Neurosurgery
- Physical medicine and rehabilitation
- Urology
- Internal medicine
- Plastic surgery
- Gastroenterology

Prognosis
- Not as good as in younger persons
  - Higher mortality and morbidity
  - Lesser functional outcomes

Helpful Hints
- Consider a power wheelchair to prevent musculoskeletal problems.
- Do not expect the same level of function as in a similar, younger person.
- Avoid narcotic medications due to gastrointestinal and respiratory side effects.
- Avoid benzodiazepines due to cognitive side effects.

Suggested Readings
Lin VW, Bono CM, Cardenas DD, et al., eds. *Spinal Cord Medicine Principles and Practice*. 2nd ed. New York, NY: Demos; 2010.

Radcliff K, Vaccaro A, Albert T, et al. Physiologic limitations and complications of spinal cord injury in the elderly population. *Top Spinal Cord Inj Rehabil*. 2010;15:85–95.

Neurologic: Stroke

Richard D. Zorowitz MD

Description
"A cerebrovascular event with rapidly developing clinical signs of focal or global disturbances of cerebral function, with signs lasting 24 hours or longer or leading to death, with no apparent cause other than of vascular origin (World Health Organization)."

Etiology/Types
- Thromboembolic: 88%.
  - Ischemic strokes occur in large vessels, while lacunar strokes occur in small vessels.
  - Embolic strokes occur as a result of atrial fibrillation, cardiac mural thrombi, paradoxical emboli through patent foramen ovale, or other remote vascular lesions.
- Intracerebral hemorrhage: 9%. These usually occur in conjunction with hypertension.
- Subarachnoid hemorrhage: 3%. These usually occur in conjunction with arteriovenous malformations or cerebral aneurysms.

Epidemiology
- Each year about 795,000 people in the United States experience a stroke. Approximately, 610,000 of these are first attacks, and 185,000 are recurrent attacks.
- Stroke is the third most common cause of death in the Western world, behind heart disease and cancer.
- Stroke is a leading cause of neurologic disability; accounts for over half of patients hospitalized for acute neurologic disease.
- 28% of strokes occur in patients under the age of 65.
- Stroke is a leading cause for admission to a nursing home or extended care facility.

Risk Factors
- Treatable
  - Hypertension
  - Diabetes mellitus
  - Coronary artery disease
  - Atrial fibrillation
  - Peripheral vascular disease
  - Hyperlipidemia
  - Smoking
  - Illicit drug and alcohol abuse
  - Obesity
- Nontreatable
  - Age (risk doubles for every 10 years above the age of 55)
  - Gender (men greater than women)
  - Race (African Americans, Mexican Americans)
  - Family history
- Other
  - Patent foramen ovale
  - Obstructive sleep apnea
  - Hormone replacement therapy

Clinical Factors
- Early symptoms
  - Change in consciousness
  - Sensory and motor impairments (e.g., weakness, ataxia)
  - Speech-language disorders (e.g., aphasia, apraxia, dysarthria), cognitive-communication impairments (e.g., memory, attention, visual-perceptual difficulties, disinhibition, impulsivity)
  - Visual disorders (e.g., field cut, hemineglect)
  - Sleep disorders
  - Dysphagia
- Late symptoms
  - Emotional problems (e.g., depression, anxiety, emotional lability, anger)
  - Spasticity
  - Fatigue
  - Seizures
  - Sexual dysfunction

Natural History
- Blood pressure may elevate early to maintain cerebral perfusion.
- Motor recovery may occur in flexor (upper limb) or extensor synergy patterns.
- Most recovery occurs over the first 6 months to 1 year. The extent of recovery varies, depending upon the location and size of the infarction.

- Research has demonstrated that further recovery can occur over the course of years. However, this depends upon the intensity of activity in which the stroke survivor participates.

Diagnosis

Differential diagnosis
- Hypoglycemia
- Cerebral mass lesions
- Seizures and postictal states
- Migraine headache

History
- Sudden paralysis or numbness, usually on one side of the face, arm, or leg
- Problems with walking or balance
- Changes in vision
- Slurred speech or drooling
- Problems with verbal expression or comprehension
- Problems with thinking, awareness, attention, learning, judgment, and memory
- Dizziness
- Swallowing problems
- Sudden, severe headache with no known cause

Examination
A detailed neurologic examination will correlate clinical findings with diagnostic testing
- National Institutes of Health (NIH) Stroke Scale:
  - Quantitative measure of stroke-related neurologic deficit.
  - Assists in determining whether the patient is a candidate for thrombolytic therapy

Testing: Immediate (Emergency Department)
- Computed tomography (CT) determines the presence of hemorrhage.
- Electrocardiogram (ECG) determines the presence of arrhythmias and atrial fibrillation.
- Blood tests
  - Complete blood count (CBC)—to evaluate for anemia or infection
    Serum electrolytes/glucose to evaluate for hyperglycemia.

Testing: Routine
Magnetic resonance imaging (MRI)—determines the amount of damage to the brain and may help predict recovery.
- Transthoracic or transesophageal echocardiography—to evaluate the anatomy of the heart and aorta
- Carotid ultrasound/Doppler—to screen the patency of the carotid arteries
- Transcranial Doppler (TCD)—to evaluate the intracerebral vasculature
- Magnetic resonance angiogram (MRA), CT angiogram, or cerebral angiogram—to evaluate the integrity of the vasculature
- Blood tests
  - Hemoglobin A1C—to check for diabetes mellitus
  - Liver/kidney function—to check for the etiology of hypertension or hemorrhage
  - Cholesterol/lipids—to check for dyslipidemia
  - Homocysteine—to check for hypercoagulable state
  - Coagulation studies—to check for hypercoagulable state
  - Anticardiolipin/antiphospholipid antibodies—to check for hypercoagulable state

Pitfalls
- Failure to recognize stroke may prevent the patient from receiving thrombolytic therapy.
- Failure to adequately assess swallowing function may result in aspiration pneumonia.

Red flags
- A decline in function, mental status, or seizure may be a sign of recurrent stroke or major depression.
- Atypical recovery of the upper limb may be a sign of brachial plexus injury (may occur if traction is placed upon a flaccid arm).

Treatment

Medical
- Tissue plasminogen activator (t-PA) within 3 hours if criteria are met
- Aspirin or aspirin/extended-release dipyridamole, except within 24 hours of t-PA for noncardioembolic ischemic stroke
- Anticoagulation for cardioembolic ischemic stroke
- Antihypertensives may be held for 7 to 10 days after ischemic stroke, unless systolic pressure is over 220 mmHg or diastolic pressure is more than 120 mmHg. In hemorrhagic stroke, blood pressure usually is treated.
- Antihyperlipidemic agent (statin) for management of lipids
- Stool softener and laxatives to prevent fecal impaction and hypertension from straining

Surgical
- Carotid endarterectomy

- Hematoma evacuation
- Craniectomy for impending herniation
- Aneurysm clipping
- Endovascular coil embolization
- Patent foramen ovale closure

Rehabilitation
- Patients who are stabilized after acute stroke may benefit from a variety of rehabilitation settings, usually involving a comprehensive team approach.

Consults
- Neurology
- Neurosurgery
- Physical medicine and rehabilitation
- Cardiology
- Nephrology
- Physical therapy
- Occupational therapy
- Speech-language pathology

Complications
- Shoulder pain
  - Traction/compression neuropathy
  - Complex regional pain syndrome (CRPS)
  - Shoulder trauma
  - Bursitis/tendonitis
  - Adhesive capsulitis
  - Rotator cuff tear
  - Shoulder subluxation
- Pneumonia
- Urinary tract infection
- Depression
- Spasticity/contracture

Prognosis
- Stroke recurs in approximately 14% of patients in the first year and in 5% annually thereafter.
- Risk factors for recurrence include: older age; evidence of coronary artery disease, peripheral artery disease, ischemic stroke, or transient ischemic attack (TIA); hemorrhagic or embolic stroke; diabetes; alcoholism; valvular heart disease; and atrial fibrillation.

Helpful Hints
- Encourage changes in lifestyle. A balanced diet, smoking cessation, moderation in alcohol, weight control, and exercise may help to decrease the risk of recurrent stroke, along with the treatment of medical risk factors.
- As stroke can be a lifetime disability, encourage lifetime follow-up. Annual physiatric visits may help to identify and prevent secondary complications.

Suggested Readings
Caplan LR. *Caplan's Stroke: A Clinical Approach*. 4th ed. Philadelphia, PA: Saunders/Elsevier; 2009.

Department of Veterans Affairs, Department of Defense, The American Heart Association/American Stroke Association. VA/DoD clinical practice guideline for the management of stroke rehabilitation. http://www.healthquality.va.gov/Management_of_Stroke_Rehabilitation.asp. Accessed February 13, 2011.

Furie KL, Kasner SE, Adams RJ, et al. Guidelines for the prevention of stroke in patients with stroke or transient ischemic attack. A guideline for healthcare professionals from the American Heart Association/American Stroke Association. *Stroke*. 2011;42:227–276.

Miller EL, Murray L, Richards L, et al. Comprehensive overview of nursing and interdisciplinary rehabilitation care of the stroke patient. A scientific statement from the American Heart Association. *Stroke*. 2010;41:2402–2448.

Stein J, Harvey RL, Macko RF, et al., eds. *Stroke Recovery and Rehabilitation*. New York, NY: Demos Medical Publishing; 2009.

Neurologic: Traumatic Brain Injury

Rani Lynn Haley MD

Description
Traumatic brain injury (TBI) is an acquired brain injury caused by an external force, resulting in the alteration of brain function with subsequent cognitive, behavioral, and/or functional impairments.

Etiology/Types
- TBI is classified based on the patient's initial presenting Glasgow Coma Scale (GCS) Score
  - Mild (13–15)
  - Moderate (9–12)
  - Severe (3–8)
- Types
  - Diffuse axonal injury
  - Focal
    - Penetrating
    - Coup-contrecoup
    - Depressed skull fracture
- Secondary
  - Edema/mass effect
  - Subdural hematoma (SDH)
  - Subarachnoid hemorrhage
  - Intracerebral hematoma
  - Epidural hematoma (usually seen with temporal bone skull fracture)
- Causes
  - Falls: most common in the elderly
  - Motor vehicle accidents

Epidemiology
- The annual estimated incidence of TBI for persons 65 years and above is 121 per 100,000.
- Falls, commonly from standing level, are the leading cause of TBI in the elderly.
- TBI sustained in motor vehicle collisions (MVC) are the second most common cause in the elderly. These MVCs are typically low-speed collisions.
- SDH is the most common pathology and is seen in approximately 55% of TBI cases in persons 65 years and above.

Pathogenesis
- Similar to younger individuals suffering TBI, the primary injury is the result of cerebral contusion and shear forces at impact.
- Secondary injury results from hemorrhage, cerebral edema, hypoxia, hydrocephalus, and neuronal death.
- Older persons have a decreased ability to autoregulate cerebral blood flow as compared to their younger cohorts and are at an increased risk for secondary injury from TBI.
- Aging-associated cerebral atrophy with stretching of the bridging veins leads to the predisposition for SDH in the elderly.

Risk Factors
- Factors contributing to fall risk, including but not limited to: neurologic disorders, hypotension, medications, and/or environmental factors
- Age-related decrease in reaction time
- Anticoagulation/coagulopathy

Clinical Features
- Acutely
  - Altered or loss of consciousness
  - Confusion
  - Memory impairment
  - Agitation
- Postacute symptoms
  - Headache
  - Fatigue
  - Decreased/poor attention span
  - Mood lability
  - Memory impairment
- Older patients may gradually develop an SDH after a fall or relatively minor trauma and may present with progressive functional and cognitive impairments days to months after the inciting event.

Natural History
- TBI outcomes are, in general, contingent on the severity of injury, post-traumatic amnesia (PTA), and loss of consciousness (LOC).
- However, in older adults, outcomes after TBI are dependent more on GCS and type of intracranial pathology than on length of coma and post-traumatic amnesia.
- Older individuals with TBI often require more time for recovery, both cognitively and physically, than younger individuals with TBI.

Diagnosis
Differential diagnosis
- Medication side effects
- Premorbid medical conditions affecting cognition
- Intensive care unit (ICU) psychosis
- Delirium
- Dementia

History
- History of fall or MVC
- Loss of consciousness
- Changes in behavior or cognition
- In the older adult, it is especially important to obtain a history concerning premorbid medical conditions, medications, cognition/function, and living environment to help with
  - Acute medical management
  - Discharge planning
  - Prevention of falls in the future

Examination
- Acutely: Emergency evaluation, including evaluation of airway, breathing, and circulation. Neurologic examination, including GCS
- Postacute: Thorough neurologic examination, including but not limited to: minimental status examination, GCS, Galveston orientation and amnesia test, and Ranchos Los Amigos Scale

Testing
- Brain/head imaging:
  - Acute computerized tomography (CT) scan for rapid diagnosis and evaluation for surgical emergencies.
  - Postacute magnetic resonance imaging (MRI) to investigate/follow sequelae of TBI
- GCS for classification of severity
- Neuropsychologic testing, postacutely

Pitfalls
- Failure to recognize delayed onset of SDH, resulting in medical and/or functional decline
- Failure to take into account the individual's premorbid cognitive and functional history, resulting in unrealistic rehabilitation goals

Red flags
- Decline in functional and/or clinical progress may indicate delayed hemorrhage (SDH), hydrocephalus, or seizures.

Treatment
Medical
- Acutely, ICU monitoring for moderate to severe injuries
- Neurostimulants to improve arousal and attention
- Judicious use of antipsychotics and antiepileptics to treat agitation and emotional lability.
- Management of comorbid medical conditions

Surgical
- Monitoring intracranial pressure
- Evacuation of hematomas causing intracranial mass effect
- Cranioplasty

Consults
- Neurosurgery for acute management
- Physical medicine and rehabilitation to assess and aid in rehabilitation needs
- Geriatrics to help with medical management
- Social worker to help with discharge options
- Neurology
- Physical therapy
- Occupation therapy
- Speech-language therapy
- Nutritionist
- Neuropsychology

Complications
- Medication side effects
- Aspiration pneumonia
- Infection of surgical site
- Exacerbation of comorbid medical condition
- Anemia

Prognosis
- Older age is a well-known predictor of worse outcome after TBI.

- Older individuals with mild brain injury are more likely to experience cognitive decline after initial injury than younger individuals, due to a number issues including, but not limited to, decreased neural plasticity, decreased cortical volume, and increased perceived/actual health problems.

Helpful Hints

- Suspect TBI in an older individual with a history of a fall or accident, even in those with a minor or remote injury.
- Premorbid cognitive and functional impairments should be considered in acute treatment and rehabilitation in the older individual with TBI.

Suggested Readings

Cifu DX, Kreutzer JS, Marwitz JH, et al. Functional outcomes in older individuals with traumatic brain injury: A prospective, multicenter analysis. *Arch Phys Med* Rehab. 1996;77:883–888.

Marquez de la Plata CD, Hart T, Hammond FM, et al. Impact of age on long term recovery from traumatic brain injury. *Arch Phys Med Rehab.* 2008;89(5):896–903.

Rakier A, et al. Head injuries in the elderly. *Brain Inj.* 1995;9(2):187–193.

Sirven JI, Malamut BL. *Clinical Neurology of the Older Adult.* Philadelphia, PA: Lippencott, Williams, and Wikins; 2008.

Timmons T, Menaker J. Traumatic brain injury in the elderly. *Clin Geriatr.* 2010;18(4):20–24.

Zasler ND, Katz DI, Zafonte RD, eds. *Brain Injury Medicine: Principles and Practice.* New York, NY: Demos; 2007.

Rheumatologic: Fibromyalgia

Brad P. Wilson DO

Description
The American College of Rheumatology defines fibromyalgia as follows:
- Widespread myalgias in the left and right side of the body, above and below the waist
- Pain in 11 of 18 tender points, with bilateral involvement
- Symptoms must be present for at least 3 months

Etiology
- Unknown

Epidemiology
- The most common cause of generalized, musculoskeletal pain in women between the ages of 20 and 55 years
- Prevalence of this disorder in the community increases with age from 2% at age 20 to 8% at age 70.
- Female to male ratio is about 10:1.

Pathophysiology
- Central sensitization (increased excitatory pain pathways and decreased inhibitory pain pathways)
- Elevated levels of substance phosphorous (P) in the cerebrospinal fluid
- Various stressors induce a heightened sense of pain and hypersensitivity to numerous stimuli
- Upregulation of opiod receptors in the periphery and reduced in the brain

Risk Factors
- May occur concurrently with any rheumatic disorder, including rheumatoid arthritis, osteoarthritis, and systemic lupus erythematosus
- Female gender
- Genetic predisposition
- Post-traumatic stress disorder
- Pain is exacerbated by overexertion, physical inactivity, sleep disturbance, and emotional stress.

Clinical Features
- Widespread chronic pain, for over a 3-month duration, involving the upper and lower body, and present on both sides of the body
- Associated symptoms include fatigue, insomnia, headache, cognitive difficulty, depression, and anxiety
- Sleep disorder
- Diffuse soft-tissue tenderness

Natural History
- Chronic course is the norm.
- Some persons improve with treatment, but the results are variable.

Diagnosis

Differential diagnosis
- Myofascial pain syndrome: myalgias in one focal region (not widespread)
- Chronic fatigue syndrome
- Obstructive sleep apnea (OSA)
- Lyme disease
- Rheumatoid arthritis
- Systemic lupus erythematosus
- Sjogren's syndrome
- Inflammatory myositis
- Metabolic myopathies
- Hypothyroidism
- Migraine headaches
- Psychiatric disorders
- Peripheral neuropathies
- Multiple sclerosis
- Myasthenia gravis
- Hypercalcemia
- Epstein-Barr virus

History
- Chronic generalized pain and tenderness
- Fatigue and poor sleep
- Problems with memory and concentration
- Positive family history

Examination
- In all 11 of 18 tender points should be positive for a diagnosis of fibromyalgia.
- A point should be considered a "tender point" if it causes pain, not just mild tenderness.

Testing
- Laboratory tests: complete blood count (CBC), erythrocyte sedimentation rate, thyroid stimulating hormone (TSH), vitamin D, calcium, and muscle enzymes (aldolase, creatine kinase, transaminases, lactate dehydrogenase)
- Neuropsychologic testing for cognitive/depressive symptoms
- Polysomnography for OSA
- Biopsy generally not needed (except to evaluate for other disease), but if done, there are normal histologic findings.

Pitfalls
- Incorrect diagnosis
- Missing a more treatable condition

Red flags
- Progressive weakness, indicative of other diagnosis
- Opioid abuse

Treatment

Medical
- Strongest evidence supports
  - Patient education
  - Cognitive behavioral therapy
  - Pharmacotherapy
  - Aerobic exercise
- Food and Drug Administration (FDA)–approved medications:
  - Duloxetine (Cymbalta)
  - Milnacipran (Savella)
  - Pregabalin (Lyrica)
- Examples of a few commonly prescribed (non-FDA approved) medications include: gabapentin, tricyclic antidepressants, selective serotonin reuptake inhibitors, and muscle relaxants.
- Monotherapy with nonsteroidal anti-inflammatories, steroids, and opioids offers little to no benefit in fibromyalgia.

Exercise
- Low-impact aerobic exercise: water aerobics, pool therapy, walking, and bicycling
- Strength training (careful not to overexert)

Other
- Sleep restoration:
  - *Continuous positive airway pressure* (CPAP) machine for OSA
  - Sleep aid medications for insomnia
- Hypnotherapy
- Biofeedback
- Therapeutic ultrasound, modalities
- Avoidance of overreliance on injections
- Multidisciplinary approach: Physical medicine and rehabilitation, physical therapy, and mental health. This is especially helpful in patients who are resistant to medications.

Consults
- Rheumatology
- Physical medicine and rehabilitation
- Psychiatry/psychology

Complications/side effects
- Chronic pain
- Disability mindset

Prognosis
- Most will have lifelong chronic pain and fatigue, however, two thirds are able to work full time.
- Patients treated by their primary care physician in the community have a better prognosis.
- Psychological and behavioral factors associated with better outcomes include
  - An increased sense of control over pain
  - Belief that one is not disabled and that pain is not a sign of damage
  - Seeking help from others
  - Exercising more

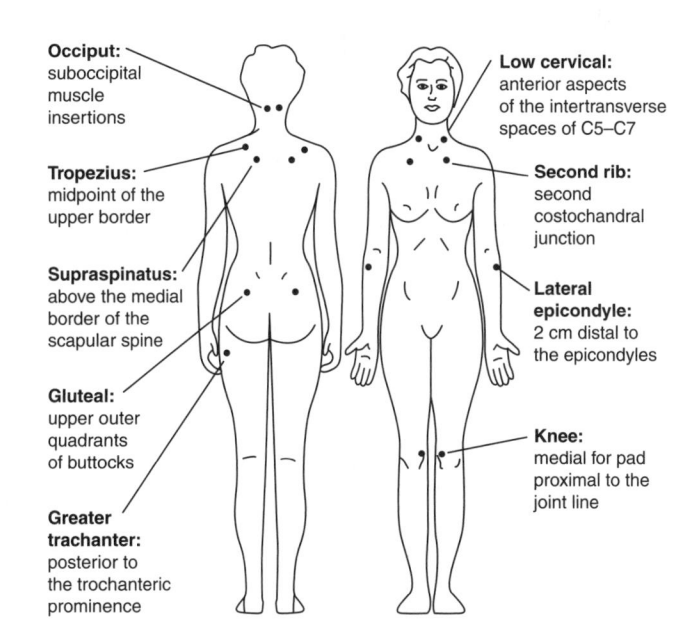

Figure 1 Fibromyalgia tender points

Helpful Hints
- Multidisciplinary approach is best.
- Avoidance of passive treatments is helpful.
- Proper sleep is important.
- Because of the long-term implications and danger of developing a chronic pain mindset, overdiagnosis should be avoided.

Suggested Readings

Busch AJ, Schachter CL, Overend TJ, et al. Exercise for fibromyalgia: A systematic review. *J Rheumatol*. 2008;35:1130.

Goldenberg DL. Fibromyalgia syndrome. An emerging but controversial condition. *JAMA*. 1987;257:2782.

Häuser W, Eich W, Herrmann M, et al. Fibromyalgia syndrome: classification, diagnosis, and treatment. *Dtsch Arztebl Int*. 2009;106(23):383–391.

Mease P, Arnold LM, Bennett R, et al. Fibromyalgia syndrome. *J Rheumatol*. 2007;34:1415.

Wolfe F, Smythe HA, Yunus MB, et al. The American College of Rheumatology 1990 criteria for the classification of fibromyalgia: Report of the Multicenter Criteria Committee. *Arthritis Rheum*. 1990;33:160.

Rheumatologic: Giant Cell Arteritis

Joseph G. Chacko MD

Description
Giant cell arteritis (GCA; aka cranial or temporal arteritis) is chronic vasculitis of large- and medium-sized blood vessels. The cranial branches of the arteries from the aortic arch are most prominently affected.

Etiology/Types
- Specific etiology is unknown.
- Certain genetic and ethnic (e.g., Northern European) factors may be associated with GCA.
- An infectious etiology, or trigger, has been proposed as well.

Epidemiology
- Rarely, if ever, occurs prior to 50 years of age; mean age of onset 72.
- Above 50 years of age, prevalence is 1:500 individuals.

Pathogenesis
- Patchy, inflammatory, vasculitic lesions are noted in the involved arteries.

Risk Factors
- Age
- Male gender
- Tobacco abuse
- Prior atheromatous disease
- Northern European descent
- Polymyalgia rheumatica (PMR); GCA is found in 15% of PMR patients, and PMR is diagnosed in 40% to 50% of GCA patients.

Clinical Features
- Classic symptoms include
  - Temporal region headaches
  - Jaw claudication (i.e., jaw muscle pain with chewing)
  - Systemic symptoms: fever, fatigue, and weight loss
  - Visual symptoms; transient or permanent monocular visual loss due to ischemic optic neuropathy (or infrequently, central retinal artery occlusion). The other eye is usually affected within days to months.
  - Polymyalgia rheumatica symptoms including aching and morning stiffness of the shoulder and hip regions.

Natural History
- Blindness is possible.
- Rare occurrence of seizure or stroke

Diagnosis

Differential diagnosis
- Large vessel vasculitides (e.g., Takayasu arteritis)
- Medium/small vessel vasculitides (e.g., Wegener's granulomatosis, polyarteritis nodosa)
- Primary angiitis of the central nervous system
- Amyloidosis

History
- See Clinical Features section.

Examination
- General: chronic illness appearance
- Vision examination: Test visual acuity in each eye with glasses on. Look for severe vision loss (20/200 or worse).
- Perform confrontational visual fields, one eye at a time. Look for altitudinal visual field defect (loss of upper two quadrants or lower two quadrants in one eye), which is consistent with ischemic optic neuropathy.
- Pulses/bruits: Assess temporal (e.g., tender or thickened), carotid, brachial, radial, femoral, and pedal pulses; depressed pulses can be seen; temporal arteries may be prominent.
- Musculoskeletal (if PMR is present); assess for tenderness and range of motion of the shoulder and hips.
  - Synovitis of the wrists and knees may be noted.

Testing
- Erythrocyte sedimentation rate (ESR); less than 50 to 100 mm/h
- C-reactive protein (CRP); often parallels ESR: an elevated ESR and CRP is 97% specific for the diagnosis of GCA.

- Complete blood count (CBC); normochromic anemia frequent
- Albumin; decreased, but increases with treatment
- Liver enzymes; moderately increased but normalize with treatment
- Temporal artery biopsy if there is an elevated ESR and/or CRP and a consistent clinical history.

American College of Rheumatology criteria
- Age greater than 50 years at disease onset
- Localized, new onset, headache
- Tenderness or decreased pulse of the temporal artery
- ESR greater than 50 mm/h
- Biopsy revealing a necrotizing arteritis with a predominance of mononuclear cells or a granulomatous process with multinucleated giant cells.

Treatment
- Glucocorticoids
  - Intravenous high-dose methylprednisolone (1,000 mg/day × 3 days), if ESR/CRP is elevated in a patient with classic symptoms and impending visual loss; this may prevent blindness.
  - Oral (40–60 mg prednisone daily); duration 2 to 4 weeks then taper.
- Antiplatelet (e.g., aspirin 81 mg) to reduce the risk of visual loss or stroke.

Complications of treatment
- Long-term steroid use complications

Prognosis
- Overall survival for GCA patients is similar to the general population.
- A substantial minority of patients may require chronic low-dose steroids to control symptoms.
- Permanent partial or complete visual loss occurs in 15% to 20% of GCA patients.

Helpful Hints
- An ophthalmologist should be contacted immediately if there is a concern about GCA. Time is of the essence.
- This is a disease of older patients and is rare in individuals under 50 years of age.

Suggested Readings
Glaser JS. *Neuro-ophthalmology.* 3rd ed. Lippincott Williams & Wilkins; 1999:162–166.

Hayreh SS, Podhajsky PA, Raman R, et al. Giant cell arteritis: Validity and reliability of various diagnostic criteria. *Am J Ophthalmol.* 1997;123:285.

Hayreh SS, Podhajsky PA, Zimmerman B. Occult giant cell arteritis: Ocular manifestations. *Am J Ophthalmol.* 1998;125:521.

Rheumatologic: Polymyalgia Rheumatica

Robert A. Ortmann MD

Description
Polymyalgia rheumatica (PMR) is diagnosed in patients who present with pain and stiffness of the neck, shoulder girdle, and pelvic girdle of at least 4 weeks duration. It is an inflammatory disorder that causes muscle pain and stiffness, primarily in the neck, shoulders, upper arms, hips, and thighs. It can be diagnosed after 4 weeks of symptoms and other causes of muscle pain (see the section on Differential Diagnosis below) are excluded.

Etiology/Types
- Considered a form of giant cell arteritis (GCA) that lacks a fully developed vasculitis

Epidemiology
- Occurs almost exclusively in patients above the age of 50; the incidence increases with age
- Frequency is highest in patients of Northern European descent.
- Incidence rates of 40 to 70 cases per 100,000 persons aged 50 or above
- Women more likely to be affected than men.

Pathogenesis
- No causative agent has yet been identified.
- Appears to be associated with global activation of the innate immune system
- Circulating monocytes produce interleukin (IL)-1 and IL-6
- Activated dendritic cells render arteries susceptible to inflammatory insult
- Interferon-gamma is absent in PMR, but abundant in GCA.

Risk Factors
- Age is the major risk factor for PMR.
- Human leukocyte antigen (HLA)-DR4 haplotype is associated with increased risk.
- Scandinavian ethnicity
- Female gender

Clinical Features
- Patients will complain of aching and pain in the muscles of the neck, shoulders, lower back, hips, thighs, and occasionally the trunk.
- Pain is usually abrupt in onset and symmetrical; the shoulders are frequently affected first.
- Weight loss, anorexia, malaise, and depression are often manifested upon presentation to the physician.
- Inflammation of periarticular structures, including bursae, is seen in a subset of patients.
- Small joint edema and inflammation, particularly in the hands, may be indistinguishable from seronegative polyarthritis.
- True joint effusions are rare, but may be seen in the knees.
- Classically, the condition will respond dramatically to low-dose steroid (15–20 mg prednisone daily) within days to weeks.
- As there is no definitive method of diagnosis, it is imperative to rule out other processes that may have a component of proximal muscle myalgia (see below).

Natural History
- Untreated, as much as 20% of patients may develop giant cell arteritis.
- Up to a third of patients may experience relapses; this frequency is increased if steroids are tapered too rapidly.

Diagnosis

Differential diagnosis
- Giant cell arteritis must be considered in patients with jaw claudication, visual complaints, and headaches.
- Inflammatory myopathy
- Hypothyroidism or hyperthyroidism
- Hyperparathyroidism
- Occult malignancy
- Subacute or chronic infection
- Fibromyalgia

Examination
- There are no specific physical findings; the muscles of the shoulders and hips may be tender to palpation.
- Pain may limit movement, but there is no true muscle weakness.
- Overt small joint synovitis is rare, but diffuse swelling of the hands may be present.
- Signs of vascular insufficiency, including extremity claudication, bruits over arteries, and discrepant blood pressure readings suggest the diagnosis of GCA.

Testing
- Although there are no specific laboratory or radiologic findings, an elevated erythrocyte sedimentation rate (ESR; often greater than 50 mm/hr) is considered to be characteristic. Although marked elevation of the ESR (greater than 100 mm/hr) is frequently seen, a small group of patients (10–15%) may have a normal or only slightly elevated ESR.

Treatment
- Dramatic response to low-dose steroids (prednisone of 15–20 mg/day) is seen in over two thirds of patients.
- Some patients may require as much as 40 mg/day for complete control; these patients are at higher risk for developing full-blown GCA.
- Once the patient reaches resolution of symptoms and the inflammatory parameters normalize, the dose can be decreased by 2.5 mg every 10 to 14 days.
- It is recommended that once the dose has been reduced to 7.5 mg/day the patients remain on this dose for a year, as there is a higher risk of recurrence in patients who are tapered off of steroids sooner.

Complications
- Long-term treatment of these patients with glucocorticoids may lead to osteoporosis, diabetes, and hyperlipidemia; a dual-energy X-ray absorptiometry (DEXA) scan should be performed upon initiation of therapy and annually thereafter; glucose and lipid levels should also be monitored periodically and treated as results dictate.

Prognosis
- Outcomes are generally good, with a majority of patients maintaining symptom-free remission after a year of treatment with glucocorticoids.
- A small subset will develop clinical features of seronegative polyarthritis and will require treatment with disease-modifying antirheumatic drug (DMARD) therapy such as methotrexate.
- The possibility of disease recurrence upon cessation of glucocorticoid treatment should be considered and patients are also warned about the potential progression of the disease into full-blown GCA.

Helpful Hints
- If a patient does not have significant clinical response in a week, consider other etiologies (i.e., giant cell arteritis).
- Be sure to offer concomitant bone preservation treatment (vitamin D, calcium) during the course of steroid treatment.
- Monitor for potential steroid-induced toxicities (hypertension, diabetes exacerbation) in at-risk patients.

Suggested Readings
Gonzalez-Gay MA, Agudo M, Martinez-Dubois C, et al. Medical management of polymyalgia rheumatic. *Expert Opin Pharmacother.* 2010;11(7):1077–1087.

Hernandez-Rodriguez J, Cid MC, Lopez-Soto A, et al. Treatment of polymyalgia rheumatica: A systematic review. *Arch Intern Med.* 2009;169(20):1839–1850.

Nothnagl T, Leeb BF. Diagnosis, differential diagnosis and treatment of polymyalgia rheumatica. *Drugs Aging.* 2006;23(5):391–402.

Spiera R, Spiera H. Inflammatory diseases in older adults: Polymyalgia rheumatica. *Geriatrics.* 2004;59(11):39–43.

Skin: Pressure Sores

Jennifer May M. Villacorta MD

Description
Pressure (decubitus) ulcers are localized areas of tissue ischemia and ulcer formation resulting from prolonged pressure and damage to skin by shear forces.

Etiology/Types
- Prolonged pressure
- Shear forces
- Skin wetness/maceration

Epidemiology
- Affects 10% to 25% of hospitalized, ill-elderly patient
- Incidence/prevalence:
  - 7.7% of hospitalized patients develop pressure sores within 21 days of admission.
  - Rates as high as 24% are seen in orthopedic and geriatric patients.
  - The rehabilitation population overall has a prevalence of pressure sores of 25% at admission from acute care settings.
  - The geriatric population has an overall prevalence of pressure sores of 17.4%; with an 83.4% prevalence among elderly patients admitted from acute care.

Risk Factors
- Cognitive deficits
- Insensate skin
- Paralysis
- Spasticity
- Older age
- Prior skin breakdown

Clinical Features

Ulcer stages

Stage 1
- Intact skin with nonblanchable erythema (redness that lasts longer than 50% of time since pressure was applied)
- Reversible

Stage 2
- Partial—loss of thickness of skin; involves epidermis and dermis
- May present as an abrasion, blister, or shallow crater
- Still reversible

Stage 3
- Full—loss of thickness of skin; involves epidermis, dermis, and subcutaneous tissue
- Presents as a deep crater with or without undermining of adjacent tissue

Stage 4
- Full—loss of thickness of skin with tissue necrosis or damage to muscle, bone, or supporting structures (e.g., tendon, joint capsule, etc.)
- Undermining sinus tract may be present.

Diagnosis

General assessment
- Sensory deficits, cognitive impairment, and hygiene
- Level of mobility and activity level of the patient
- Nutritional assessment
- Level of continence
- Presence of diabetes or vascular disease
- Assessment of smoking

Wound assessment
- Classification of the site, shape, and depth of the wound, including any undermining sinus tract (tracing graph, photograph, volume measure)
- Classification of the stage of the ulcer
- Description of the general appearance of the wound: open versus closed, color, drainage, and covering
- Assessment of the presence of infection: wound culture or culture of biopsy, if indicated

Treatment

Prevention: understanding etiologic factors
- Duration and intensity of pressure
  - Maintain skin pressure support of less than 32 mmHg to allow good capillary inflow pressure.
  - Reactive hyperemia (bright red flush to area) characterizes appropriate pressure relief.
- Shear
  - Occurs when there is movement of underlying tissue, while the skin is adherent or stationary

- Common causes: poor sitting position, poor bed positioning, spasticity, and sliding transfers versus lifting transfers
- "Shear ulcer" is a wide undermining around the base of a visible ulcer resulting from skin ischemia.
- Secondary factors
  - Immobility
  - Malnutrition
  - Old age
  - Incontinence/moisture
  - Diabetes
  - Smoking
  - Elevated body temperature
  - Impaired mental status

Primary prevention
- Focus on relief from prolonged static positional pressure
- Common areas of involvement include areas of bony prominences: ischial tuberosity, sacrum, greater trochanter, heels, ankles, elbows, scapula, and occiput
- Whenever necessary, lift instead of sliding patients during transfers
- Reposition patients every 2 hours
- Frequently inspect and assess skin with each turning
- Utilize appropriate support surfaces (mattresses with built-in relief systems, or cushions that allow appropriate pressure mapping for chronic wheelchair users)

Wound management
- Reduction/elimination of causative factors
- Systemic support for wound healing
- Proper tissue perfusion and oxygenation
- Nutritional and fluid support
  - Nutritional assessment with baseline serum albumin (half-life 15–19 days) and prealbumin levels (half-life 1.9 days)
  - Indicators of poor nutrition: abnormal levels of total protein, cholesterol, triglyceride, creatinine, blood urea nitrogen (BUN), total lymphocyte count, and beta-carotene levels
  - Supplemental vitamins and trace elements: zinc for protein synthesis and repair and vitamin C for collagen synthesis
  - Control of compounding systemic conditions: diabetes, hematopoietic abnormalities, immunosuppression, and renal failure

Wound care
- Good skin care and hygiene
  - Cleanse skin with normal saline or pH neutral cleanser
  - Keep skin dry
  - Apply skin emollients and lubricants to help eliminate friction and mechanical forces
  - Maintain clean, dry linen and clothing
- Debridement
  - Autolytic debridement: autodigestion of eschar by wound fluid enzymatic action
  - Not as effective in patients with impaired immune function
  - May involve application of dressings that promote moisture retention: transparent film, hydrocolloid, hydrogel, and moist gauze
- Mechanical debridement: removal of necrotic tissue by physical forces
  - Modalities: Whirlpool
  - Wet-to-dry dressing
  - Wound irrigation: pulse lavage
- Chemical debridement: topical application of enzymes that dissolve dead tissues
  - Concurrent use of Polysporin powder decreases risk for infection as necrotic tissue separates from wound.
- Surgical debridement: removal of nonvital tissue by instruments such as scalpels or surgical scissors.
  - Sharp debridement is most effective for removing thick eschars and heavy coagulum.
  - Large wounds may require extensive debridement in the operative setting.
  - Grade IV lesions may require bone biopsy to rule out the presence of osteomyelitis.
  - Sharp debridement may cause pain. Treat appropriately.

Wound dressing

Goals
- Maintain moist wound bed
- Maintain dry surrounding skin margins without evidence of maceration
- Control drainage
- Eliminate dead spaces to avoid abscess formation
- Frequency: 1 to 3x/day, aseptic technique
- Dressing types and characteristics
  - Hydrogel—transparent and nonadhering
  - Hydrocolloid (*DuoDERM*)
- With hydrophilic (absorbent) particulate and hydrophobic adhesive matrix covered by an outer film or foam layer
- Adherent dressing that allows absorption of excess exudates, while maintaining a moist wound environment
- Polymeric

- Nonadherent, absorbent, semipermeable that allows evaporation of exudates
- Appropriate for wounds with macerated wound margin or hypergranulating wound beds
- Transparent adhesive (*Tegaderm*)
  - Semipermeable membrane allows water vapor to escape and oxygen to diffuse into wound bed
- Absorptive dressing
  - Fills wound, absorbs excessive exudates, and maintains moist wound environment
  - Includes wound gels, copolymer starch/beads, alginates, and gauze
- Enzymatic debriding agents (*Santyl*)

Surgery indications
- Noninfected, nonhealing Grade III or IV ulcers
- Medically stable and well-nourished patient willing to participate in a surgical wound care program preoperatively and postoperatively (smoking cessation, meticulous wound care, sitting protocol)
- Good control of bowel/bladder incontinence

Other new treatment options

Electrotherapy
- Hypothesized to
  - Improve transcutaneous partial pressure of oxygen
  - Have bactericidal properties
  - Increase protein and adenosine phosphate synthesis
  - Increase calcium uptake

Ultrasound
- Reportedly heralds early healing by facilitating the inflammatory phase and enhancing chemotaxis and the cellular secretion/release of growth factors

Ultraviolet light
- Consider a short-term application of ultraviolet light C (UVC) if traditional therapies fail

Hyperbaric oxygen
- Has been used but evidence of effectiveness is insufficient

Growth factors
- Platelet-derived growth factors (PDGF) are chemotactic to fibroblasts, mononuclear cells, and smooth muscle cells that direct cell and tissue repair.
- Sources: autologous from patient's platelet-rich plasma or recombinant DNA
- Precipitates inflammatory response and matrix synthesis

Suggested Readings
Ramundo J, Gray M. Enzymatic wound debridement. *J Wound Ostomy Continence Nurs*. 2008;35(3):273–280.

Smith R. Enzymatic debriding agents: An evaluation of the medical literature. *Ostomy Wound Manage*. 2008;54:16–34.

Braddom RL. *Physical Medicine and Rehabilitation*. 3rd ed. Philadelphia, PA: W B Saunders Co; 2006.

Brammer CM, Spires MC. *Manual of Physical Medicine and Rehabilitation*. Philadelphia, PA: Hanley & Belfus Inc; 2002.

Skin: The Problem Wound

Joseph Canvin MD

Description
- As there is no specific time frame for wound healing, a problem wound may be defined as any wound that does not continue to heal as expected.

Etiology/Types
- Most common chronic wounds include
  - Pressure ulcers
  - Vascular ulcers (i.e., arterial and venous)
  - Neuropathic

Epidemiology
- In all 70% of pressure ulcers occur in the geriatric population.
- Chronic nonhealing wounds most frequently affect the lower extremities.
- The prevalence of chronic nonhealing wounds is 0.18% to 1.3% of the adult population.

Pathogenesis
Wounds should normally heal in the following sequential process:
- Hemostasis
- Inflammation
- Epithelialization
- Fibroplasia
- Maturation

When this process is disrupted, a problem wound may develop.

Common etiologies for delayed healing include
- Peripheral arterial disease
  - The rate-limiting step in wound healing is the oxygen supplied by the arterial system.
- Venous insufficiency
- Pressure; unrelieved
- Insensate skin
- Diabetes
- Renal insufficiency
- Nutritional deficiency
- Aging
- Sickle cell disease
- Chemotherapy
- Radiation therapy
- Chronic corticosteroids
- Wound toxins (e.g., peroxide, iodine)

Risk Factors
- History of poor wound healing
- Diabetes
- Peripheral vascular disease
- Heart failure
- Venous insufficiency
- Peripheral neuropathy
- Chemotherapy
- Radiation therapy
- Medications (e.g., anticoagulants, antibiotics, immunosuppressants)
- Tobacco use; current or previous

Diagnosis

History

Key questions
- Mechanism of injury/wound onset (e.g., trauma, pressure)
- Duration of wound
- Size (e.g., increasing or decreasing)
- Drainage present
- Pain; severity, if present
- Edema of involved region or extremity
- Infectious symptoms
  - Fever
  - Spreading erythema
  - Warmth
  - Purulence
- Current treatment
- Prior treatment/treatments
- Comorbid medical conditions
  - Diabetes
  - Vascular disease
  - Heart failure
  - Venous insufficiency
  - Peripheral neuropathy
  - Chemotherapy
  - Radiation therapy

- Medications (e.g., anticoagulants, antibiotics, immunosuppressants)
- Prior wounds
- Wound healing history (e.g., surgery)
- Tobacco use; current or previous

Examination

Normal wound
- Base is moist, with red granulation tissue (i.e., raw hamburger meat appearance).
- Edges should be pink, dry, and flat with translucent epithelium advancing onto the base.
- Granulation tissue should be at, or below the level of the skin.
- Surrounding skin should be dry.

Wound evaluation
- Measurement:
  - Length (longest distance)
  - Width (longest distance)
  - Depth (deepest point)
- Undermining; noted as on a clock face (e.g., 3 cm undermining at 12 o'clock)
- Granulated base present
- Erythema
- Drainage, exudate, or purulence present
  - Purulence not necessary for infection to be present
- Odor
  - Foul or characteristic (e.g., pseudomonas) smell may indicate infection
- Foreign bodies
  - Especially in patients with neuropathy

Vascular evaluation
- Pulses (i.e., large vessel evaluation)
- Capillary refill (i.e., small vessel evaluation)
- Edema present; pitting or not
- Skin thickness (e.g., atrophic)
- Hair growth (e.g., absent)
- Nails (e.g., hypertrophic)

Testing
- Laboratory studies
  - Complete blood count (CBC)
  - Albumin/prealbumin
- Vascular studies; if poor perfusion by examination.
  - Ankle-Brachial Index (ABI); ankle systolic blood pressure divided by brachial systolic blood pressure (see Table 1)
    - Measure of large vessel perfusion
    - In all 95% sensitive/99% specific compared to angiography
    - Normal: 0.95 to 1.2
    - If greater than 1.2, likely false negative due to calcified vessels (e.g., diabetic) or moderate aortoiliac stenosis
  - Toe-Brachial Index (TBI)
    - Toe systolic blood pressure divided by brachial systolic blood pressure (see Table 1)
      - For apparent vessel calcification (e.g., diabetic patient)
- Ultrasound; including Doppler pulse waveform analysis
- Angiography
- Magnetic resonance angiography (MRA)
- Transcutaneous oxygen measurement (TcPO2)
  - Measures tissue oxygen saturation (see Table 2)
  - Evaluates small vessel perfusion
- X-ray has good sensitivity but poor specificity for osteomyelitis.
- Elevated erythrocyte sedimentation rate (ESR) is sensitive but nonspecific for osteomyelitis.
- Magnetic resonance imaging (MRI) has high sensitivity but poor specificity for osteomyelitis.

Treatment

General principles of wound care
- Clean with soap and water only
- Wounds need to be evaluated frequently
- Avoid cytotoxins (e.g., peroxide, iodine, antibiotic ointment)
- Optimize perfusion
  - Vascular surgery referral for abnormal ABI/TBI
- Sharp debridement down to bleeding tissue is required for removal of nonviable tissue, eschar, and tissue slough

Table 1 Vascular Perfusion Studies

	Normal	Mild arterial disease	Moderate arterial disease	Severe arterial disease
ABI	0.95–1.2	0.7–0.95	0.3–0.7	Less than 0.3
TBI	Less than 0.75	0.75–0.5	0.5–0.25	Less than 0.25

Table 2 Healing Probability and Tissue Oxygenation

TcPO2	Less than 40 mmHg	30–40 mmHg	Less than 30 mmHg
Probability of healing	Good	Gray zone, probability drops rapidly	Poor

- Confirm adequate vascular perfusion prior to sharp debridement
- Avoid exposure of bone, tendon, or connective tissue
- All wounds are colonized with bacteria
- Wounds with excessive drainage/exudate may be infected
  - Edges may be raised and pink/inflamed
  - Debride exudate and gently scrub with soap and water
  - Antibiotic ointment, or acetic acid wash (once only), may decontaminate the wound but can slow healing.
  - Ionic silver kills bacteria and is not cytotoxic, but dressings are expensive.
- Edema effectively decreases blood supply
  - Treatment of edema is compression.
  - Compression must be adjusted to the amount of concomitant arterial disease by ABI (see Table 3).
  - For limb edema, compression is applied to the entire limb not just to the wound.
  - Improperly applied compression can cause pressure ulcers.
  - Exercise great care with compression on an insensate limb.

Wound dressings
- The goal of a wound dressing is to create the ideal healing environment for the wound.
- Be familiar with the dressings available to you.
  - Wound care handbooks can explain each of the dressings.
- Simple dressings are usually better.
  - If a wound is wet, use a dressing designed to remove the moisture.
  - If the wound base is dry, use a dressing, or wound moisturizer, to moisten the base.
  - If the dressings are adhering to the wound edges, use a nonadherent dressing.
  - Under most conditions you will use a nonocculsive dressing.
  - Occlusive dressings
    - Moisten a very dry base
    - Help with autodebridement
    - Risk macerating wound edges and enlarging the wound.
    - Should be avoided in an infected wound

Table 3 Recommended Edema Compression Adjustments for Arterial Disease

ABI	Less than 0.8	0.5–0.8	Less than 0.5
Allowable compression	Full (35–40 mmHg)	Reduced (23–30 mmHg)	None

- Ionic silver dressings are best for long term (e.g., weeklong) and/or compression dressings.
- Ionic silver is not cost effective for dressings requiring frequent changes.
- Areas of undermining needed to be packed.
- Debridement ointments can keep a wound clean, but will not significantly debride the wound.
- If granulation tissue is above the level of the skin (i.e., hypergranulation) consider debridement or weekly application of silver nitrate.

Hyperbaric oxygen
- Supplies oxygen at greater than atmospheric pressure
- Beneficial for
  - Small vessel disease
  - Diabetic foot ulcers
  - Osteomyelitis

Infected wounds
- Characterized by redness, swelling, and heat.
- Usually have an increased exudate and possible foul smell; it is not necessary to see pus.
- Abscesses and fluid-filled cavities must be drained and packed as necessary.
- Avoid mistaking infection for inflammation.
- Diabetics frequently have infections caused by multiple organisms.
- Start with wide-spectrum antibiotic and adjust treatment according to culture results.
- All chronic wounds are colonized with bacteria. So swab culture identifies colonized bacteria.
- The best culture results will be obtained by sending a piece of infected tissue for culture.
- A frequent cause of nonhealing wound is underlying osteomyelitis.
- Osteomyelitis is common in nonhealing diabetic foot ulcers.
- If a wound has a history of infection and is close to underlying bone, osteomyelitis should be suspected.
- Exposed bone is indicative of osteomyelitis.
- Consider surgical debridement of infected bone.
- Appropriate antibiotics for 6 to 8 weeks.
- Hyperbaric oxygen can be used with refractory osteomyelitis and necrotizing infections.

Treatment of wound trauma
- Look for and eliminate the cause of the wound.
- Pressure is the most common cause (e.g., tight shoes).
- Look for wound pickers; excoriations around the wound edges.
- Weight-bearing must be eliminated 100% of the time.

Foreign bodies
- At each evaluation, the wound needs to be carefully inspected for foreign objects.
- Foreign bodies are common in diabetic foot wounds.

Nutrition
- Protein malnutrition is seen frequently in the elderly and obese (check prealbumin).
- Multivitamin with minerals, and vitamin C aids healing.
- Look at skin as a sign of nutrition; thin, fragile skin is often a sign of malnutrition.

Tobacco
- No one should smoke, but with wounds it decreases oxygen supply, worsening ischemia.
- Smokers need to know that the wound may never heal due to their smoking alone.

Treating metabolic comorbidities
- Diabetes (blood sugar must be optimally controlled)
- Renal disease
- Liver disease
- Hereditary disorders
- Malignancy
- Systemic infection
- Connective tissue disease
- Immunological disorders
- Chemotherapy
- Steroids both topical and systemic

Suggested Readings

Broughton G II, Janis JE, Attinger CE. The basic science of wound healing. *Plast Reconstruct Surg.* 2006; 117:12S–34S.

Hess CT. *Clinical Guide: Skin and Wound Care.* 6th ed. Philadelphia, PA: Lippincott Williams & Wilkins; 2007.

Mustoe T. Understanding chronic wounds: A unifying hypothesis on their pathogenesis and implications for therapy. *Am J Surg.* 2004;187:65S–70S.

Sheffield PJ, Fife CE. *Wound Care Practice.* 2nd ed. Flagstaff, AZ: Best Publishing; 2007.

Special Senses: Hearing

Samuel R. Atcherson PhD

Description
Hearing impairment (or hearing loss) is defined as total or partial inability to hear sound in one or both ears. It can be congenital, acquired, or genetic and can have a debilitating impact on communication, psychosocial status, and quality of life.

Etiology/Types
- Sensorineural hearing loss (SNHL; cochlear)
- Conductive hearing loss (CHL; outer or middle ear)
- Mixed hearing loss (combination of SNHL and CHL)
- Retrocochlear/neurologic hearing loss
- Unilateral or bilateral hearing loss
- Presbycusis: slow, progressive hearing loss associated with aging
- Severity of hearing loss: pure tone average of 0.5, 1, and 2 kHz in decibel hearing level (dB HL)
  - Mild (26–40 dB HL)
  - Moderate (41–55 dB HL)
  - Moderate to severe (56–70 dB HL)
  - Severe (71–90 dB HL)
  - Profound (less than 90 dB HL)

Epidemiology
- It is estimated that 10% of the U.S. population has a hearing impairment.
- In all 3 of 10 people above the age of 60 have hearing loss.
- Hearing loss is highly associated with aging (presbycusis) after age 65 (35% of the population).

Pathogenesis
- Cochlear insult (hair cell)
- Cochlear fluid disturbance (Meniere's disease/endolymphatic hydrops)
- Auditory nerve disease, neuropathy, or trauma
- Conductive abnormality
  - Excessive cerumen
  - Cholesteatoma
  - Exostoses
  - Tympanic membrane perforation
  - Atelectasis
  - Stapes fixation
  - Ossicular chain disarticulation
  - Otitis media with effusion

Risk Factors
- Age above 65 years, but presentation may begin as early as the fifth decade.
- Hereditary (e.g., aging-related autosomal dominant, nonsyndromic hearing loss gene, DFNA18)
- Vocational or lifestyle noise exposure (i.e., high-frequency hearing loss)
- Aminoglycoside (nonreversible) or medication ototoxicity (reversible or irreversible)
- Smoking (appears to interfere with inner ear recovery process as a result of chronic noise exposure) and alcohol (over 4 drinks/day)

Clinical Features
- Behavioral manifestations:
  - Difficulty hearing in noisier environments
  - Greater fixation on the speaker's face
  - Head turning to sound
  - Mishearing
  - Complaints that others are not speaking clearly
  - Understanding men's voices better than female or children's voices
  - Changes in voice output (too soft or too loud) or speech quality
- Increased feelings of isolation, depression, loneliness, fear, frustration, and disappointment
- May have tinnitus in conjunction with hearing impairment

Diagnosis

Differential diagnosis
- Central auditory processing disorder (CAPD)
  - Poorer than expected speech understanding that is inconsistent with hearing sensitivity; usually associated with the decline of the central auditory nervous system; however, may indicate cognitive impairment.
- Traumatic brain injury affecting the auditory central nervous system

- Vestibular schwannoma
- Stria vascularis atrophy (i.e., K+ pump for hair cell function)
- Cognitive impairment

Examination
- Otoscopic examination
  - Observation of pinna, external auditory canal, and tympanic membrane for signs of cerumen impaction, disease, or trauma
- Tympanometry
  - Assessment of the tympanic membrane and ossicular chain function
- Acoustic reflex battery
  - Assessment of the auditory nerve, lower brainstem nuclei, facial nerve, and stapedius muscle function
- Puretone air- and bone-conduction
  - Assessment of hearing sensitivity thresholds at various audiometric frequencies
- Speech audiometry
  - Assessment of functional hearing sensitivity and performance involving speech materials in a quiet environment, as well as with competing/background noise; results are influenced by type, degree, and severity of hearing loss.
- Dichotic listening screening
  - Cursory assessment of auditory cortex and corpus callosum function using different numbers presented to each ear

Testing
- Otoacoustic emission (OAE) testing
  - Assessment of outer hair cell function objectively using clicks or tones presented to the ear; poor or absent OAEs correlate well with hearing sensitivity and can signal cochlear damage due to chemotherapy, before hearing loss sets in
- Evoked potential testing
  - One or more tests that assess auditory nerve and central auditory nervous system function objectively with surface electrodes and clicks or tones when poor auditory function cannot be explained by hearing sensitivity alone.
- Imaging of head/brain, that is, computerized tomography (CT) and magnetic resonance imaging (MRI)
  - Provide radiologic information regarding the external and internal auditory canals, as well as the auditory structures in the temporal bone; also useful in detecting mass lesions and/or structural abnormalities of the auditory nervous system
- Central auditory testing
  - Behavioral assessment of central auditory function for age-related structural deficits and/or cognitive declines; can be paired with evoked potential measures
- Vestibular testing
  - To determine the site of a lesion for balance difficulties, whether unilateral or bilateral, central or peripheral; can assist in the management/treatment of the disorder; sometimes hearing and vestibular complaints are comorbid as a result of the close proximity of end organs.

Pitfalls
- Cognitive impairment may impede audiometric testing

Red flags
- Sudden hearing loss, tinnitus, or any drastic noticeable change: suspicion of autoimmune, viral, or vascular causes
- Hearing and vestibular complaints
- Head injury
- Aminoglycoside or medication ototoxicity
- Cerumen impaction (sedentary lifestyles or regular hearing aid use)

Treatment

Hearing technology
- Hearing aids (consider built-in telecoil add-on that aids in telephone and assistive listening device use)
- Cochlear implants (for severe to profound SNHL)
- Bone-anchored hearing aid (for bilateral CHL or unilateral SNHL)
- Assistive listening devices (frequency modulation, FM, system)
- Other assistive technology (captioned TV, amplified telephones, vibrating or flashing alarms, etc.)

Rehabilitation
- In addition to technology, group rehabilitation may be helpful in using a facilitator-led, self-help support approach.
- Communication compensatory strategies

Consults
- Otology or otolaryngology
- Psychology or psychiatry for socioemotional issues

Complications of treatments
- Noncompliance with technology use
- Unrealistic expectations of technology

Prognosis
- Hearing aids or implantable devices, along with assistive technology can greatly improve quality of life; however, motivation to use them is key.
- Conductive hearing impairments may be surgically corrected in part or in whole, but may still require hearing technology.

Helpful Hints
- Maintain face-to-face communication with elderly patients and avoid "Elderspeak."
- Dementia/Alzheimer's can be mistaken for hearing loss.
- Short self-report questionnaires or a properly conducted whisper test can be used to screen for hearing loss.
- Spousal input of communication difficulties can often be helpful.
- Some patients may actually do better with one hearing aid, but the majority of patients with symmetric hearing losses benefit from two.

Suggested Readings
Humes LE. Aging and speech communication: Peripheral, central-auditory, and cognitive factors affecting the speech-understanding problems of older adults. *ASHA Lead*. 2008;13:10–13.

Lin FR, Thorpe R, Gordon-Salant S, et al. Hearing loss prevalence and risk factors among older adults in the United States. *J Gerontol A Biol Sci Med Sci*. 2011;66:582–590. Doi:10.1093/gerona/glr00.

Weinstein BE, ed. *Geriatric Audiology*. New York, NY: Thieme Medical Publishers; 2000.

Yueh B, Shekelle P. Quality indicators for the care of hearing loss in vulnerable elders. *J Am Ger Soc*. 2007;55(Suppl. 2):S335–S339.

Special Senses: Vision—Cataracts

Romona LeDay Davis MD

Description
A senile cataract is an age-related opacity of the crystalline lens or the lens membrane, which causes vision impairment.

Etiology/Types

Nuclear cataract
- Yellow or brown discoloration of the central part of the lens; most common type

Cortical cataract
- "Spoke like" opacities extending into the visual axis of the lens

Posterior subcapsular cataract
- Granular/plaque-like lesion in the center of the visual axis near the posterior aspect of the lens
- Usually seen in diabetics, steroid use, intraocular inflammation, or radiation exposure

Epidemiology
- Over 350,000 new, visually disabling cataracts are diagnosed yearly in the United States.
- Leading cause of reversible blindness in the United States.

Pathogenesis
- Multifactorial
- The lens increases in thickness and weight with age as the nuclear fibers are compressed by the continued addition of concentric cortical fibers.
- The nucleus discolors and hardens, forming nuclear cataracts, the most common type.

Risk Factors
- Age (half of the patients are older than 65)
- Chronic steroid use (topical or systemic)
- Previous ocular surgery
- Trauma to the eye

Clinical Features
- A slowly progressive, painless decline in visual acuity
- May be asymmetric
- Decreased color perception
- Cortical cataracts cause glare with night driving or with bright light sources.
- Nuclear cataracts cause blurred distance vision more so than near vision.

Natural History
- Slow, progressive deterioration of the patient's visual function
- Untreated, it may lead to reversible blindness.
- The lens may swell, causing secondary glaucoma
  - Elevation in intraocular pressure and nerve damage
  - May lead to permanent blindness

Diagnosis

Differential diagnosis

Secondary cataracts (related to medical condition, injury, or exposure)
- Traumatic cataract
- Intraocular inflammation
- Toxic cataract
  - Medications—steroids and antipsychotics
- Intraocular tumor-related
- Diabetes
  - Age-related cataracts develop at a younger age in diabetics.
- Radiation

History
- Decreased visual acuity
- Increased glare and monocular diplopia (vacuoles or opacifications within a lens may scatter or refract light)

Examination
- Distance and near vision
- Pupillary examination—no relative afferent pupillary defect (RAPD) should be seen.
- Direct ophthalmoscopy at 3 ft—opacities in the cornea, lens, or vitreous may cause a blemish in the red reflex as seen through the scope aperture.

Pitfalls
- Ideally visual function should be established prior to cataract development.
  - Poor vision may be pre-existing
    - Amblyopia
    - Macular degeneration
    - Glaucoma
    - Trauma

Treatment
- Correction of refractive error if patient declines surgical correction or if cataract does not meet criteria for surgery.
- Cataract surgery
  - To improve vision
  - To facilitate management of other ocular conditions such as
    - Diabetic retinopathy
    - Glaucoma

Surgical complications
- Endophthalmitis (early)
- Bullous keratopathy (late)
- Dislocated intraocular lens (late)
- Macular edema

Prognosis
- Modern cataract surgery is the most common elective surgical procedure performed in the United States.
- In all 90% of patients undergoing cataract surgery experience improved quality of life and improved vision.
- Pre-existing eye disease limits potential improvement
  - ARMD and diabetic retinopathy

Helpful Hints
- Patients, aged 65 and above, should receive yearly dilated examinations from an ophthalmologist who can monitor the progression of their disease.
- Generally, cataracts do not require urgent action unless a secondary complication arises, such as lens-related glaucoma.

Suggested Readings
Age-Related Eye Disease Study Research Group. Risk factors associated with age-related nuclear and cortical cataracts: A case-control study in the Age-Related Eye Disease Study. AREDS report no. 5. *Ophthalmology*. 2001;108:1400–1408.

Miglior S, Marighi PE, Musicco M, et al. Risk factors for cortical, nuclear, posterior subcapsular and mixed cataract: A case-control study. *Ophthalmic Epidemiol*. 1994;1(2):93–105.

Rosen PN, Kaplan RM, Davis K. Measuring outcomes of cataract surgery using the Quality of Well-Being Scale and VF-14 Visual Function Index. *J Cataract Refract Surg*. 2005;31(2):369–378.

West SK, Valmadrid CT. Epidemiology of risk factors for age-related cataract. *Surv Ophthalmol*. 1995;39(4):323–334.

Special Senses: Vision—General

Romona LeDay Davis MD

Description
Vision impairment in the elderly is a major health care problem. Impairment may lead to
- Difficulty with instrumental activities of daily living (reading or driving)
- Increased risk of falls and hip fractures
- Increased risk of depression (seen in 13%, compared to 5% of 75-year-olds with good vision)

Etiology/Types
The four most common causes are as follows:
- Age-related macular degeneration (ARMD); two types: dry or wet
- Glaucoma
- Cataract
- Diabetic retinopathy

Epidemiology
- There are over 40 million people above the age of 65 in the United States.
  - One third are affected by vision impairment.

Pathogenesis

Age-related macular degeneration
- Oxidative stress leads to retinal pigment epithelial damage and choroidal vascular damage, which may predispose the macula to deterioration.
- In all 90% of patients have the dry (nonexudative) form. They have difficulty adapting to changes in varying light conditions, speed reading, and a gradual loss of central vision.
- In all 10% of patients develop subretinal neovascularization, causing an acute loss of central vision (exudative or wet ARMD).

Glaucoma
- Multifactorial: Primary open-angle glaucoma (POAG) is most common.
- Intraocular ischemic insult to the optic nerve head versus a mechanical insult leading to optic nerve damage and associated visual field loss.

Cataract
- Multifactorial
- The lens nucleus discolors and hardens, forming nuclear cataracts (most common type).

Diabetic retinopathy
- Microvascular retinal changes lead to the loss of blood–retinal barrier, macular edema or retinal ischemia, and vision loss.

Risk Factors

Age-related macular degeneration
- Advanced age
- Family history
- Hypertension
- Smoking

Glaucoma
- Family history
- Advanced age
- Diabetes
- Myopia
- Hypertension

Cataracts
- Advanced age
- Steroid use
- History of trauma
- Intraocular inflammation

Diabetic retinopathy
- Poor glucose control
- Increased duration of diabetes
- Hypertension

Clinical Features

Age-related macular degeneration
- Central scotoma
- Image distortion

Glaucoma
- Loss of peripheral vision

Cataracts
- Blurred vision, glare
- Loss of color contrast

Diabetic retinopathy
- Blurred vision
- Poor night vision

Natural History

Age-related macular degeneration
- Central scotoma

Glaucoma
- "Tunnel vision"
- Blindness

Cataract
- Progressive loss of vision
- Reversible blindness

Diabetic retinopathy
- Blurred or distorted central vision
- Poor night vision
- Blindness

Diagnosis

Differential diagnosis
- ARMD (nonexudative or dry—90%)
- ARMD (exudative or wet—10%)
- Glaucoma (POAG)
- Cataract
- Diabetic retinopathy
- Retinal vein occlusions
- Hypertensive retinopathy
- Radiation retinopathy

History
Each condition increases in prevalence with advanced age. A thorough medical and family history review may be helpful in determining the etiology of the vision loss.

Examination
- Visual acuity
- Pupillary function
  - Relative afferent pupillary defect (RAPD) may be present if ARMD, glaucoma, or diabetic retinopathy are severe and asymmetric.
- Direct ophthalmoscopy at 3 ft—allows the examiner to shine a bright light into the patient's pupil. Opacities in the lens, cornea, or vitreous will cause a darkening or change in the red reflex.
- Confrontational fields
  - ARMD—central scotoma with sparing of the peripheral field
  - POAG—peripheral field loss (in early disease); "tunnel vision"—a small island of remaining vision in late disease; complete blindness in end-stage disease.

Testing
- Visual field testing
- Optical coherence topography (OCT)
  - A noncontact imaging technology that produces cross-sectional images of the retina or other tissue using the backscattering of light.
- Central corneal thickness
  - Measurement in micrometers of the cornea using ultrasound (contact method) or OCT (noncontact) methods.
- Gonioscopy
  - Assessment of the anterior chamber angle using a goniolens and slit lamp
- Fluorescein angiography
  - Technique for assessing the circulation of the retina and choroid.
  - A fluorescent dye is injected into the systemic circulation.
  - A camera with special filters is used to capture photographs of the retinal images through the pupil as the dye illuminates the retinal vasculature and pathology.

Pitfalls
- Elderly patients need yearly dilated eye examinations.
- Vision loss is painless and may go unnoticed until late.

Red flags
- A RAPD will likely indicate significant damage to the affected eye.
- A RAPD may not be present if the damage is symmetric.

Treatment

Medical
- ARMD
  - Antioxidant vitamins (Age-Related Eye Disease Study, AREDS, formulation) shown to have a 25% reduction in progression in high-risk patients from dry ARMD to wet ARMD (should be recommended by an ophthalmologist). See risk association in the section titled Complications of treatment.
  - Smoking cessation
  - Intravitreal injection of antiangiogenic agents for wet ARMD.

- Glaucoma
  - Topical and/or oral medications to lower intraocular pressure
- Cataract
  - Smoking cessation
  - Sun protection
- Diabetic retinopathy
  - Intensive blood glucose control with oral glucose lowering medication
  - Insulin
  - Diet and exercise

Surgical
- ARMD
  - Selective dye-enhanced laser photocoagulation
  - Low-dose radiation therapy
  - Retinal transplantation/translocation
- Glaucoma
  - Laser trabeculoplasty
  - Incision surgery
- Cataract
  - Phacoemulsification with lens implantation
- Diabetic retinopathy
  - Focal argon laser for macular edema
  - Panretinal photocoagulation for proliferative diabetic retinopathy

Consults
- Ophthalmology
  - Subspecialty referrals to glaucoma or vitreoretinal specialists may be needed

Complications of treatment
- Side effects from medications
- Infection from invasive surgical procedures
- Scotoma from laser procedures
- Increased risk of lung cancer for AREDS vitamins used in patients who currently smoke

Prognosis
- Worse if dry-ARMD progresses to wet-ARMD
- Worse if RAPD is present in any condition.
- Worse in diabetics with long-standing, poorly controlled disease or who are experiencing proliferative diabetic retinopathy and chronic renal failure.

Helpful Hints
- Suspect vision loss in the elderly if the quality of their daily life is compromised by depression and loss of independence.
- Consider poor vision as a cause or contributor to frequent falls in the elderly.

Suggested Readings
Abdelhafiz AH, Austin CA. Visual factors should be assessed in older people presenting with falls or hip fracture. *Age Ageing*. 2003;32(1):26-30.

Evans JR, Fletcher AE, Wormald RP. Depression and anxiety in visually impaired older people. *Ophthalmology*. 2007;114(2):283-288.

Harvey PT. Common eye diseases of elderly people: Identifying and treating causes of vision loss. *Gerontology*. 2003;49(1):1-11.

Pizzarello LD. The dimensions of the problem of eye disease among the elderly. *Ophthalmology*. 1987;94:1191-1195.

Quillen DA. Common causes of vision loss in elderly patients. *Am Acad Fam Physician*. 1999;60:99-108.

Special Senses: Vision—Glaucoma

Romona LeDay Davis MD

Description
Glaucoma is a group of disorders with characteristic optic neuropathy and visual field loss. There is usually an associated elevated intraocular pressure (IOP).

Etiology/Types

Primary open-angle glaucoma—most common
- IOP is above normal (greater than 22 mm Hg; normal 10–22)
- Normal anterior chamber angle for aqueous outflow
- No structural abnormality of the eye

Normal tension glaucoma
- May be on the same continuum as primary open-angle glaucoma (POAG), but with IOP remaining below 22 mmHg.

Secondary open-angle glaucoma
- Identifiable blockage to aqueous outflow, leading to a rise in IOP and causing nerve damage
  - Pseudoexfoliative glaucoma
  - Steroid-induced glaucoma
  - Trauma (debris, blood, pigment)
  - Pigment dispersion

Epidemiology
- POAG causes 10% of blindness in the United States.
- Women and men are equally affected.
- Most common cause of blindness in Black Americans.

Pathogenesis

Multifactorial
- POAG
  - Intraocular ischemic insult to optic nerve head versus
  - Mechanical insult from high IOP leading to optic nerve damage and associated visual field loss
- Secondary open-angle glaucoma
  - Obstruction of aqueous outflow at the trabecular meshwork leading to elevated IOP. Some causes of obstruction include blood, pigment, and debris.

Risk Factors
- Elevated intraocular pressure
- Age above 40
- Race (more common in Black Americans)
- Family history

Clinical Features
- Early POAG—asymptomatic
- Advanced POAG—loss of peripheral vision
- End-stage POAG—complete blindness

Natural History
- Early POAG
  - Asymptomatic
  - Elevated IOP
  - Cupping of optic nerve
- Advanced POAG
  - Loss of peripheral vision ("tunnel vision")
  - Decline in central vision
  - Optic nerve pallor
  - Severe constriction of visual fields
  - Loss of independence
- End-stage POAG—complete blindness

Diagnosis

Differential diagnosis
- Ocular hypertension
- Physiologic optic nerve cupping
- Secondary open-angle glaucoma
- Secondary angle-closure glaucoma
- Chronic angle-closure glaucoma (CACG)

History
- POAG—a possible history of steroid use and positive family history; no symptoms early. Loss of peripheral vision late.
- Secondary OAG—trauma, "haloes" around lights

Examination
- Confrontational fields
- Vision testing

Testing
- Formal visual field testing
- Optical coherence tomography
- Central corneal thickness measurements
- Gonioscopy

Consults
- Ophthalmology

Pitfalls
- Patients may not be aware of vision loss in one eye, since visual fields of the two eyes overlap considerably.

Red flags
- Vision loss in glaucoma is slow and painless. Sudden vision loss in the elderly warrants immediate attention and is not likely due to glaucoma (consider giant cell arteritis or other vascular etiologies).

Treatment

Goal: lower IOP

Medical
- Topical drops
  - Beta-blockers: decrease aqueous production
  - Alpha-agonists: decrease aqueous production
  - Prostaglandin analogues: increase uveoscleral outflow
  - Carbonic anhydrase inhibitors: decrease aqueous production
  - Miotic agents: increase trabecular outflow
- Oral agents
  - Systemic carbonic anhydrase inhibitors: decrease aqueous production
  - Hyperosmotic agents: dehydrate vitreous

Surgery
- Laser trabeculoplasty—applied to trabecular meshwork
  - Argon laser trabeculoplasty (ALT)
  - Selective laser trabeculoplasty (SLT)
  - Diode laser trabeculoplasty
- Incisional surgery—creation of a surgical defect in the sclera to allow aqueous flow from the anterior chamber into the subconjunctival space.

Complications of treatment
- Side effects from medications
- Infection from invasive surgical procedures

Prognosis
- Vision loss is greatly reduced with early detection and aggressive management.
- Untreated, POAG may progress to blindness.

Helpful Hints
- Suspect vision loss in the elderly, if they are not participating fully in their normal activities or if they experience depression.

Suggested Readings
Chaudhry I, Wong S. Recognizing glaucoma. A guide for the primary care physician. *Postgrad Med.* 1996;99(5):247–248, 251, 252, 257–259.

Inatani M, Iwao K, Inoue T, et al. Long-term relationship between intraocular pressure and visual field loss in primary open-angle glaucoma. *J Glaucoma.* 2008;17(4):275–279.

Special Senses: Vision—Macular Degeneration

Sami Uwaydat MD

Description
Progressive degeneration of the retina leading to loss of central vision in an elderly patient.

Etiology/Types
- Dry Age-Related Macular Degeneration (ARMD; most common; 90% of patients)
  - Drusen: lipid-rich deposits seen on eye examination as yellow subretinal lesions
  - Pigment abnormalities: dark spots on the retina
  - Geographic atrophy: loss of retinal tissue
- Wet ARMD (less common)
  - Abnormal blood vessels that grow under the retina and can bleed or leak fluid

Epidemiology
- 6.4% of patients aged 65 to 74 and 19.7% of patients older than 75 years have signs of ARMD.

Pathogenesis
- Aging changes in the retina lead to
  - Accumulation of lipofuscin in the retinal cells
  - Thinning of the choriocapillaris
  - Loss of photoreceptors

Risk Factors
- Aged above 55 years
- Family history of ARMD
- Hypertension
- Smoking
- Caucasian race
- Others: ultraviolet light exposure, atherosclerosis, and increased Body Mass Index

Clinical Features
- Dry ARMD
  - Can be asymptomatic
  - Difficulty reading in dim light
  - Mild decrease or distortion of central vision
- Wet ARMD
  - Sudden onset of central vision loss or distortion

Natural History

Dry ARMD
- Slow progression to the more advanced forms
- Risk of progression depends on the size, morphology, and extent of the drusen and pigment anomalies.
- Central vision is lost when the fovea is involved.

Wet ARMD
- Progressive irreversible loss of central vision

Diagnosis

Differential diagnosis
- Inherited retinal dystrophies
- Retinal vascular diseases (diabetes, vein occlusion, macroaneurysm)
- Retinal inflammations/infections

History
- Progressive worsening of central vision
- Sudden onset of scotoma (partial alteration of vision) or metamorphopsia (distorted vision)

Examination
- Fundus examination
- Dry ARMD
  - Subretinal yellow deposits
  - Pigmented scars
  - Loss of retinal layers
- Wet ARMD
  - Subretinal hemorrhage
  - Macular exudates
  - Gray membrane under the macula

Testing
- Amsler grid: 3-inch square grid of horizontal and vertical lines
- New changes noted by a patient on the grid may indicate a progression in the macular degeneration.
- Fluorescein angiography: detects growth of new blood vessels. Done when the patient notes changes on the Amsler grid or if the eye examination reveals blood or fluid under the retina.

- Optical coherence tomography: specialized imaging technique that gives high-resolution cross-sectional images of the retina. Detects intraretinal or subretinal fluid that comes from leaky vessels.

Pitfalls
- Always consider giant cell arteritis in an elderly patient who presents with sudden loss of vision.

Red flags
- Higher incidence of depression in patients with poor vision
- Charles Bonnet syndrome: visual hallucinations in patients with profound visual loss. No auditory component (differentiates this from psychosis)

Treatment
- Dry ARMD
  - Educate about modifiable risk factors (smoking cessation, blood pressure control, avoidance of ultraviolet light, weight control)
  - Vitamins: Age-Related Eye Disease Study (AREDS): high doses of vitamins C, E, beta-carotene, zinc, omega-3 fatty acids, lutein, and zeaxanthin can delay the progression of the dry form of ARMD.
- Wet ARMD
  - Intravitreal injections of anti-*vascular endothelial growth factor* (anti-VEGF) medication: bevacizumab and ranibizumab: office procedure
  - Monthly injections. Vision improves in around 40% of patients and stabilizes in around 90% of patients.
  - Photodynamic therapy: intravenous administration of a photosensitizing agent (verteporfin) followed by the application of a low-energy laser to the leaky vessels found on fluorescein angiography: stabilizes, but does not improve, vision.
  - Low-vision aids: magnifiers and loupes: for patients with advanced ARMD and poor central vision

Complications of treatment
- Beta-carotene: increased risk of lung cancer in smokers
- Vitamin E: slight increase in the risk of hemorrhagic strokes
- Photodynamic therapy: patients should avoid bright lights for 3 days after the treatment. Severe skin burns can result from direct sun exposure.
- Intravitreal injection:
  - Ocular complications
- Retinal detachment
- Cataract
- Infection
  - Nonocular complications
- Potential increase in ischemic cerebrovascular and cardiac events
- Increase in blood pressure

Prognosis
- Dry ARMD: Vision is usually maintained, until late in the disease.
- Wet ARMD: Intravitreal injections stabilize vision loss and may improve vision, but patients require monthly injections.
- Patients lose their central vision from the advanced forms of ARMD, but do not become "completely blind" from this condition.

Helpful Hints
- Any patient with sudden onset of metamorphosia or vision loss should be promptly referred for a complete eye examination.

Suggested Readings
American Society of Retina Specialist. www.amdawarness.org.
Casten RJ, Rovner BW, Tasman W. Age-related macular degeneration and depression: A review of recent research. *Curr Opin Ophthalmol.* 2004;15:181–183.
Klein R, Klein BE, Knudtson MD, et al. Fifteen-year cumulative incidence of age-related macular degeneration: The Beaver Dam Eye Study. *Ophthalmology.* 2007;114(2):253–262.
Krishnadev N, Meleth AD, Chew EY. Nutritional supplements for age-related macular degeneration. *Curr Opin Ophthalmol.* 2010;21:184–189.
National Eye Institute. www.nei.nih.org/amd.

Urinary Incontinence

Nabil K. Bissada MD ■ Ayman Mahdy MD

Description
Urinary incontinence (UI) is defined by the International Continence Society as "the complaint of any involuntary leakage of urine."

Etiology/Types

Acute incontinence: DRIP
- **D**ehydration/**D**elirium/**D**iapers
- **R**etention/**R**estricted mobility
- **I**nfection (urinary-symptomatic), **I**mpaction (fecal), **I**nflammation (vaginitis, urethritis)
- **P**olypharmacy/**P**olyuria

Transient incontinence: DIAPPERS
- **D**elirium/confusion
- **I**nfection/urinary (symptomatic)
- **A**trophic urethritis/vaginitis
- **P**harmaceuticals
- **P**sychologic, especially depression
- **E**xcess urine output
- **R**estricted mobility
- **S**tool impaction

Established incontinence
- Bladder related: detrusor overactivity/low bladder compliance
- Sphincter related: urethral hypermobility (females)/intrinsic sphincter deficiency

Functional urinary incontinence
- In patients with physical disability and restricted mobility. The patient cannot reach the bathroom on time.

Epidemiology
- UI is much more prevalent in the elderly compared with other age groups.
- Affects 15% to 30% of older people living at home
- Affects one third of the elderly in acute-care settings
- Affects half of those in nursing homes

Pathogenesis
- Age-related changes in the bladder: decreased bladder sensation, contractility, and ability to postpone voiding
- Deficits outside the urinary tract
- Prostate enlargement in men may result in bladder outlet obstruction with subsequent detrusor overactivity and urgency urinary incontinence (UUI).
- Decreased urethral length, urethral closure pressure, and cells of the rhabdosphincter in women precipitate stress urinary incontinence (SUI).

Risk Factors
- Advanced age
- Gender: higher incidence in females
- Obstetric history: pregnancy and childbirth
- Menopause
- Prostate disorders in men
- Pelvic floor muscle weakness in women
- Depression
- Pelvic surgery
- Polypharmacy
- Smoking
- Obesity
- Physical and occupational force and activity
- Childhood incontinence
- Family history of incontinence

Clinical Features
- In UUI: patient complaints of urine leakage with urgency.
- In SUI: leakage occurs with cough, sneeze, lifting heavy objects, and/or physical activity.
- In mixed urinary incontinence (MUI): Patient has the symptoms of both UUI and SUI.
- Patient might leak without awareness
- Leakage only at night (nocturnal enuresis)
- Associated lower urinary tract symptoms: frequency, urgency, difficulty, weak stream, and/or interrupted stream
- Associated bowel symptoms: constipation, diarrhea, and/or fecal incontinence

Natural History
- Acute and transient incontinence usually resolve with treatment of the underlying conditions.

Diagnosis

Differential diagnosis
- SUI
- UUI
- MUI
- Unconscious (unaware) incontinence
- Continuous urinary incontinence
- Nocturnal enuresis
- Postmicturition dribble
- Overflow incontinence
- Extraurethral incontinence
- Dual (fecal and urinary) incontinence

History
- Onset and duration: acute, transient, and established
- Type of incontinence
- Severity and degree of bother
- Underlying conditions
- Other urinary symptoms
- Previous related surgeries

Examination
- Neurologic
- Pelvic examination in women:
  - Bladder stress test
  - Pelvic organ prolapse
  - Atrophic vaginitis
- Digital rectal examination in men:
- Enlarged prostate
- Prostate cancer

Testing
- Urinalysis
- Postvoid residual urine measurement:
  - Bladder scan
  - Straight catheter
- Pad testing: The patient wears a preweighed pad for certain period of time. The pad is reweighed and the amount of increase of pad weight in grams is recorded. An increase of 1.3 g pad weight after 24 hours is a positive test.
- Urine flow studies
- Urine cytology and cystoscopy: in patients with urgency and frequency, especially smokers (who are at high risk for bladder cancer).
- Urodynamic studies:
  - If invasive treatment option is pursued
  - In case of poorly characterized urinary incontinence
  - In case of failed conservative management
  - In case of failed previous surgery for urinary incontinence
  - In case of known or suspected neurogenic bladder
  - In case of MUI
  - In case of high residual volume

Pitfalls
- Diagnosis and treatment of underlying conditions is critical when managing urinary incontinence in the elderly.

Red flags
- Elderly patients with urinary incontinence are at increased risk of falls:
  - Wet floor
  - Drug effects (confusion and postural hypotension)
  - Urgency: patient hurries to void
  - Disturbed sleep pattern: due to nocturia
- Perineal skin complications of urinary incontinence may include severe infections and even sepsis in the frail elderly.
- When using antimuscarinics in treating UUI: the patient should be evaluated for central nervous system and gastrointestinal side effects, interaction with other medications, and effect on bladder emptying.

Treatment
- *Transient incontinence*
  - Treatment of the underlying condition
- *Functional incontinence*
  - Behavioral therapy
  - Environmental manipulation
  - Absorptive products
  - External collection devices
  - Bladder relaxants (selected patients)
  - Indwelling catheter (selected patients)
- *Bladder related*
  - Treatment of the underlying condition: stones, infections, tumors, and so on.
  - Behavioral modification
  - Pelvic floor muscle exercise
  - Estrogen therapy
  - Bladder relaxants
  - Neuromodulation
  - Bladder augmentation
  - Bladder denervation
  - Urinary diversion: using the small or large bowel.
- *Sphincter related*
  - Pelvic floor muscle (Kegel) exercise
  - Estrogen therapy: to replenish the vascularity of the urethra and periurethral tissues and to re-establish the urethral mucosal folds

- Alpha-agonists: induce smooth muscle contraction at the bladder neck area
- Bulking agents: reduce the urethral lumen and increase the bladder outlet pressure
- Surgery: slings/artificial sphincter
- *Overflow incontinence*
  - Surgical correction
  - Clean intermittent catheterization (CIC)
  - Indwelling catheter in patients who cannot self-catheterize, and who are not good candidates for surgical correction
- *General*
  - Perineal skin care
  - Absorptive products such as diapers and pads; must they be frequently changed

Consults
- Urology
- Neurosurgery
- Neurology
- Physical medicine and rehabilitation
- Psychiatry

Helpful Hints
- Determining the type of incontinence is the key to correct management.
- The underlying nonurologic causes of incontinence in the elderly should always be addressed.
- Consider other disease conditions and review thoroughly the patient's medication list before prescribing antimuscarinics. An example is a patient with dementia who is treated with one of the cholinesterase inhibitors (antagonize the effect of antimuscarinics). Memantine can be considered as an alternative to cholinesterase inhibitors in those patients.

Suggested Readings
Johnson T, Ouslander JG. Lower urinary tract disorder in the elderly female. In: Raz S and Rodríguez L, eds. *Female Urology* 3rd ed. Philadelphia, PA: WB Saunders; 2008:948–960.

Newman DK, Wein A. *Managing and Treating Urinary Incontinence.* 2nd ed. Baltimore, MD: Health Professions Press; 2008.

Resnick N, Yalla S. Geriatric incontinence and voiding dysfunction. In: Wein AJ, Kavoussi LR, Novick AC, Partin AW, and Peters CA. *Campbell-Walsh Urology.* 9th ed. Philadelphia, PA: Saunders; 2007:2330–2321.

III

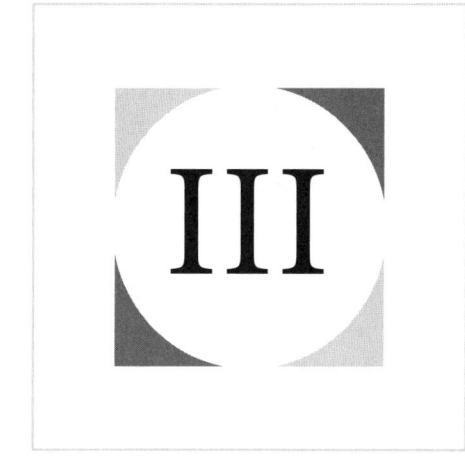

Special Topics

Aging With a Developmental Disability

Tamara Zagustin MD

Description
Aging with a disability is a multifactorial and dynamic phenomenon, where impairments are often exacerbated. As people age with a disability, there are changes in physical, sensory, and/or mental function that may result in difficulties in activities of daily living and changes in social interactions.

Common Disabling Disorders Present From Childhood Into Adulthood
- Down syndrome
- Neuromuscular diseases:
  - Cerebral palsy (CP)
  - Friedreich's ataxia
  - Hereditary sensory motor neuropathy
  - Poliomyelitis and postpoliomyelitis syndrome
  - Muscular dystrophies
- Traumatic brain injury
- Spinal cord injury
- Myelomeningocele
- Juvenile idiopathic arthritis
- Cystic fibrosis

Epidemiology
- A majority of children with a congenital or early acquired disability are surviving to older ages and are therefore experiencing the process of aging.
- Declines in function may begin earlier than for nondisabled adults ("premature aging process").
- Mortality declines as survival time increases.
- The more severe the disability with respect to mobility and cognitive function, the greater the impact on quality of life and life expectancy.
- Individuals living with a disability encounter substantial new medical, functional, and psychosocial problems later in life.
- Over 90% of people with a disability acquired early in life do not receive preventative general health evaluations as adults.
- Adults with disabilities have very fragmented medical care compared to the pediatric disabled population.

Pathophysiology
- Disabled people age differently than the nondisabled.
- The physiological reserve capacity of disabled individuals is reduced, as is their recovery capacity, and they have an increased propensity for illness. When combined with the aging process, they are more challenged in life and require more care and attention.
- The exact cause of premature aging in disabled individuals is unknown but is felt to be multifactorial.
- People with disabilities have higher rates of medical and functional problems 20 or more years earlier, as compared to the nondisabled.
- People with disabilities have three to four times the number of secondary health problems compared to their age-matched peers without disabilities.
- Rates of respiratory illnesses are much higher in the disabled, aged population.
- Diabetes is seen five to six times more often in individuals aging with a disability and with associated activity limitation (e.g., Down syndrome population).
- Cardiovascular disease is more relevant as a cause of death in the disabled as they have a higher incidence of hypertension, hypercholesterolemia, and heart disease.
- Musculoskeletal problems, including osteoarthritis and osteoporosis are more prevalent in the disabled, and onset is at a much younger age compared to age-matched peers without disabilities.
- Depression is more common in disabled adults than in adults without a disability.

Risk Factors
- Severity of disability: The greater the disability, the greater the impact of premature aging.
- Time of onset of disability and how it impacts individual development: Individuals with a history of traumatic brain injury at an early age (less than 5 years of age) have a poorer prognosis for functional outcomes. For adults with childhood-onset spinal cord injury, a younger age at injury and longer time with physical disability are associated with increased hip subluxation and/or spine scoliosis.

- Years with a disability
- Type and number of disabilities in an individual: The more complex the disability and the greater the number of systems involved, the greater the risk of premature aging.

Clinical Features
- Chronic pain
- Peripheral neurologic compression may occur due to the use of crutches, propelling manual wheelchairs, and/or transfer techniques. The median nerve at the wrist is most commonly affected, with the ulnar nerve at the wrist and elbow being less frequently involved.
- Overuse injuries to the shoulders are common in individuals who depend on manual wheelchairs for mobility.
- Decreased flexibility, pain, and spasticity can lead to contractures.
- Osteoarthritis is commonly seen in CP due to altered biomechanics, poor motor control, and muscle imbalance. Total hip and knee replacements are an option for pain management in adults with CP.
- Balance deficits
- Osteoporosis: Bone mineral density (BMD) testing and fall prevention are important for women and men with disabilities. Current recommendations are to use the BMD scan results for the distal femur in children with CP and contractures. Bisphosphonates are recommended, but long-term effects are not known.
- Depression
- Social isolation
- Weakness, with loss of mobility and function
- Increased functional dependence
- Hypertension
- Dyslipidemia is very common in persons with spinal cord injury; especially elevated serum low-density lipoprotein cholesterol and reduced serum high-density lipoprotein cholesterol level. This results in a higher cardiovascular risk.
- Gastroesophageal reflux disease, stasis in the duodenum, and gastrointestinal dysmotility worsen in CP, spinal cord injury, spina bifida, and traumatic brain injury patients when transitioning from childhood to adulthood.
- Dementia/cognitive deficits: At least one third of people with Down syndrome can expect to develop Alzheimer disease by middle age.
- Cervical spondylotic myelopathy; common in adults with athetoid CP.
- Respiratory deficits; frequently due to central nervous system dysfunctions and/or severe motor disabilities with aging, regardless of whether the primary cause of the disability is progressive or nonprogressive.
- Pressure ulcers/skin breakdown
- Bowel/bladder dysfunction
- Nephrolithiasis; especially in individuals with neurogenic bladders (e.g., spinal cord injury, spina bifida)
- Dysphagia
- Communication deficits
- Hearing loss; may develop in adult Down syndrome patients.
- Medication hypersensitivity due to reduced metabolic clearance. Drug responses are usually stronger than in younger subjects, and the rate and intensity of adverse effects is higher.

Prevention
- Conservative techniques and strategies should be implemented early on.
- Comprehensive multidisciplinary care.
- Musculoskeletal, skin, gastrointestinal, cardiovascular, and respiratory functions should be monitored early on in management and then throughout adulthood.
- Preventative general health evaluations should be facilitated.

Treatment
- Management should be individualized and specific to aging symptoms.
- Prevention with early treatment/treatments and intervention/interventions is encouraged.
- Counseling and support from a multidisciplinary team should be performed throughout the treatment process, including how daily life for the patient and the family may be positively and negatively influenced by a particular treatment plan.
- Psychotherapy to help with appropriate coping and management skills related to aging with a disability.

Red Flags
- Any health change in a disabled person should not be attributed to aging alone, until a complete evaluation is performed to rule out other treatable conditions and illnesses.
- Aged, disabled patients are at risk for abuse.

Prognosis
- Variable, depending on the extent of disability, coping skills, and each individual's available support system.

Helpful Hints
- Aging with a disability presents many challenges, including the successful transition to an adult-centered health care system with age-appropriate services (e.g., routine health promotion and screening).
- Create awareness of the common medical, physical, and functional needs associated with aging for the disabled.
- More research is needed examining the area of aging with a disability in order to optimize resource utilization, as well as the long-term care and outcomes of these patients.

Suggested Readings
Binks JA, Barden WS, Burke TA, et al. What do we really know about the transition to adult-centered health care? A focus on cerebral palsy and spina bifida. *Arch Phys Med Rehabil.* 2007;88(8):1064–1073.

Greco SM, Vincent C. Disability and aging. *J Gerontol Nurs.* 2011;13:1–10.

Haak P, Lenski M, Hidecker MJC, et al. Cerebral palsy and aging. *Dev Med Child Neurol.* 2009;51(S4):16–23.

Klingbeil H, Baer HR, Wilson PE. Aging with a disability. *Arch Phys Med Rehabil.* 2004;85:68–73.

Aging With a Spinal Cord Injury

Thomas S. Kiser MD

Description
The life span of someone with a spinal cord injury (SCI) has significantly improved since 1936, when Dr Donald Munro started the first SCI service in the United States. As a result, the life span of people with SCIs is approaching normal, and aging in this population is becoming an important issue.

Key Principles
- The effects of aging appear more quickly in the individual with SCI, so it is important to be proactive with preventative strategies to minimize these effects.
- Individuals with SCI who have a higher neurologic level of injury, complete SCI, and who are older at the time of injury have a higher mortality rate.
- Aging has an effect on medication metabolism. A good review of medications used is important. Slowly tapering the dosage and frequency of use must be considered.
- Depression is common among individuals with SCI and is greater in those who have been injured for a long time and in those who are older.
- Individuals with SCI have a relatively good and stable life satisfaction over time, even after many years of living with a SCI.
- Routine medical and rehabilitation follow-up is important. Attention to the patient's complaints, functional activity, equipment, medication, and a good review of systems is important to mitigate the myriad of secondary complications that can develop with aging and a SCI.

Contraindications
- The chronic use of narcotics should be avoided if at all possible, due to the effect of narcotics on the gastrointestinal tract and respiratory system. There is also a significant risk of habituation and, thus, the need to increase doses over time. Medication diversion by caretakers is also a potential issue.
- If unable to avoid, the lowest narcotic dose possible should be used, and it should not be increased over time.
- The chronic use of benzodiazepines for spasticity should be avoided. It is difficult to wean patients from benzodiazepines after they have used them chronically for years. There are medications with less risk factors and complications that can be used for the treatment of spasticity.
- Benzodiazepines exhibit slow cognition and reaction time, even in patients who deny side effects.
- Medications that are relatively contraindicated in a general geriatric practice (soma, valium, etc.) should also be avoided in older SCI patients; as the person with SCI ages more quickly, it makes sense to avoid these medications in the first place.

Conditions That the SCI Patient Is at Risk for
- Pressure sores
  - Incidence increases with age from about 15% in the first year after injury to about 30%, 20 years after injury.
  - The odds ratio for developing pressure ulcers has been shown to increase every year after injury.
  - Prevention efforts, periodic skin assessments, and reinforcement of prevention strategies are all important.
- Arm pain
  - Reported by more than 50% of SCI subjects
  - There is a positive association between aging and shoulder pain.
  - Poor sitting posture, increased use, and abnormal stresses with transfers, wheelchair use, and bed mobility put the shoulder at risk of a rotator cuff tear.
- Urologic issues
  - Persons with an indwelling catheter have a higher rate of bladder stones, urinary tract infections, and bladder cancer.
  - Screening cystoscopy is recommended in these patients.
  - In patients with bladder stones consideration should be given to changing the catheter more often.

- Prostate cancer in SCI is usually diagnosed at a more advanced grade and stage; screening in this population should be considered at age 50.
- Osteoporosis
  - One third of the original bone mass is lost in the initial 16 months after injury; bone mass then stabilizes.
  - Thus, bone fracture risk is a major concern.
  - Measures to prevent falls and aggressive forces across the paralyzed limbs need to be encouraged to prevent fracture.
- Neurologic problems
  - 11% to 20% of individuals with SCI who have had SCI for more than 20 years experience some deterioration of neurologic function, such as a loss of one or more neurologic levels of spinal cord function.
  - Up to 63% of those with paraplegia show evidence of entrapment neuropathies, with the most frequent site being the median nerve at the wrist or hand. Power wheelchairs should be considered to prevent this problem.
  - Post-traumatic cystic myelopathy, or syrinx, can occur from several months to several decades after the initial SCI, but most commonly within the first 5 to 10 years after injury. It can present as increased spasticity, pain, or worsening of functional abilities.
- Heterotopic ossification
  - Heterotopic ossification usually presents early after a SCI.
  - It is clinically significant in 20% to 30% of patients, but only proceeds to ankylosis in less than 10%.
  - However, when present, deceased joint range of motion needs to be managed to accommodate good sitting and adequate function.
- Autonomic dysfunction
  - Seen in SCI with an injury above the T6 level
  - More severe in higher level SCI subjects
  - More prevalent in complete SCI as compared to incomplete SCI.
- Neuropathic pain
  - Neuropathic pain is characterized by burning, stabbing, and/or electric shock-like symptoms and can occur at or below the level of SCI.
  - The treatment is difficult and the pain is mitigated, but not removed, with the use of antiseizure, antidepressants, and/or narcotic medications.
  - Narcotic medication should be used with care, as described above.
- Coronary artery disease
  - Heart disease is the leading cause of death in long-term SCI. Risk factors include
    - Higher level SCI
    - Greater completeness of SCI
    - Low HDL
    - Increased prevalence of diabetes mellitus
- Respiratory problems
  - Respiratory disorders are the leading causes of rehospitalization and death in acute and chronic SCI.
  - Vital capacity should be measured periodically.
  - Annual immunization against influenza and pneumococcus, as appropriate, is recommended.
  - Sleep disorder breathing has a prevalence ranging from 25% to 35%.

Preventing/Treating Problems

- Routine skin checks by care givers and the treating physician are important; frequent pressure relief is essential for all individuals with SCI, and even more so in the elderly.
- Shoulder exercises to address the posterior shoulder girdle and good wheelchair mechanics should be addressed. Consideration should be given to the use of power wheelchairs to prevent overuse and degenerative problems.
- If heterotopic ossification severely limits function, a wedge resection of the bone followed by irradiation, bisphosphonates, and passive range of motion can be considered.
- When the symptoms of a syrinx are progressive, surgical treatment with untethering, duraplasty, and, in some cases, shunting of the syrinx is warranted.

Helpful Hints

- Schedule routine medical and rehabilitation follow-up to address issues as they come up. A good review of systems is important to mitigate the myriad of secondary complications that can develop with aging and SCI.
- Attention should be paid to patient complaints
  - A decline in function should not be accepted just because patients are getting older.
- Technology and advances in equipment and medication have provided new management options.
- If at all possible, the chronic use of narcotics should be avoided.
- The chronic use of benzodiazepines (such as valium for spasticity) should be avoided; better medications for the treatment of spasticity are now available.
- For a list of medications to avoid in the elderly, see

- http://archinte.ama-assn.org/cgi/content/full/163/22/2716
- www.dcri.org/trial-participation/the-beers-list/

Suggested Readings

Charlifue S, Jha A, Lammertse D. Aging with spinal cord injury. *Phys Med Rehabil Clin N Am.* 2009;21:383–402.

Krassioukov A, Waburton DE, Teasell R, et al. A systematic review of the management of autonomic dysfunction after SCI. *Arch Phys Med Rehabil.* 2009;90:682–695.

Teasell RW, Mehta S, Aubut JL, et al. A systematic review of the therapeutic interventions for heterotopic ossification after spinal cord injury. *Spinal Cord.* 2010;48:512–521.

Whiteneck GG, Charlifue SW, Gehart KA, et al., eds. *Aging with Spinal Cord Injury.* New York, NY: Demos Publications; 1993.

Alternative Medicine

Lisa Merritt MD

Description

- Complementary and alternative medicine (CAM) has come into great favor over the last two decades.
- The 2007 National Health Interview Survey (NHIS) indicated that 38% of American adults use CAM, spending $33.9 billion a year out of pocket (a 14% increase since 2002). CAM is becoming more and more sought after by patients.
- The president of the American Academy of Anti-Aging Medicine Dr Ronald Katz notes that the worldwide antiaging market is valued at $115 billion.
- In the United States, this consumer-driven surge of interest in alternative and complementary practices is driven by the large demographic of aging post-World War II "Baby Boomers."
- From Harvard to the Mayo Clinic, most major universities and medical centers have to some degree incorporated what was once considered "alternative" practices into mainstream or "conventional" medicine.
- This pairing of services has come to be known as "complementary medicine," where different approaches are combined for the optimal benefit of the patient and patient care outcomes.
- Practitioners who incorporate both conventional and complementary approaches are known as "integrative medicine" (IM) practitioners.
- Alternative medicine is when practitioners use CAM instead of conventional medicine.
- Complementary medicine is defined by the National Center for Complementary and Alternative Medicine (NCCAM) as "A group of diverse medical and health care systems, practices, and products that are not generally considered part of conventional medicine."
- CAM practitioners have varied levels of training and experience, ranging from allopathic medical doctors (MD) and osteopathic doctors (DO) to acupuncturists (LAc), Naturopath (ND) herbalists, and many other disciplines.
- There is no standardized, national system for credentialing CAM practitioners. The extent and type of credentialing vary widely from state to state and from one CAM profession to another.

Key Principles

- Practitioners may use CAM to treat many conditions such as
  - Arthritis/inflammatory processes
  - Autism
  - Adrenal support/stress management
  - Brain support/cognitive enhancement
  - Cancer/immune dysfunction
  - Cellular support/mitochondrial dysfunction
  - Environmental toxicities
  - Fatigue
  - Fibromyalgia
  - Gastrointestinal health
  - Glucose management
  - Male health issues
  - Female health issues
  - Mental health issues/depression/anxiety
  - Nutritional support
  - Pain management
  - Sleep disorders
  - Weight management
  - Vascular health
- There are many different approaches, techniques, and philosophies in CAM. Some may be regional, and some are influenced by certain traditional healing or cultural beliefs.
- A common philosophy in CAM is the attempt to consider the "whole person"; hence, the prior terminology of "holistic" clinicians. This philosophy differs somewhat from conventional medicine. However, the difference may be primarily due to the organization of conventional medicine into primary care (with a more holistic focus) versus specialty care (more disease or organ system oriented).
- In addition, there is often a strong emphasis on prevention of imbalance leading to disease, as opposed to the medical model of diagnosing and treating a disorder once it has occurred.
- The broad classes of CAM may include
  - Natural products and supplements
  - Topical or specially compounded agents

- Specialized delivery systems using intravenous therapies, inhalation therapies, or other delivery systems
- Energy or "mind–body" medicine

Treatments

Natural products and supplements
- May include herbs, homeopathic agents, tinctures, nutritional supplements or combinations, vitamins, and essential minerals
- A popular example is the use of echinacea for early cold symptoms.
- Many detoxification protocols such as chelation therapy use intravenous approaches or suppositories, with a specialized cocktail of vitamins and other agents.
- The trial to assess chelation therapy (TACT) sponsored by the National Heart, Lung, and Blood Institute (NHLBI) and National Center for Complementary and Alternative Medicine (NCCAM) will soon have results of a prospective study that they are carrying out on this modality.

Topical or specially compounded agents
- May include a wide variety of crèmes, lotions, oils, or poultices that are applied to the body, injected, or inhaled for their reported therapeutic benefits.
- For example, many athletes find use of Arnica crème helpful for minor aches and pains and lavender has been incorporated into numerous formulations for its reported calming effect.
- Mesotherapy is used widely in Europe for tendonitis and myofascial pain syndrome.

Energy or mind–body medicine
- May include hands-on therapies such as acupuncture, manipulative therapies, craniosacral therapy, massage, and "no touch" techniques such as Reiki, qi-gong, yoga, guided imagery, and various meditative practices.
- Electrotherapy and biofeedback are sometimes also included in this category.
- Mind–body approaches have been found to be useful adjuncts for patients under great stress, for example, patients in pain, cancer survivors, and cardiac patients.

Research and CAM
- Many alternative therapies have been tested, but the results have varied.
- Rigorous, well-designed clinical trials for many CAM therapies are often lacking.
- Accordingly, the safety and effectiveness of many CAM therapies is uncertain.
- According to a 2005 U.S. Institute of Medicine report, the number of randomized controlled trials focused on CAM has risen dramatically since 1998. However, many of the CAM-related clinical trials that have been conducted are not published in conventional medical journals and are not available in MEDLINE.
- There is now in the National Institutes of Health, the NCCAM, which is dedicated to conducting evidence-based research in a variety of CAM practices.
- The NCCAM is attempting to fill the knowledge gap by funding research studies designed to build a scientific evidence base for CAM therapies—whether they are safe, and whether they work for the conditions for which people use them, and, if so, how they work.

Criticism of CAM
- Because of the differences between conventional medicine and CAM, and because of the largely unproven efficacy and safety, CAM and integrative medicine are still viewed by many within the mainstream medical community as controversial.
  - For example, Dr Arnold Relman, editor-in-chief emeritus of *The New England Journal of Medicine* wrote: "There are not two kinds of medicine, one conventional and the other unconventional, that can be practiced jointly in a new kind of 'integrative medicine.'"
  - References to CAM as "pseudoscience," "illegitimate" therapy," and "a new kind of snake oil" can be found on recent journal editorial pages and scientific blogs.
- Despite this criticism, courses on CAM and IM are being introduced into a growing number of U.S. medical schools—perhaps an acknowledgement that even conventional physicians will need more knowledge of therapies that more and more of their patients are exploring.

CAM Awareness
- The NCCAM in the National Institutes of Health has launched an educational campaign, "Time to Talk," to encourage older patients and their health care providers to openly discuss the use of CAM.
- The goals of this campaign are: more effective management of patient health by providers who

are more aware of CAM, and better information for patients to facilitate fully informed health care decisions.
- NCCAM has posted the following consumer information:
  - As with any medical treatment, there can be risks with CAM therapies. The following general precautions can help to minimize risks:
    - Select CAM practitioners with care. Find out about the practitioner's training and experience.
    - Be aware that some dietary supplements may interact with medications or other supplements, may have side effects of their own, or may contain potentially harmful ingredients not listed on the label.
    - Also keep in mind that most supplements have not been tested in pregnant women, nursing mothers, or children.
    - Tell all your health care providers about any complementary and alternative practices you use. Give them a full picture of what you do to manage your health. This will help ensure co-ordinated and safe care.

Helpful Hints
- Caution is advised to evaluate the credentials of practitioners, the source of natural products, and the potential for adverse interactions with conventional pharmaceuticals.
- Good communication with one's primary care physician or an integrative practitioner will help to best determine the optimal approach to seeking CAM modalities.

Suggested Readings

American College for the Advancement of Medicine, www.acam.org

American Academy of Anti-aging Medicine (A4M). www.worldhealth.net

American Association of Integrative Medicine. www.aaimedicine.com/about/

Brown D: Scientists speak out against federal funds for research on alternative medicine. *The Washington Post.* March 17, 2009.

Consumer Labs. www.consumerlabs.com/

Institute of Medicine. *Complementary and Alternative Medicine in the United States.* Washington, DC: National Academy Press; 2005.

National Center for Complementary and Alternative Medicine. http://nccam.nih.gov

Perlman A, Stagnaro-Green A. Developing a complementary, alternative, and integrative medicine course: One medical school's experience. *J Alternat Complement Med.* 2010;16:601–605.

Thomson PDR. *PDR for Nonprescription Drugs, Dietary Supplements, and Herbs.* 28th ed. Montvale, NJ: Thomson Healthcare; 2007.

Driving Evaluation

Florian S. Keplinger MD

Key Principles
- People 65 and above are the fastest growing segment of the driving population. As the number of elderly drivers increases, the competence of the elderly to drive becomes a growing concern for health care providers, caregivers, and the public in general.
- Having a driver's license symbolizes autonomy and competence. For many older adults, losing the ability to drive is almost equivalent to losing the ability to walk. Their need to be able to continue driving becomes even more evident as they grow older, because of their increasing physical limitations (e.g., joint problems, diminished walking endurance, and vulnerability to extremes of environmental temperature).

Epidemiology
- The National Highway Traffic Safety Administration driving statistics show that in 2006, when the last data was computed, there were nearly 30 million elderly drivers driving on the streets of America. The statistics further showed that in 2006, 6,017 elderly people were killed in road accidents and this figure is around 14% of total people killed by road accidents.
- It is predicted that by 2030, the elderly will comprise nearly 25% of the total people driving and they will be involved in nearly 25% of fatal vehicular accidents.

Risk Factors for Traffic Accidents
- Medical diagnoses that are inherently unpredictable or episodic
  - Syncope
  - Hypoglycemia
  - Seizure
  - Transient ischemic attack
  - Angina
  - Narcolepsy
- Acute medical conditions
  - Recent stroke
  - Acute myocardial infarction
  - Surgery
- Chronic medical conditions, which can affect driving ability
  - Vision disorders—cataracts, diabetic retinopathy, macular degeneration, and glaucoma
  - Cardiovascular disease—congestive heart failure, valvular disorders, arrhythmias, unstable angina, peripheral vascular disease, and anemia
  - Pulmonary disease—sleep apnea and chronic obstructive/restrictive lung disease
  - Metabolic disease—uncontrolled diabetes mellitus, hypothyroidism, and renal failure requiring dialysis
  - Musculoskeletal disorders—arthritis, disc disease, contractures, joint replacement/repair, and amputation
  - Neurologic disease—dementia, stroke, Parkinson's disease, and peripheral neuropathy
  - Psychiatric disease—psychosis, alcohol/substance abuse, anxiety, and depression

Assessment
- Functional History provides information on the patient's ability to perform activities of mobility and daily living; can be considered as an indirect evidence for driving abilities and cognitive status.
- Social History will reveal if a patient's lack of social support is the reason a patient is reluctant to give up driving, even if the patient is aware of difficulties.
- Vehicular Factors reveal if the vehicle being driven has safety features (seatbelts, airbags, antilock brakes) known to decrease injury. Power steering, automatic transmission, and larger mirrors (side and rear view) can compensate for the problems with which the elderly have most difficulty: turning and braking.
- Assessment of environmental factors can help to determine if a patient merely needs to limit driving to low-risk conditions, namely
  - Rural versus urban
  - Daytime versus nighttime
  - Short versus long distances
- Medication profile
  - Many prescription and nonprescription medications have the potential to impair driving ability, either inherently or when interacting with other drugs.
- Review of systems
  - This can reveal symptoms, which can impair driving abilities, such as

- Vision difficulties
- Fatigue and dizziness/vertigo
- Chest pains
- Palpitations
- Shortness of breath
- Decreased balance
- Joint pains
- Numbness
- Weakness
- Memory loss

Physician Evaluation

- Physician assessment of driving-related skills (ADRS)
  - Vision
    - Visual fields (confrontation testing)
    - Visual acuity (Snellen E chart)
  - Motor function
    - Rapid pace walk (patient is asked to walk on a 10-ft path, turn around and walk back to the starting point as quickly as possible; a walker or cane may be used if the patient normally walks with it)
    - Active joint range of motion (neck, fingers, shoulder, elbow, and ankle)
    - Motor strength—manual muscle testing
  - Cognition
    - Trail-making test, Part B (involves timing the ability to connect encircled numbers 1 to 12, and letters A to L, in alternating order; a score greater than 180 seconds is considered abnormal)
    - Clock-drawing test (checks the ability to properly draw a clock, with proper placement of numbers and hands)

Driver Rehabilitation Specialist Evaluation

- Predriving evaluation, including a clinical assessment similar to that of the physician's
- Functional on-road assessment
- Communication of results and recommendations to patient
- Passenger vehicle evaluation
- Treatment and intervention
- Follow-up with physician to discuss results of driving evaluation
- Counseling patient who is no longer safe to drive, and recruitment of family and friends to come up with alternate means of transportation.

Ethical and Legal Responsibilities of the Physician

- Once you have identified an impaired driver, you have the primary responsibility of protecting the patient's mental and physical health.
- You should advise and counsel the patient and, if necessary, the family about driving cessation.
- Assist the patient with determining resources for transportation (enlisting the help of a social worker is recommended).
- Familiarize yourself with your state's Llicensing and reporting laws; certain states have mandatory reporting requirements, which place a physician in danger of both civil and criminal liability for failure to report.
- Before reporting to the State Department of Motor Vehicle (DMV), tell the patient what you are about to do; assure the patient that you will provide only the minimum information required, and keep all other information confidential.
- Document thoroughly all assessments and encounters, which provide evidence that you made efforts to assess and maintain the patient's safety and privacy.
- If your state has no reporting laws, your priority is to ensure that an unsafe driver does not drive; you may not need to report the patient if you can accomplish this by discussing it with the patient.
- If your impaired patient refuses to stop driving, then you have to decide which is more important: the potential for injury versus patient confidentiality (AMA Policy E-2.24 "in situations where clear evidence of substantial driving impairment implies a strong threat to patient and public safety, and where the physician's advice to discontinue driving privileges is ignored, it is desirable and ethical to notify the Department of Motor Vehicles.")
- If your state has a Medical Advisory Board (MAB), you may be able to ask for its assistance; an MAB is usually composed of locally licensed physicians, who work with the driver-licensing agency to determine whether mental and/or physical conditions may impair an individual's ability to drive safely.

Helpful Hints

- Carefully observe the patient throughout the clinical encounter for signs which can indicate an impaired driver (red flags).
- Impaired mobility, such as poor balance, difficulty walking, or problems transferring from different surfaces should be assessed.

- Poor hygiene and/or grooming should be noted.
- Difficulty with visual tasks should be assessed.
- Impaired attention, memory, language, comprehension, or expression should be evaluated.
- Be alert to any medical condition, medication, or symptom which can affect driving skills (see the section titled Risk Factors for Traffic Accidents).
- Advise elderly patients to take a driver safety class (e.g., AARP 55 Alive Driver Safety Program, AAA Safe Driving for Mature Operators Program, National Safety Council Defensive Driving Course).
- Each state's reporting laws vary—make sure you know them; if you fail to follow them, you may be liable for patient and third-party injuries.
- Document diligently and thoroughly, in the event of a crash injury.

Suggested Readings

Carr DB, Schwartzberg JG, Manning L, et al. Physician's guide to assessing and counseling older drivers. 2nd ed. Washington, DC: NHTSA; 2010. http://www.ama-assn.org/ama1/pub/upload/mm/433/older-drivers-guide.pdf

Baby Boomer Care. www.babyboomercaretaker.com/Law/Elderly-Driving-Statistics.html

Keplinger FS. The elderly driver: Who should continue to drive. *Phys Med Rehabil: State Art Rev.* 12(1). Philadelphia, PA: Hanley & Belfus, Inc.; 1998:147–154.

National Highway Traffic Safety Administration (NHTSA). Family and friends concerned about an older driver; August 2001. www.nhtsa.dot.gov/people/injury/olddrive/FamilynFriends/state.htm

Ethics

Kimberly A. Curseen MD ■ Sarah E. Harrington MD

Description
Ethics is defined as the rules or standards governing the conduct of a person or the conduct of members of a profession. Medical ethics is the moral construct governing the set of ethical principles by which practitioners communicate and provide care to patients.

Principles Governing Practitioner/Patient Interactions
- Beneficence: to act in the best interest of the patient; patient welfare and benefit are the first considerations.
- Nonmaleficence: do no harm; respect for the worth of the patient and avoid treatments that knowingly cause harm; respect for the sanctity of life.
- Autonomy: respect for the right of self-determination; a patient with capacity may accept or reject any form of medical therapy.
- Justice: protect vulnerable populations and provide fair allocation of resources; actions should be consistent, accountable, and transparent.
- Veracity: truth telling, obligation to full and honest disclosure.
- Confidentiality: except when legally or ethically required, confidentiality of all personal and medical treatments must be maintained; basis of loyalty and trust.
- Virtue: relates to the professional's moral character which guides behavior; these includes fidelity, compassion/empathy, effacement of self-interest, respect for personhood, intellectual honesty, and prudence.

Informed Consent
Informed consent is the process of communication between a patient/surrogate decision maker and the practitioner that results in the patient's voluntary authorization or refusal of a specific medical intervention. Informed consent must include the following:
- Explanation of the procedure/treatment and reasonable alternatives
- Explanation of risk and benefits of procedure and alternatives
- Assessment of understanding of procedure/treatment and risks/benefits
- Agreement or decline of proposed procedure/treatment

Preconditions for informed consent
- *Decisional capacity*: The patient must have the ability to understand, deliberate, and decide on information.
- *Voluntariness*: Decisions must occur without coercion by others or highly coercive conditions.

Capacity and competence
- Capacity requires that a patient is given adequate information, can understand the relevant risks and benefits of the presented treatment/procedure, and, based on this understanding, communicate a choice to the persons obtaining the consent. Any physician can assess capacity.
- Competency is a legal determination by a legal authority, which refers to a patient's ability to make decisions and understand the consequences and complexity of those decisions.
- If a patient lacks decisional capacity, the health care team will call upon a surrogate decision maker.
- Patients with an advance directive will usually appoint a Durable Healthcare Power of Attorney (DHPOA) or heath care proxy to serve in this role.
- In the absence of an advance directive, there is a hierarchy of family decision makers that is defined by each state, which usually starts with the spouse of an adult patient.
- Surrogates have the right to consent to treatment *and* the right to refuse treatment for the patient.
- Surrogate decision makers are guided by the following principles:
  - Best interest: to act in the medical interest of the patient, weighing the benefits and burdens of therapy
  - Substituted judgment: an attempt to make the decision the patient would have made under the circumstances

End-of-Life Care Issues

Many ethical issues surround end-of-life care for patients.

- Cessation of life-sustaining treatments (LSTs) is an act where a physician, after a request from a patient or surrogate, either *withholds or withdraws* resuscitation efforts, medication, ventilation, artificial hydration, or nutrition, which is helping to sustain the biological functions of the patient.
- The underlying disease that is allowed to run its natural course would be the cause of death.
- It is ethically and legally acceptable for patients with capacity or their surrogates to decide to forgo or withdraw LSTs.

Controversial Issues

- Euthanasia—An act by a medical professional where both the means necessary are provided and the final act of causing death is performed by said-professional for merciful or beneficial reasons; illegal in the United States.
- Suicide—Act of a person intentionally causing his/her own death. Attempted suicide is *not* illegal, but is grounds for immediate, involuntary psychiatric evaluation.
- Physician-assisted suicide (PAS)—An act where a patient intentionally takes his/her own life through means (typically prescribed drugs) provided by a licensed physician. The controversy around PAS concerns primarily the role that physicians should be allowed to (or are expected to) play in end-of-life care. PAS is legal in three American states—Oregon, Washington, and Montana.

Suggested Readings

American Medical Association. *Code of Medical Ethics*. Council on Ethical and Judicial Affairs; 2010–2011. Beaucheamp TL. Principlism and its alleged competitor. *Kennedy Inst Ethics U*. 1995;5(3):181–198.

Ethics in medicine. University of Washington School of Medicine. http://depts.washington.edu/bioethx/topics/consent.html

Gillion R. Medical ethics: Four principles plus attention to scope. *BMJ*. 1995;310(6974):261–262.

Jonsen AR, Siegler M, Winsland WJ. *Clinical Ethics*. New York, NY: Macmillan; 1982.

Pellegrino ED. Toward a virtue-based normative ethics for the health care professions. *Kennedy Inst Ethic J*. 1995;5(3):253–277.

Exercise

Patrick M. Kortebein MD

Description
Physical activity is defined as bodily movement that is produced by skeletal muscle contraction and that substantially increases energy expenditure. *Exercise* (a type of physical activity) is a planned, structured, and repetitive bodily movement done to improve or maintain one or more components of physical fitness (e.g., muscle strength, flexibility, balance). Both have known positive benefits for older adults, including prolonged life expectancy and improved quality of life.

Age-Related Changes in Physical Capability
- Aerobic capacity declines by 1% to 2% per year after age 40, with a more precipitous decline after age 70.
- Muscle strength declines 10% to 15% per decade after about age 40.
- Maximum heart rate declines with aging and may be estimated with standard equations (220 minus age; 164 minus [0.7 × age] for individuals on beta-blockers).
- Only 39% of adults above age 65 perform the minimum recommended amount of physical activity.
- The prevalence of asymptomatic coronary artery disease is much greater in older individuals.
- The relative risk of a myocardial infarction in the first hour after vigorous exertion in an older individual is approximately twice that of a younger subject.
- The risk of cardiac arrhythmia during exercise is approximately 1:30,000 and death 1:150,000.

History
- Prior to initiating a physical activity/exercise program, older adults should review their individual risks and benefits with their physician.
- As per standard guidelines (see the American College of Sports Medicine Guidelines for Exercise Testing and Prescription), cardiac risk factors and symptoms at rest or with exertion (e.g., chest pain, palpitations, dyspnea, orthopnea, dizziness/syncope) should be evaluated.
- Although formal exercise or pharmacologic stress testing could be recommended for virtually all sedentary older adults prior to initiating a physical activity/exercise program, it seems more prudent to assess potential risk using simple functional tasks (see the following section titled Physical Examination), due to the increased morbidity and mortality associated with stress testing.

Physical Examination
The following should be evaluated during the screening evaluation for an older adult prior to initiating an exercise program.

Vital signs
- Elevated heart rate (greater than 100 bpm) or abnormal rhythm requires further investigation
- Blood pressure (exercise is contraindicated if systolic pressure exceeds 200 mmHg or diastolic pressure exceeds 110 mmHg)

Cardiopulmonary evaluation
- Evaluation for murmurs, rales, and pedal edema

Neuromusculoskeletal evaluation
- Joint examination and range of motion
- Neurologic examination focused on motor/sensory/reflex function
- Gait evaluation (for safety)

Vascular evaluation
- Foot pulses and capillary refill

Functional activities
- Recommended functional stress testing activities may include climbing one flight of stairs and walking 15 m; exercise is contraindicated if there is angina or significant shortness of breath.
- A 400-m corridor walk may be used to estimate peak oxygen consumption in healthy older adults.

Testing
- Electrocardiogram (ECG); evaluation for new Q waves, ST segment depression, or T wave inversion.
- Laboratory studies (e.g., complete blood count, electrolytes, blood urea nitrogen/creatinine, BUN/Cr, if warranted)

Contraindications to Exercise
- Myocardial infarction in past 6 months (See also Suggested Readings by American College of Sports Medicine; Bean; and Williams)
- Angina or signs/symptoms of heart failure (e.g., bilateral rales, shortness of breath with/without pedal edema)

Recommended Types of Physical Activity/Exercise
Below are the recommended minimum amounts and types of physical activity/exercise for all older adults (i.e., all individuals above age 65 and those aged 50 to 64 years with clinically significant chronic medical conditions and/or functional limitations). Individuals unaccustomed to exercise are advised to start at a low intensity and gradually increase, if they remain asymptomatic.

Aerobic/cardiovascular
- Duration/frequency:
  - Moderate intensity: 30 minutes cumulative (minimum 10 minutes per session), 5 days per week
  - Vigorous intensity: 20 minutes, 3 days per week.
- Intensity (rating of perceived exertion, RPE: 0—rest/sitting, 10—maximal effort)
  - Moderate (5–6/10)
  - Vigorous (7–8/10)
  - Moderate and vigorous intensity activities may be combined

Resistance exercise/muscle strengthening
- Frequency: two nonconsecutive days per week
- Mode: 8 to 10 exercises, including all major muscle groups of the upper and lower extremities
- Intensity: Moderate to high intensity/10 to 15 repetitions per exercise
- Valsalva maneuver should be avoided during resistance exercise.

Flexibility
- Stretching of the major muscle groups 2 days per week for 10 minutes each day (10–30 seconds per stretch).

Balance
- Individuals who have fallen or who are at risk for falls should perform balance exercises.

Older adults should develop an activity plan to include the above elements in consultation with their physician or a qualified fitness professional.

Anticipated Problems/Complications
- Individuals with asymptomatic cardiac disease may become symptomatic; these individuals require evaluation and possible cardiac testing.
- Previously, sedentary individuals initiating a physical activity/exercise program are at the greatest risk of a cardiac event and should be monitored closely.
- Older individuals are at a greater risk of musculoskeletal injuries related to exercise.

Benefits of Physical Activity/Exercise
- Physical activity has been found to be beneficial for virtually every organ system, although the cardiopulmonary and musculoskeletal systems derive the greatest benefits.
- Adhering to the aforementioned recommendations regarding physical activity can reduce the risk of chronic disease, functional limitations, disability, and premature mortality.

Suggested Readings
American College of Sports Medicine. *Guidelines for Exercise Testing and Prescription*. 7th ed. Baltimore, MD: Lipincott Williams and Wilkins; 2006.

Bean JF, Vora A, Frontera WR. Benefits of exercise for community-dwelling older adults. *Arch Phys Med Rehabil*. 2004;85(Suppl. 3):S31–42.

Brawner CA, Ehrman JK, Schairer JR, et al. Predicting maximum heart rate among patients with coronary heart disease receiving beta-adrenergic blockade therapy. *Am Heart J*. 2004;148:910–914.

Gill TM, DiPietro L, Krumholz HM. Role of exercise stress testing and safety monitoring for older persons starting an exercise program. *JAMA*. 2000;284:342–349.

Nelson ME, Rejeski WJ, Blair SN, et al. Physical activity and public health in older adults: Recommendation from the American College of Sports Medicine and the American Heart Association. *Circulation*. 2007;116:1094–1105.

Simonsick EM, Fan E, Fleg JL. Estimating cardiorespiratory fitness in well-functioning older adults: Treadmill validation of the long distance corridor walk. *J Am Geriatr Soc*. 2006;54:127–132.

Williams MA, Haskell WL, Ades PA, et al. Resistance exercise in individuals with and without cardiovascular disease: 2007 update. *Circulation* 2007;116:572–584.

Home and Environment Modifications

Kevin M. Means MD

Key Principles
- The physical environment can either enhance or impede the independence and mobility of older people. Since people spend a significant part of their lives in homes, the physical environment of the home is an important factor in their daily function.
- More than 80% of older Americans prefer to remain in their homes rather than move to an assisted living or nursing home setting, even in the presence of a disabling condition.
- Home should represent a familiar setting and a source of comfort and security. Newer homes are often designed to maximize functional independence.
- Older residences may lack structural features that can assist older persons (who are more likely to have disabling conditions) in safe mobility and performance of their activities of daily living (ADLs).
- The two most frequently studied issues related to the home environment of older persons are home safety hazards and home physical barriers. Both of these issues can be addressed by modifications and assistive technology.

Home Hazards
- Many home environment hazards have been reported in the geriatric rehabilitation and falls prevention literature.
- In one large in-house study of community-living older persons
  - The prevalence of home hazards ranged from 22% for dim lighting to 61% for no grab bars in the tub/shower.
  - Two or more hazards were found in most bathrooms and in some other rooms.
  - Almost all homes had at least two potential hazards.
  - Half of the homes with stairs had two or more stair hazards.
  - Of the 20 potential hazards studied, 9 were significantly less common in senior housing than in community housing.
  - Two hazards (unsafe chair and light switches not clearly marked) were significantly more common in senior housing than in community housing.
  - Grab bars in the tub/shower were absent in 77% of community housing, but in only 9% of age-restricted housing.

Home Environment Barriers
- Homes may present several physical barriers to independence and safe mobility.
- Barriers are relative and emerge as the motor, sensory, or cognitive ability of the older individual declines.
- A home environment once considered to be safe can present barriers after hospitalization, or after acquisition of a new illness or impairment.
- Examples of barriers include
  - Absent or unsteady entrance or stairway railings
  - Poor lighting
  - Slippery bathroom or kitchen floors
  - Low toilet seats
  - Unstable furniture
  - Clutter
  - Inaccessible light switches, telephones, or cabinets
- 25% of older adults have a lower body impairment and an unmodified barrier in their home and may be considered in need of a home modification.

The Physician's Role in Home Assessment and Modifications
- Physicians caring for older patients living at home can help by identifying potential needs and by proposing and prioritizing possible home adaptations.
- Help can be provided directly by the physician or more typically, through referral to an occupational therapist.
- Other rehabilitation team members who may assist in this important assessment include the physical therapist, home health nurse, or social worker.
- Several home assessment tools are available for use by clinicians.
- A home visit will provide direct information about the home environment and will lead to more specific interventions. Unfortunately, home visits are increasingly rare, primarily due to limited reimbursement.

Home Modifications

- The modifications and priorities for individual homes depend on the patient's current and anticipated future medical conditions, environmental restrictions, and available resources.
- Some older persons may decide to move to homes built on universal design standards or within communities developed to meet the needs of disabled seniors.
- For others who live in general or older housing, home modification may allow them to stay in their homes and neighborhoods and remain engaged in existing social networks and activities.
- Home modification cost varies with the features required. For example, bathroom modifications can range from a few hundred dollars (raised toilet seat, nonslip tub mat, tub bench, grab bar) to several thousand dollars (widen doorway, wheelchair accessible shower). Patient resources should be considered in modification planning.
- In a 2006 survey of older adults asking about assistive home features, the most common features were entrance railings (36%), grab bars in shower/tub (30%), and a shower/tub seat (27%).
- Home owners were more likely than renters to add assistive features to their home.

Efficacy of Home Modifications

- The efficacy of home environment modifications in improving functioning and quality of life has been demonstrated in several studies.
- Home modification efficacy has been shown in disability prevention and reduction in personal care expenditures that would be used for institutional care; however, evidence regarding the economic benefits of care in the home environment is still mixed.
- A Cochrane review found little evidence that home environment modification prevents fall-related injuries; however, it did not show that home modifications were ineffective.
- Other evidence-based reviews report that environmental assessment and home modification are most successful in preventing falls in older adults, when conducted as part of a multidimensional risk assessment.

Home Assessment and Modification Resources

- Examples of home safety checklists are available at www.cdc.gov/ncipc/falls/default.htm.
- The American Association of Retired Persons offers free and low-cost publications on housing plans, home safety features, and modifications (www.aarp.org/home-garden/home-improvement/info-09–2009/what_is_universal_design.html).
- Local chapters of national organizations provide lists of reputable home remodeling contractors: National Association of Area Agencies on Aging (www.n4a.org/) and National Association of Home Builders (NAHB; www.nahb.org) (see also Table 1 below).

Table 1 Home Assessment Tools

Assesment Tool	Source	Online
Assessment and Intervention of the Home Environment for Older Persons	Center for Therapeutic Applications of Technology, University of Buffalo, Buffalo, New York	http://wings.buffalo.edu/academic/department/hrp/ot/cat/
Check for Safety: A Home Fall Prevention Checklist for Older Adults	Department of Health and Human Services, Centers for Disease Control and Prevention	www.cdc.gov/HomeandRecreationalSafety/pubs/English/booklet_Eng_desktop-a.pdf
Adapting Your Home for More Accessible Living	Janie Harris The Texas A&M University System	https://agrilifebookstore.org/tmppdfs/viewpdf_1389_63953.pdf?CFID=15506639&CFTOKEN=214dde57065a817b-5F4E5978-DFEC-01D0-1B9989B6C309D1A7&jsessionid=9030cf571ae594e3fd19486f116967426562
Designing Homes for Function and Safety	Janie Harris The Texas A&M University System	https://agrilifebookstore.org/tmppdfs/viewpdf_1388_12508.pdf?CFID=15506837&CFTOKEN=38d428a2b27a751b-5F558B95-CED9-561F-56675DBF96404F8B&jsessionid=9030cf571ae594e3fd19486f116967426562
Steps to Making Your Home and Community Safer and Better	American Association of Retired Persons	www.aarp.org/home-garden/livable-communities/info-05–2010/ho_order_form.html

Helpful Hints

- Older patients may not anticipate or recognize home environment hazards or barriers, especially after recent physical or functional changes.
- Home environmental assessment and modification needs should be addressed prior to discharge from the hospital.
- State and local aging or housing agencies may be able to provide home modification technical or funding assistance.
- Medicare Part B beneficiaries may be eligible for home occupational therapy assessment and training in the use of home modifications.
- Medicare pays for some durable medical equipment used in the home, but usually not the cost of home modification.
- Medicaid services vary by state, but some patients may qualify for home modifications through waiver programs.
- Other funding options include funding via reverse mortgages, long-term care insurance policies, and Veterans Affairs benefits.

Suggested Readings

Lyons RA, John A, Brophy S, et al. Modification of the home environment for the reduction of injuries. *Cochrane Database Syst Rev.* 2006;4:CD003600. Doi: 10.1002/14651858.CD003600.pub2.

Pynoos J, Steinman BA, Nguyen AQD. Environmental assessment and modification as fall-prevention strategies for older adults. *Clin Geriatr Med.* 2010;26:633–644.

Unwin BK, Andrews CM, Andrews PM, et al. Therapeutic home adaptations for older adults with disabilities. *Am Fam Physician.* 2009;80:963–968, 970.

Wahl HW, Fänge A, Oswald F, et al. The home environment and disability-related outcomes in aging individuals: What is the empirical evidence? *Gerontologist.* 2009;49:355–367.

Medicolegal Concerns

Hugh H. Gregory MD JD

Description
Medicolegal issues that are pertinent in rendering health care to the general population also are relevant to the geriatric population, but with particular focus on proactively addressing patient autonomy in health care treatment and end-of-life decision making.

Key Principles
- Chronological age should not be the only consideration for treatment options.
- Patient–family planning needs to be encouraged to maximize autonomy and to minimize disputes and legal interventions.
- Physicians need to be knowledgeable of local standards and precedents, as legal definitions and requirements are state-specific.

Autonomy and Beneficence
- Each person is best able to direct their own self-determination and preferences for health care.
- Generally, an informed person is able to best judge what sort of treatment is in their best interest.
- Informed consent protects patient autonomy.
- Patients have a right to promotion of their welfare and protection from harm.
- Physicians should practice nonmalfeasance, "first, do no harm."

Assessment of Patient Decision-Making Capacity
- The legal presumption is that adults are mentally competent.
- Competent patients are able to make their own informed decisions, including making an advance care directive and appointing a health care agent.
- Patient decision-making capacity is both time-specific and task-specific and must be evaluated at the time the decision is made and by the complexity of the decision.
- Patients must be able to understand information relevant to a health care decision.
- Patients must be able to appreciate the anticipated benefits, and the reasonably foreseeable risks of obtaining or declining a particular treatment.
- Patients must be able to communicate that choice to others.
- Competent people are allowed to make bad decisions; agreement with recommendations is not a requirement.
- Lack of decision-making capacity must be properly documented.
- Individual state legal requirements should be consulted regarding the physician's role in assessments and responsibilities.

Advance Care Directives and Health Care Agents
- Advance care directives document an individual patient's preference for health care treatments to be followed if the patient is no longer mentally competent.
- Patients may designate a health care agent to make health care decisions if the patient becomes cognitively incapacitated.
- The authority of the health care agent is defined by the patient.
- Decisions must be made consistent with the patient's wishes, and if unknown, then in the patient's best interests.
- The health care agent may decide to forgo life-sustaining procedures without physician certification of presence of persistent vegetative state, terminal condition, or end-stage condition.
- When no health care agent has been appointed, decisions may be made by a patient's surrogate, who is usually a family member or, if no family is identified, a close friend who is familiar with the patient's wishes.
- Conflicts between surrogates that involve critical decisions are best resolved through discussion led by a health care provider. Conflicts that cannot be resolved should be referred to the Ethics Committee.
- Patients without a health care agent or an identifiable surrogate need to have a court-appointed guardian, as per state law.

Medically Nonbeneficial (Futile) Treatment

- Definition: Medical intervention that has no pathophysiologic benefit and has no realistic chance of permitting survival without continuing an acute level of care, and is contrary to generally accepted medical standards.
- Physicians need not provide treatment that is medically ineffective ("futile") or inappropriate.
- Physicians must certify that treatment, to a reasonable degree of medical certainty, will neither prevent nor reduce the deterioration of health.
- Certification that treatment is ineffective must be confirmed by a second physician, as per state law.
- Patients or their representatives must be informed.
- Patients and families must be given the opportunity to transfer to another provider or facility.
- The physician must continue treatment to prevent death during the transfer period.

Ethics Committees

- Serve to establish guidelines and procedures, whereby biomedical and ethical issues and questions can be identified and addressed.
- Requests for Ethics Committee review may be initiated by any patient, family member, surrogate, or member of the treatment team.
- All proceedings and discussions in Ethics Committee meetings are protected confidential information.
- After investigation, the Ethics Committee report becomes part of the medical record.
- Ethics Committee recommendations are advisory only, and adherence to recommendations remains voluntary.

Elder Abuse

- Definition: An act or omission that results in harm or potential harm to the health or welfare of a person 65 or older.
- It can be divided into three main categories:
  - Abuse or neglect by another at home
  - Abuse or neglect at an institution
  - Self-neglect
- Laws that address elder abuse are categorized into three groups:
  - Adult protective services
  - Laws governing institutional abuse
  - The Long-Term Care Ombudsmanship Program (LTCOP)
- Rates of elder abuse range from 4.5 to 14.6 per 1,000 elders but are under-reported.
- Types of abuse include neglect, abandonment, physical abuse, diversion of medication, sexual abuse, financial abuse, and psychological abuse.
- Self-neglect is one of the largest categories of abuse and is reportable.
- State laws governing the reporting of elder abuse vary, but most states have enacted laws requiring mandatory reporting by health care workers.

Driving

- The majority of patients above 70 depend on automobile transportation.
- Older persons can be at an increased risk due to impairments in cognition, reaction time, arthritis, and visual and sensory dysfunction or effects of medication.
- Physicians should evaluate and intervene when driving capability is impaired.
- Formal driving simulation testing should be obtained, when appropriate.
- State Department of Motor Vehicles (DMV) medical advisory boards can provide specific information regarding physician assessment and reporting responsibilities.

Suggested Readings

Barbas NR, Wilde EA. Competency issues in dementia: Medical decision making, driving, and independent living. *J Geriatr Psychiatry Neurol.* 2001;14:199–212.

Brown BB. *Mental Capacity: Legal and Medical Aspects of Assessment and Treatment.* 2nd ed. Eagan: West; 1997–2011.

Elder Abuse Laws By State – (American Bar Association Commission on Law and Aging (2007) Research conducted on Westlaw compliments of West Group). www.ncea.aoa.gov/NCEAroot/Main_Site/Library/Laws/APS_IA_LTCOP_Citations_Chart_08-08.aspx

Kapp MB. *Legal Aspects of Elder Care.* 1st ed. Sudbury: Jones and Bartlett Learning; 2009.

U.S. Administration on Aging—National Center on Elder Abuse, 2011. http://ncea.aoa.gov/NCEAroot/Main_Site/Find_Help/State_Resources.aspx

Pain Management

William L. Doss MD MBA

Description
Geriatric pain management refers to treating chronic pain—pain lasting 3 months or longer—in the elderly population. Chronic pain management usually refers to musculoskeletal or somatic pain.

General Concepts in Geriatric Pain Management
- The objective of pain management is not to alleviate pain completely, as this is often unrealistic, but to improve the function of the individual going through the pain experience.
- The geriatric population is often untreated or undertreated compared to their nongeriatric counterparts.
- Mismanaged musculoskeletal pain in the geriatric population can lead to systemic illness. For example,
  - *Endocrine*: increased release of cortisol, thus increasing blood sugars
  - *Protein catabolism*: up to 40% reduction in protein synthesis following surgery
  - *Cardiovascular*: increased catecholamine release, thus increasing heart rate and myocardial oxygen consumption
- Depression may be the initial pain presentation in the geriatric population.
- The main indication is to reduce pain symptoms and behavior in order to improve physical function, including activities of daily living, and improve mood.

Red Flags
- Metastatic cancer (breast, lung, prostate) should be considered in any patient with a sudden increase in musculoskeletal pain, especially in a patient with a previous cancer history or family history of cancer.
- Compression fractures should be considered as a source of musculoskeletal pain in anyone with a history of osteoporosis.
- Fractures can occur even in the absence of a fall, especially at the hip.

Potential Problems
- Geriatric patients may be reluctant to take pain medications.
- Geriatric patients may be reluctant to changing their lifestyles in order to reduce musculoskeletal pain (weight loss, smoking cessation).
- Pain may be under-reported by the geriatric patient.
- Interference by family and/or caregivers may complicate the clinician's ability to provide effective musculoskeletal pain management for the geriatric patient.
- Depression may accompany musculoskeletal pain complaints.
- Sleep disorders may be associated with musculoskeletal pain.
- Constipation can be caused by pain medicines, especially opioids.

Helpful Hints
- Address chronic musculoskeletal pain as any other disease entity and treat appropriately
- Use a Visual Analog Scale (VAS) to assist the geriatric patient in identifying pain complaints
- Explain the preference of "scheduled" dosing of pain medicines versus "prn" dosing
- The clinician should be prepared to explain differences of "true addiction" versus "pseudo-addiction" regarding pain medicines.
- *Avoid* using Demerol as a chronic pain medicine.
- Consider obtaining a sleep study on the patient taking an opioid, as opioids can lead to respiratory depression. This, coupled with apneic episodes that occur with sleep apnea, can lead to respiratory arrest.
- Anticipate constipation with opioids and provide patients with appropriate laxatives on initial dosing.
- When prescribing methadone, start dosing low and increase slowly. Its half-life is variable and can be as long as 72 hours.
  - An initial electrocardiogram (ECG) should be obtained to rule out underlying cardiac

arrhythmias; Methadone alone can cause *torsades de pointes*.
- Consider topical analgesics for pain management
- Consider aquatic physical therapy as an alternative to standard physical therapy

Suggested Readings

Neurologic Disorders. Chapter 43. Pain. The Merck Manual of Geriatrics. n.d. www.merck.com/mkgr/mmg/sec6 (2010, October 26).

Sirven JI. *Clinical Neurology of the Older Adult.* 2nd ed. Philadelphia, PA: Lippincott Williams & Wilkins; 2008.

Cavalieri T. Managing pain in geriatric patients. *J Am Osteopath Assoc.* 2007;107(Suppl. 4):10–16.

Burris J. Pharmacologic approaches to geriatric pain management. *Arch Phys Med Rehabil.* 2004;85(Suppl. 3):S45–51.

Pargeon K, et al. Barriers to effective cancer pain management: A review of the literature. *J Pain Symptom Manage.* 1999;18(5):358–368.

Pharmacology: General

Lisa C. Hutchison PharmD MPH

Description

Use of medications in the older adult is most challenging due to the changes in physiology, economic issues, and the concurrent use of multiple agents which frequently interact.

Key Principles

- Medication doses must be adjusted to address pharmacokinetic and pharmacodynamic alterations associated with aging.
- Assessment of adverse drug–drug interactions is necessary due to the use of multiple medications.
- Periodic review of the medication list to identify and remove unnecessary medications is recommended.

Pharmacokinetics

Absorption

- Transit time through the gastrointestinal tract slows with aging; this causes a delay in the time of onset and a lower maximum concentration of medications, because most drugs are absorbed in the small intestine. However, the total absorption of oral drugs is not altered.

Water-soluble drugs distribution

- In older persons, a decrease in the volume of distribution for water-soluble drugs is seen, and correlates with decreased total body water and muscle mass for these individuals.
- Lower doses are required to fill-up body stores of a water-soluble medication.

Lipid-soluble drugs distribution

- In older persons, lipid-soluble medications will have a larger volume of distribution, because older individuals have a higher percentage of body fat; therefore, it will take more medication to fill-up the body stores for lipid-soluble medications.
- However, clearance of lipid-soluble medications will be decreased by a similar degree causing drug accumulation.
- Therefore, it is not recommended to give larger doses of lipid-soluble medication.
- Instead, small doses should be given more frequently, until body stores are filled.

Protein binding

- In frail elderly patients, a low serum albumin level is common.
- Highly protein-bound medications will not have as many binding sites, thus leaving a higher percentage of unbound medication.
- The unbound medication is the active medication, and exerts therapeutic and toxic effects.

Metabolism

- Liver size and blood flow decrease with aging.
- Drugs with high extraction rates with the first pass through the liver will have increased serum concentrations.
- Also, medications which undergo oxidation, reduction, or hydrolysis may have a reduced elimination rate.
- Metabolism through glucuronidation, sulfation, or acetylation is unchanged with aging.

Excretion

- Kidney size and blood flow decrease with aging.
- This results in reduced excretion of drugs that are renally cleared.
- The Cockcroft–Gault estimation of creatinine clearance is the most recognized and validated equation for use in adjusting the dose of medications cleared by the kidney.
- The estimated creatinine clearance is calculated with the formula below; the package insert or other drug reference should be consulted for recommended dosing adjustment, if creatinine clearance is less than 50 mL/min.

Pharmacodynamics

- Even when dosing has been properly adjusted, many older adults respond differently to medications, likely due to changes in cell receptors or barriers.
- Elderly patients are more sensitive to agents affecting the central nervous system—such as benzodiazepines,

- opiates, and anticholinergic medications—and exhibit an increased risk for delirium.
- In addition, the blood–brain barrier has increased permeability, thus increasing drug concentrations within the central nervous system.
- There is a down-regulation of beta-adrenergic receptors associated with aging. This reduces the response to both beta-adrenergic receptor agonists and blockers.
  - However, receptors will up-regulate with continued exposure to these medications, so older patients will respond to them, just not as briskly.
- Older adults may be at a higher risk for toxicity from medications that prolong the QT interval, especially when they are used in combination with each other.
- Decreased total body water and alterations in hormonal response increase the risk for dehydration; electrolyte abnormalities are more difficult to correct in the elderly.
- Constipating agents are more problematic in older adults due to a physiologic slowing of gastrointestinal transit time.
- Elderly patients, especially those above the age of 75, are more susceptible to gastrointestinal bleeding induced by nonsteroidal anti-inflammatory agents.

Key Procedural Steps in Prescribing
- Before adding a new medication, appropriate nonpharmacologic treatments should be maximized.
- Medications with the least potential for interaction with current treatments should be chosen.
- The indication for the medication should be included in the instructions for the prescription and explained to the patient. This has been shown to improve adherence.
- It is best to start with the lowest effective dose and increase slowly, with frequent monitoring for therapeutic and toxic responses.

Table 1 Pharmacokinetic Dosing Suggestion in Older Adults

Cockcroft–Gault Formula for Estimation of Creatinine Clearance

$[(140 - \text{age in years}) \times (LBW)] / [(SCr) \times 72] = \text{estCrCl}^*$

*Result is multiplied by 0.85 in females

estCrCl = estimated creatinine clearance in mL/min
LBW = lean body weight in kilograms (or actual weight, whichever is less)
SCr = serum creatinine in mg/dL

Common Examples of Medications Affected by Pharmacokinetic Changes in Aging

Absorption:
Pain medications and antihypertensives
Recommendation—avoid readministering a dose too quickly; may give antihypertensives at bedtime to reduce the risk of orthostatic hypotension

Water-soluble drug distribution: Antibiotics
Recommendation—use smaller doses

Lipid-soluble drug distribution:
All benzodiazepines except Lorazepam and Oxazepam; all antipsychotics
Recommendation—avoid benzodiazepines except for Lorazepam and Oxazepam; for others, give small doses more frequently with monitoring, until effects seen

Protein binding:
Diazepam, Lorazepam; Ibuprofen, Naproxen; Phenytoin, Valproic acid; Furosemide, Warfarin
Recommendation—give smaller doses, especially when used concurrently with other protein-bound drugs

Metabolism:
Chlordiazepoxide, Diazepam; Diphenhydramine; Amitriptyline, Fluoxetine; Meperidine, Tramadol; Warfarin
Recommendation—avoid use when possible; when used, use smaller doses with frequent monitoring

Excretion:
Antibiotics; antigout medications; Digoxin; histamine-2 blockers; Gabapentin; Meperidine, Tramadol
Recommendation—estimate creatinine clearance and adjust doses per drug reference

Anticipated Problems
- When reviewing a patient's medication list, the following problems are often found:
  - No current indication exists for a medication the patient is taking.
  - A medication is an unnecessary duplication, contributing to polypharmacy.
  - A medication is prescribed to treat side effects of another medication.
  - Doses were started too high, or increased too rapidly considering pharmacokinetic and pharmacodynamic variables or potential drug–drug interactions.

Helpful Hints
- Medications should be reviewed regularly to identify and correct problems.
- The patient and/or caregiver should be counseled to maintain a current medication list.
- The indication for each medication and how it should be taken should be reinforced frequently.
- Common contributors to noncompliance include
  - Cognitive impairment
  - Multiple doses/frequencies during the day
  - Economic barriers
- Methods to improve adherence include
  - Enlisting the help of a caregiver to monitor medications
  - Switching to medications that can be dosed once or twice daily, or using combination of products
  - Providing pillboxes or other compliance aids

Suggested Readings
Delafuente JC. Pharmacokinetic and pharmacodynamic alterations in the geriatric patient. *Consult Pharm.* 2008;23:324–334.

Hutchison LC, O'Brien C. Changes in pharmacokinetics and pharmacodynamics in the elderly patient. *J Pharm Prac.* 2007;20(1):4–12.

Hutchison LC, Sleeper-Irons RB, eds. *Fundamentals of Geriatric Pharmacotherapy: An Evidence-Based Approach.* Bethesda, MD: American Society of Health-system Pharmacists; 2010.

Pharmacology: Management of Polypharmacy

Andrew Geller MD ■ Dale C. Strasser MD

Description
Polypharmacy is often defined as the use of multiple medications or the use of a medication that is not (or is no longer) indicated. Polypharmacy is associated with an increased risk of geriatric syndromes including cognitive impairment, falls, hip fractures, and urinary incontinence. More appropriate medication use, including the elimination of unnecessary or inappropriate medications, is associated with improved functioning and decreased hospitalization among the elderly.

Etiology/Types
- Inappropriate prescribing, where a medication is prescribed whose risks outweigh the benefit
- Drug–drug interactions
- Drug–disease interactions
- Adverse drug effects, resulting from the above, can increase the risk of falls and hospital admissions and can cause a deterioration of health status.

Epidemiology
- In the United States, 100,000 excess deaths per year are attributed to inappropriate medication prescriptions.
- Morbidity and mortality associated with drug-related problems cost an estimated $177.4 billion per year in U.S. outpatients and an estimated $4 billion per year in nursing home residents.
- Polypharmacy (using over 8 drugs) incidence approaches 60% in U.S. skilled nursing facilities.
- 20% of people above 70 are taking 5 or more medications.
- Inappropriate prescribing occurs in up to 92% of elderly U.S. ambulatory patients.
- Adverse drug events in the elderly account for 10% of Emergency Department visits, and up to 17% of hospital admissions.
- Studies of ambulatory elderly patients have documented an average of 1 unnecessary drug per patient, including drugs with no identifiable indication or that provide little benefit for the indication for which they were prescribed.
- In older adults, up to 28% of hospital admissions are drug related.

Key Principles
- Elderly patients are more likely to have multiple comorbidities and to have more than one physician involved in their care.
- Changes in drug metabolism, excretion and receptor sensitivity in the elderly put them at increased risk for the effects of polypharmacy (see chapter on Pharmacology: General).
- Elderly patients have been under-represented in premarketing clinical drug trials, making it more difficult to anticipate the effects of medications in this population.

Risk Factors
- Multiple medications
- Older age
- Multiple medical comorbidities
- Multiple physicians treating the patient, and transitions of care (hospital discharge)
- Use of medications which cause additive hypotension, sedation, or anticholinergic effects
- Use of medications with narrow therapeutic thresholds, or with susceptibility to interact with other medications

Clinical Features
- Clinical presentation is variable, depending on the medication side effect profiles and individual patient comorbidities.
- Examples of side effects include impaired cognition, gastrointestinal/genitourinary disturbances, and renal insufficiency.

Complications of Polypharmacy
- Polypharmacy can significantly impact morbidity and mortality by contributing to geriatric syndromes such as delirium, falls, and urinary incontinence.
- Polypharmacy may impair cognitive function, which is an independent predictor of functional decline in the elderly.
- Inappropriate prescribing may mimic or worsen preexisting disease.
- Unrecognized medication side effects can trigger the "prescribing cascade," where a drug is added to treat a side effect of another medication (for example, drug-induced parkinsonism).

Diagnosis
History
- Complete medication list, including over-the-counter medications, to ascertain potentially problematic medications such as common psychoactive drugs (sedatives, antipsychotics, antidepressants), anticonvulsants, and antihypertensives
- Falls (or near falls) in the previous 12 months
- Altered cognition, consciousness, or behavior
- Decline in functional independence measures and activities of daily living performance
- Urinary incontinence and constipation
- Lightheadedness upon standing

Examination
- Orthostatic vital signs
- Cognitive assessment
- Anticholinergic signs (dry mouth)
- Assessment of gait and balance

Pitfalls
- Under use of beneficial drug therapy by older adults may also be associated with increased morbidity, and decreased mortality and quality of life (for example, treatment of osteoporosis).

Red flags
- In evaluating virtually any symptom in an older patient, the possibility of an adverse drug event should be considered in the differential diagnosis.

Treatment
Medical
- "Brown bag" medication review of the prescription bottles to confirm accuracy of medication list, rather than relying on the list provided by the patient/caregiver; making sure to clarify indication/diagnosis is appropriate; clarifying prescribing physician and actual compliance with scheduled medications.
- Discontinuing potentially unnecessary or inappropriate therapy (see chapter on Pharmacology: General).
- "Starting low and going slow," when starting medications.
- Educating patient and caregiver on potential medication side effects.
- When new medications are introduced, following up laboratory panels as indicated (for example, liver, kidney, blood).
- Monitoring compliance; simplifying regimens; and collaborating with caregivers/family to ensure drug regimen and indication are understood.
- For treatment of pain, nonpharmacologic agents (physical/occupational therapy, exercise, topical heat) along with local therapies (for example, corticosteroid injection, transdermal anti-inflammatory) should be used where possible rather than adding an oral agent.
- A "medication debridement" can be useful in any elderly patient with functional loss.
- When "debriding" a medication list, it may be helpful to refer to one of the various discontinuation guidelines.
  - One such guide, the "FORTA" classification, guides the clinician in ranking medications from the most indispensable and safe, to those medications that are easily discontinued and/or harmful in the elderly.
  - Another tool that has been shown useful is the Good Palliative-Geriatric Practice (GP-GP) algorithm for discontinuing elderly patients' unneeded medications, which employs a slightly different approach to the same end.
- Look out for commonly encountered inappropriate regimens (proton pump inhibitors at maximum therapeutic dosage for over 8 weeks; nonsteroidal anti-inflammatories for over 3 months; long-acting benzodiazepines for over 1 month, and/or duplication of therapy within the same drug class).
- Recall key medication interactions (see chapter on Pharmacology: General).

Complications of Treatment
- Discontinuation of multiple medications is generally well tolerated in the elderly.
- However, possible withdrawal syndromes from discontinuation of psychoactive/centrally

acting medications are possible (especially benzodiazepines, antidepressants, antiparkinsonian, and antihypertensive medications), with resulting insomnia, agitation, and irritability.
- Therapeutic failure is possible (important to educate patients on trial-and-error approach and goals of treatment).

Prognosis
- Residents of skilled nursing facilities, patients with cognitive impairment, and those with multiple comorbid conditions are especially vulnerable to polypharmacy.

Suggested Readings

Garfinkel D, Mangin D. Feasibility study of a systematic approach for discontinuation of multiple medications in older adults. *Arch Intern Med.* 2010;170:1648–1654.

Gloth FM III. Pharmacological management of persistent pain in older persons: Focus on opioids and nonopioids. *J Pain.* 2011;12:S14–S20.

Hayes BD, Klein-Schwartz W, Barrueto F Jr. Polypharmacy and the geriatric patient. *Clin Geriatr Med.* 2007;23(2):371–390, vii.

Lin JL, Armour D. Selected medical management of the older rehabilitative patient. *Arch Phys Med Rehabil.* 2004;85(7, Suppl. 3):S76–82.

Rochon P, Tjia J, Gill S, et al. Appropriate approach to prescribing. In: Hazzard WR, Halter JB, eds. *Hazzard's Geriatric Medicine and Gerontology.* 6th ed. New York, NY: McGraw-Hill Medical; 2009:289–301.

Prescription Writing: Drugs and Therapy

Danielle L. Hinton MD

Description
The combination of disease presentation and physiologic changes of aging is of great consideration when prescribing medications and rehabilitation programs. Changes in absorption and metabolism accompany organ-system aging, while adverse drug events may go unrecognized in the elderly because they are nonspecific. Limitations in aerobic capacity, muscle strength, and range of motion may exist. Pharmacologic and therapeutic prescriptions can be integral to the rehabilitation of older persons.

Pharmacologic Prescriptions
- Prescriptions are a method of communicating with pharmacists.
- Several categories of medications are commonly used to treat conditions affecting the rehabilitation program. Adverse side effects of these medications should be considered when prescribing.

Analgesics/nonsteroidal anti-inflammatory drugs
- May be used for acute or chronic pain management of musculoskeletal disorders
- Acetaminophen toxicity is the most common cause of acute hepatic failure and the second leading cause of liver transplantation in the United States.
- Nonsteroidal anti-inflammatory drugs (NSAIDs) may exacerbate acute or chronic kidney injury.
- Narcotic side effects include constipation, sedation, nausea, vomiting, orthostatic hypotension, and diminished respiratory rate.
- Tramadol may lower the seizure threshold and should be avoided with concomitant use of tricyclic antidepressants (TCAs), monoamine oxidase inhibitors (MAOIs), and selective seratonin reuptake inhibitors (SSRIs).

Anticonvulsants
- May be used for neuropathic pain
- Common side effects are sedation and cerebellar dysfunction.
- Chronic clonazepam use, often for movement disorders such as restless leg syndrome and myoclonic jerks, may lead to psychologic addiction and physical tolerance.
- Monitoring of phenytoin serum levels is recommended; toxic effects include sedation, ataxia, and nystagmus.

Antidepressants
- Off-label use in the treatment of chronic nonmalignant pain syndromes and neuropathic pain is common.
- Common TCA side effects include orthostatic hypotension, anticholinergic effects, and sedation.
- SSRI side effects include nausea, vomiting, and drowsiness.

Anticoagulants
- Often indicated for stroke prophylaxis, deep vein thrombosis treatment/prophylaxis, and atrial fibrillation
- Bruising, petechiae, epistaxis, and gastrointestinal (GI) bleeding are common adverse effects

Cardiovascular medications
- May be used for hypertension and cardiac arrhythmias
- Beta-blockers may cause orthostatic hypotension or bradycardia and can exacerbate chronic obstructive pulmonary disease, asthma, or congestive heart failure.
- Alpha-blockers may lead to dry mouth, sedation, GI symptoms, and orthostatic hypotension.

GI medications
- Promotility agents (e.g., metoclopramide) may help diabetics and other patients with slow GI transit, but can lead to central nervous system side effects such as sedation, agitation, or tardive dyskinesia.
- H2 blockers and proton pump inhibitors used to prevent stress ulcers and to treat gastroesophageal reflux disease may cause dizziness, diarrhea, or nausea.

Hypnotics
- May be used for treatment of insomnia

- Benzodiazepines most frequently cause daytime drowsiness, headache, and fatigue; dependence and rebound insomnia may occur.

Traumatic brain injury related
- Common sequelae of traumatic brain injury potentially helped with medications include agitation, impaired concentration, decreased attention, and hypoarousal.
- SSRIs have been used to treat insomnia, agitation, aggression, and impaired arousal; side effects are nausea, vomiting, and drowsiness.
- Amantadine may improve arousal, attention, concentration, and decrease agitation; side effects include orthostatic hypotension, renal dysfunction, and anorexia.
- Methylphenidate is used for impaired initiation, concentration, and attention; weight loss, tachycardia, and insomnia are the side effects.
- Modafinil has been used to treat hypoarousal and fatigue; side effects include nausea, nervousness, and insomnia.

Genitourinary
- Anticholinergics (e.g., oxybutynin, tolterodine, solifenacin) are used for overactive bladder and may cause urinary retention, dry mouth, or sedation; contraindicated with uncontrolled glaucoma.

Therapy Prescriptions
- A method of communication with other clinicians, including physical therapists, occupational therapists, and speech-language pathologists
- Therapy prescriptions should be individualized in order to address any functional limitations caused by medical problems.

Composition
- Prescriptions should, at a minimum, include the patient's demographic information, diagnosis relevant to the physical findings and medical conditions, the therapy discipline requested, frequency and duration of each session, and total treatment period, as well as the treating physician's name.
- The intensity of therapeutic exercise and specific therapy techniques/modalities may be included when relevant.

- Importantly, precautions and risks essential to patient safety during therapy must be stated. These may be related to specific diagnoses or effects of medications.

Precautions
- Cardiovascular precautions, often necessary with myocardial infarction, pacemaker placement, and cardiac transplantation, typically require identification of target heart rate ranges and blood pressure monitoring with specific parameters.
- Pulmonary precautions for obstructive or restrictive lung disease may indicate the use of oxygen supplementation.
- Diabetic precautions should be noted to alert clinicians of potential complications from high or low blood sugars, including diaphoresis, syncope, or cognitive changes.
- Weight-bearing restrictions after a fracture or joint replacement must be clarified, as the rehabilitation program may require accommodations with assistive devices or aquatic therapy.
- High falls risk precautions are commonly applicable in the elderly population.

Additional Considerations
- Patients with low endurance or limited exercise tolerance should have recommendations for flexible therapy scheduling intervals, decreased duration of treatment when indicated, and inclusion of frequent rest periods.
- Potential complications of inappropriate or excessive exercise programs include sudden death, hyperthermia, myocardial infarction, excessive fatigue, musculoskeletal problems, and respiratory compromise.
- Aquatic therapy may be an attractive option in the elderly.

Suggested Readings
Hajjar ER, Caflero AC, Hanlon JT. Polypharmacy in elderly patients. *Am J Pharmacother.* 2007;5(4):345–351.

Potentially harmful drugs in the elderly: Beers list and more. *Pharmacist's Letter/Prescriber's Letter.* 2007;23(9):230907.

Rehabilitation Settings: Evaluation for Postacute Rehabilitation

Audra Arant APN

Description
In the United States, several options are available for patients ready for transition from the acute care hospital setting. These include acute inpatient rehabilitation, nursing home/subacute rehabilitation, long-term care hospitals (LTCHs), and home; home health or outpatient therapy are often provided to patients transitioning home.

Epidemiology
- In all 30% or more of older adults admitted to an acute care hospital experience a functional decline.
- Older patients experiencing a functional decline may require some form of postacute care rehabilitation.

Characteristics of Postacute Care Options
- The primary goal of postacute care rehabilitation is to maximize the functional recovery, while providing the requisite medical care for each patient.
- Social work/case coordination can assist with determining what is available/covered by an individual patient's insurance.
- Acute inpatient rehabilitation
  - Close physician supervision; evaluation required every 3 days
  - 24-hour nursing care
  - Multiple therapy disciplines; minimum of two required
    - Physical therapy
    - Occupational therapy
    - Speech-language pathology
    - Recreational therapy
    - Psychology
  - Minimum 3 hours of therapy, 5 days per week
  - Laboratory testing and radiologic imaging available
  - In all 60% of patients must have 1 of 13 medical diagnoses (see Table 1).
  - Patients on ventilators may be admitted, depending upon the facility.
  - Patients must remain medically stable and continue to make functional progress.
- Nursing home/subacute rehabilitation
  - Infrequent physician evaluation; required every 30 days
  - 24-hour nursing coverage not required
  - Therapy services generally available but not required
  - Laboratory and radiologic services not generally available
- LTCH
  - Average length of stay greater than 25 days
  - Close medical supervision required
  - 24-hour nursing coverage
  - Therapy services generally available
  - Patients have long-term medical needs (e.g., ventilator dependence, intravenous antibiotics).
- Home health
  - Patient considered home bound and unable to travel to therapy
  - All therapy disciplines may be available
  - Skilled nursing care or a nursing aide may be available
- Outpatient therapy
  - All therapy disciplines may be available
  - Transportation is generally provided by family or friends.

History
- Patients are evaluated by a physician, or a nurse supervised by a physician, regarding the most appropriate transfer setting.
- Key factors include
  - Prehospitalization functional status (e.g., independent, use of gait aid)
  - Living situation (e.g., alone, with family)
  - Social support available (e.g., family, friends)
  - Living setting (e.g., single-level or multilevel home, stairs)
  - Current functional status (from therapy or nursing evaluations)
    - Mobility (e.g., bed mobility, ambulation)
    - Activities of daily living (e.g., dressing, bathing)
    - Use of gait aid or assistive devices
    - Therapy tolerance (e.g., fatigue, shortness of breath)
    - Ability to follow instructions/retain information

Table 1 60% of Patients in an Acute Rehabilitation Setting Will Have One of These 13 Diagnoses

1	Stroke
2	Spinal cord injury
3	Congenital deformity
4	Amputation
5	Major multiple trauma
6	Femur fracture (hip fracture)
7	Brain injury
8	Neurologic disorders (included multiple sclerosis, muscular dystrophy, myopathy, Parkinson's disease)
9	Burns
10	Active polyarticular rheumatoid arthritis, psoriatic arthritis, and seronegative arthritides resulting in significant functional impairment that has not improved after a sustained course of outpatient therapy or other less-intensive rehabilitation immediately preceding the inpatient rehabilitation admission or that results from a systemic disease activation immediately before admission but has the potential to improve with more intensive rehabilitation
11	Systemic vasculitides with joint inflammation, resulting in significant functional impairment that has not improved after a sustained course of outpatient therapy or other less-intensive rehabilitation immediately preceding the inpatient rehabilitation admission or that results from a systemic disease activation immediately before admission but has the potential to improve with more intensive rehabilitation
12	Severe or advanced osteoarthritis involving two or more major weight-bearing joints (not including a joint with a prosthesis) with joint deformity or substantial loss of range of motion, muscle atrophy surrounding the joint, significant functional impairment not improved after a sustained course of outpatient therapy, or other less-intensive rehabilitation immediately preceding the inpatient rehabilitation admission but has the potential to improve with more intensive rehabilitation
13	Hip or knee joint replacement, or both, during an acute hospitalization immediately preceding the inpatient rehabilitation stay, and also meets one or more of the following specific criteria: a. Bilateral knee or hip joint replacement surgery b. Extreme obesity with body mass index of at least 50 c. Age 85 or above

- Active medical problems and required physician supervision
  - Medications (e.g., intravenous)
  - Future treatments and timing (e.g., chemotherapy, radiation therapy)
- Financial resources/insurance coverage
- Patient/family preferences

Examination

- Physical examination is focused on the following:
  - Vital signs
  - Musculoskeletal system
    - Joint range of motion and contractures
  - Neurologic system
    - Cognition/mental status
    - Motor
    - Sensory
    - Reflexes
    - Co-ordination
    - Gait/station
  - Cardiac
  - Pulmonary
  - Skin/pressure sores
  - Other relevant organ systems (e.g., vascular)

Rehabilitation Considerations

- The decision as to whether a patient is medically stable and/or appropriate for inpatient rehabilitation (as opposed to another setting) should be made by a physiatrist or other physician familiar with postacute care settings.
- Other key factors to be taken into consideration when determining the most appropriate discharge setting/location for an individual patient include
  - Patient motivation
  - Potential for functional recovery
  - Planned ultimate discharge location (e.g., home with family, nursing home)
  - Facility characteristics (e.g., availability of a spinal cord injury program)

Prognosis

- Approximately, 70% to 85% of patients in acute inpatient rehabilitation are discharged to home.
- Discharge rates for nursing home/subacute rehabilitation and LTCH are not as well characterized.

Suggested Reading

American Academy of Physical Medicine and Rehabilitation. Standards for assessing medical appropriateness criteria for admitting patients to rehabilitation hospitals or units; February 2011. www.aapmr.org/zdocs/hpl/MIRC0906.pdf.

Rehabilitation Settings: Home Health Care

Andre Taylor MD MBA ■ Junell Taylor RN MA ■ Kevin M. Means MD

Description
Home health care rehabilitation of the geriatric patient is not limited to one organ system, disease process, or set of medical conditions; it encompasses all medical conditions that a geriatric patient have that may benefit from rehabilitative services in the home setting.

Home Health Missions
- The primary rehabilitation mission for geriatric patients in the home health care setting is to maintain the patient's ability to function safely in the community environment.
  - Home health care seeks to maintain a geriatric patient's ability to perform activities of daily living (ADLs) with or without assistance and to ambulate with or without assistance in the community environment.
  - An unusual (the primary) aspect of the home health care setting is that registered nurses (RNs) are the (primary) managers of patient care with physicians playing a strong supportive role in the geriatric patient's care.
  - RNs employ the services of many allied health care professionals and paraprofessionals in order for geriatric patients to remain in the community environment safely.

Home Health Care-Allied Health Care Professionals and Paraprofessionals
The home health care-allied health care professionals and paraprofessionals include, but are not limited to, the following:
- RNs
- Physical therapists (PTs)
- Occupational therapists (OTs)
- Speech pathologists (SPs)
- Medical social workers (MSWs)
- Respiratory therapists (RTs)
- Home health aides (HHAs)
- Personal care aides (PCAs)

- Each professional brings a unique set of skills, and all of them function as a team to help the geriatric patient remain at home safely.
  - The services a geriatric patient will require are determined by several factors: diseases, severity of diseases, response of the geriatric patient to treatment and therapy, cognitive function, conditions within the geriatric patient's home, and conditions in the community environment.
- The secondary rehabilitation mission for the home health care setting is to assist patients in their recovery from acute conditions.
  - For example: if a geriatric patient has received a knee replacement, but has been sent home instead of to an acute rehabilitation facility or nursing home
  - The PT's rehabilitation goal is to help the geriatric patient improve the range of motion, both passive and active, within the limitations set by the orthopedic surgeon.
  - These therapeutic interventions should continue until the short-term acute rehabilitation goals have been attained.
  - An OT may work in collaboration with the PT to assist the geriatric patient with limited ambulatory ability to adapt to his home and community.
  - A HHA may be assigned to assist the patient in ADLs. The HHA provides assistance with positioning, transfers, and prevention of falls.
  - The MSW visits the geriatric patient to determine their psychosocial needs during rehabilitation therapy and to assure that the patient has the financial and social support needed to return to their previous health status.
- With the advent of telemedicine and mobile health, conditions that would have normally been treated in an acute rehabilitation facility, rehabilitative nursing home, or outpatient rehabilitation facility can now be treated in a home or community-based setting.

Funding Criteria for Home Health Care

- For many geriatric patients, maintenance within the home setting is facilitated by informal unpaid caregivers who provide a significant quantity and quality of services.
  - The work that these caregivers perform is not directly reimbursed or rewarded by the health care system.
  - If the indirect costs of providing these services to elderly parents, relatives, and others could be calculated, including actual lost wages and productivity and forsaken opportunities for paid employment, they would be substantial.
- For formal care, in the most common model of home health care, a HHA certified to provide care under Medicare reimbursement rules employs the home health care workers and assigns them to individual patient cases.
  - A physician must certify that the patient is homebound and has a "skilled need" in order for a Medicare-certified HHA to provide care for a 60-day certification period.
  - A skilled need is a condition that requires part-time, intermittent care provided by a specially trained person (i.e., nurse or therapist).
  - Unskilled personal care for ADL assistance is covered by Medicare during the certification period, but not in the absence of a skilled need. A patient can be recertified for multiple 60-day periods, as long as a skilled need exists.
  - HHAs can also be paid privately by the care recipient.
- A relatively small number of older adults have privately funded long-term care insurance policies that can also pay for home health care costs. This option appears to be increasing among employers, and such funding may become more prevalent in the future.

Program of All-Inclusive Care for the Elderly

In the future, more elderly patients will be enrolled in Program of All-Inclusive Care for the Elderly (PACE) programs.

- PACE is a Medicare program and Medicaid state option that provides community-based care and services to frail people aged 55 or above, who otherwise would need a nursing home level of care.
- Most PACE programs have a diverse group of health care providers providing co-ordinated health care to geriatric patients in the community.
- PACE provides care and services covered by Medicare and Medicaid, and authorized by the health care team—including rehabilitation services.
- PACE also covers additional medically necessary care and services not covered by Medicare and Medicaid.
- PACE provides coverage for prescription drugs, physician care, transportation, home care, hospital visits, and nursing home stays, when necessary.
- As of 2010, there were over 75 PACE programs operating in 29 states.
- Several PACE programs have demonstrated
  - The ability to provide health care cost savings by reducing hospital and nursing home admissions.
  - Improvement in quality of life measures of geriatric patients.
  - For example, in Texas, PACE enrollees have had fewer hospital admissions than the overall Medicare population (2,399 per 1,000 per year vs. 2,448), even though PACE enrollees are far more frail than the average Medicare patient.
- Nursing home admissions in PACE are lower—only 7.6% of PACE enrollees live in nursing homes, although all meet the criteria and are eligible for institutional care.
- Rehabilitative services are one of the factors in attaining these results in the PACE setting.

For consumers, PACE provides
- The option to continue living in the community as long as possible
- One-stop shopping for all health care services

For health care providers, PACE provides
- A managed care arrangement with capitated funding that rewards providers who are flexible and creative in providing the best care possible
- The ability to co-ordinate care for individuals across settings and medical disciplines
- The ability to meet increasing consumer demands for individualized care and supportive service arrangements

For those who pay for care, PACE provides
- Cost savings and predictable expenditures
- A comprehensive service package emphasizing preventive care that is usually less expensive and more effective than acute care
- A care model for older individuals, focused on keeping them at home and out of institutional settings

For information on PACE, see www.medicare.gov/Nursing/Alternatives/Pace.asp.

Helpful Hints
- Geriatric patients often exhibit periods of depression because of their limited ability to ambulate and provide for their ADLs.
- Discharging the geriatric patient home where family, friends, and community support is available allows the patient to focus less on physical limitations.
- A well-planned rehabilitation program has proven to positively affect the geriatric patient's quality of life.

Suggested Readings

Golden AG, Roos BA, Silverman MA, et al. Home and community-based Medicaid options for dependent older Floridians. *J Am Geriatr Soc.* 2010;58:371–376.

Kadushin G. Home health care utilization: A review of the research for social work. *Health Soc Work.* 2004;29:219–244.

Levine SA, Boal J, Boling PA. Home care. *JAMA.* 2003;290:1203–1207.

Meyer RP. Consider medical care at home. *Geriatrics.* 2009;64:9–11.

Russell T, Buttrum P, Wootton R, et al. Internet-based outpatient telerehabilitation for patients following total knee arthroplasty: A randomized controlled trial. *J Bone Joint Surg Am.* 2011;93:113–120.

Rehabilitation Settings: Inpatient Rehabilitation, Acute

LaTanya Lofton MD

Description

Geriatric inpatient rehabilitation is designed to maximize function and minimize disability associated with hospitalizations due to medical conditions or catastrophic events.

Key Principles

- It is estimated that up to 35% of elderly patients admitted to acute care hospitals demonstrate functional decline, as evidenced by loss of independence in one or more areas of activities of daily living. This may be due to complications from the medical illness, bed rest, medications, or a variety of other factors related to the hospitalization.
- Inpatient rehabilitation has been shown to provide improvements in function, independence, pain, balance, and general well-being in the aging population.
- Older adult patients admitted to inpatient rehabilitation often have multiple medical comorbidities and conditions that require concurrent treatment and close medical supervision.
- Physiologic changes in the elderly may affect a patient's endurance and performance and the overall ability to tolerate a standard regimented program. Thus, the rehabilitation program should be tailored to the individual patient, while taking into account the physiological alterations that may accompany normal aging.
- The inpatient rehabilitation setting may be appropriate to assist in facilitating appropriate environmental modifications in the home, education of family and caregivers, and identification of resources for support in the home after discharge.
- The most common diagnoses in the geriatric patient population for inpatient rehabilitation include stroke, fractures, debility, and Parkinson's disease.

Key Procedural Steps

- Patient selection. Patients must be able to tolerate at least 3 hours of therapy per day and must require 24-hour supervision by a physician and rehabilitation nursing staff.
- Patients should be expected to make functional gains in the rehabilitation program.
- A thorough physical examination and assessment of medical comorbidities should be done on admission to inpatient rehabilitation to assess the patient's current medical status and to address any pertinent medical issues. This may ultimately reduce the impact of the patient's medical issues on their ability to tolerate the therapy program.
- A review of all medications, including over-the-counter medications, prescription drugs, and herbs or vitamins, should be done on admission in order to simplify the medication regimen, eliminate unnecessary medications, and reduce polypharmacy and potential drug interactions.
- Reconciliation of home medications and hospital medications should be completed on admission and prior to discharge.
- Patients and families should be educated regarding the purpose of medications and possible adverse effects of all medications.
- Adjustments to therapy protocols should be considered in order to facilitate compliance and participation with the rehabilitation program. This may include initiating therapies earlier during the day to accommodate the patient and allowing for more frequent rest breaks to prevent fatigue. Further adjustments may include avoidance of hyperflexion exercises to reduce the risk of vertebral body fractures and increasing duration of exercise prior to increasing intensity of exercise to reduce risk of further injury and promote strengthening.
- The therapy program should consist of progressive resistance training and aerobic exercise. Both types of exercise are important to improving and maintaining independent function in the elderly patient population, and they may be important in reducing cardiac risk factors, improving physiologic impairments due to coronary heart disease, and enhancing the quality of life.

- The intensity of the therapy program may need to be adjusted in order to maximize participation and functional recovery; rest breaks must be incorporated into the patients' schedules. Concurrent treatment with physical and occupational therapies may be considered in order to encourage participation.
- Cognitive assessment with psychology or speech therapy should be considered to formally assess the patient's cognitive performance.
- Delirium is a common reversible complication in elderly hospitalized patients, and it is characterized by waxing and waning of attention and performance. More than 50% of cases of delirium are thought to be underdiagnosed, especially in the elderly patient population. Evaluation for common causes of delirium include medications, electrolyte imbalances, infection, drug withdrawal, intracranial process, fecal impaction, urinary retention, myocardial problems, and pulmonary issues.
- Depression can mimic cognitive dysfunction in the aging population.
- Treatment of any medical or psychiatric condition that may contribute to cognitive impairments should be addressed.
- Falls are common in the inpatient setting, and special attention should be given to assess the patient's risk of falling.
- Gait assessments can be done to evaluate each patient's individual gait abnormalities and to determine appropriate assistive devices, when warranted.
- Assessment of bowel and bladder continence should be done on admission and throughout the hospitalization. Various management options are available to treat incontinence, and maintenance of continence may be essential to the patient's ability to be discharged home.
- Adequate nutrition is important for overall health maintenance. An assessment of nutritional status should be completed on admission.
- Special consideration should be given to address dysphagia, potential for aspiration pneumonia, impaired cognitive ability, and limitation in access to meals and meal preparation due to disability.
- Elderly patients frequently have caregivers who are also aging. This may potentially limit the amount of assistance available to the patient at the time of discharge. Consideration for caregivers and their potential limitations should be integral to the overall plan of care for this patient population.
- Due to limited life expectancy of the older, disabled patient; the rehabilitation program should be facilitated in a manner to expedite discharge home with family.

Benefits of Inpatient Rehabilitation
- In all 18% reduction in functional decline
- Potentially reduces admissions to nursing home
- Higher likelihood of living at home in 6 months
- Maintenance of quality of life for the elderly
- Improvement in mortality
- Improvement in functional status

Anticipated Problems
- Polypharmacy
- Falls
- Multiple medical comorbidities
- Cognitive impairment
- Depression
- Dementia
- Pain
- Incontinence
- Malnutrition
- Frailty

Helpful Hints
- Inpatient rehabilitation in the elderly patient population should be individualized for each patient. However, the basic rehabilitation program should consist of aerobic exercise, progressive resistance training, and flexibility.
- Elderly patients often have lower muscle mass, which may result in muscle weakness and decreased aerobic capacity. The effect of these changes must be considered prior to the initiation of the rehabilitation program and throughout the hospitalization.
- Attainment of patient goals is often used to determine successful rehabilitation outcomes. The patient should actively participate in goal setting in order to optimize functional recovery and to personalize the rehabilitation program.
- Studies to determine cost effectiveness of inpatient geriatric rehabilitation have been inconclusive.

Suggested Readings
Bachman S, Finger C. Inpatient rehabilitation specifically designed for geriatric patients: Systematic review and meta-analysis of randomized controlled trials. *BMJ*. 2010;340:c1718.

Baztán JJ, Suárez-García FM, López-Arrieta J, et al. Effectiveness of acute geriatric units on functional decline, living at home, and case fatality among older patients admitted to hospital for acute medical disorders: Meta-analysis. *BMJ*. 2009;338:b50.

Bean JF, Voara A. Benefits of exercise for community-dwelling older adult. *Arch Phys Med Rehabil.* 2004;85(Suppl. 3):S31–S42.

Dechamps A. Effects of exercise programs to prevent decline in health related quality of life in highly deconditioned institutionalized elderly person: A randomized controlled trial. *Arch Intern Med.* 2010;2010(2):162–169.

Heath JM, Stuart MR. Prescribing exercise for frail elders. *J Am Board Fam Pract.* 2002;15(3):218–228.

Hubbard RE. The aging of the population: Implications for multidisciplinary care in hospital. *Age and Ageing.* 2004;33:479–482.

Kus S, Müller M, Strobl R, et al. Patient goals in post-acute geriatric rehabilitation: Goal attainment is an indicator for improved functioning. *J Rehabil Med.* 2011;43:156–161.

Ottenbacher K, Smith PM, Illig SB, et al. Trends in length of stay, living setting, functional outcome, and mortality following medical rehabilitation. *JAMA.* 2004;292(14):1687–1748.

Rehabilitation Settings: Long-Term Acute Care Hospital and Adult Day Care

Deepthi S. Saxena MD ■ Stephanie Hansen DO

Description
Older patients with high medical complexity often require "Transitions of care," that is, movement between levels of care as their needs change.
- In the Long-Term Care Continuum, individuals may, either transiently or permanently, transit to a nursing home (NH)/skilled nursing facility (SNF) and/or adult day care setting.

Definitions
- NHs provide care to frail adults with physical disabilities, who need continuous nursing care and/or low-intensity rehabilitation for chronic medical conditions and declines in activities of daily living (ADLs) and function (e.g., ambulation).
- The primary goal of these programs is to assist the individual in achieving and maintaining the highest level of function.
- Patients in NHs and long-term acute care hospitals (LTACHs) do not have the requirement for 3 hours of therapy per day like those in acute inpatient rehabilitation facilities (IRF).

Differences in Rehabilitation Settings
- LTACHs admit patients who are acutely ill, and who require continued medical treatment (e.g., ventilators).
- IRFs admit patients who are medically stable after a new acute condition or after an exacerbation of a chronic condition.
- NHs admit individuals with chronic illnesses. NHs provide two types of care:
  - SNF care or subacute rehabilitation, with nursing and/or low-intensity rehabilitation; SNFs or subacute rehabilitation can also be provided in free-standing facilities or in units within hospitals.
    - Patients are classified into resource utilization groups (RUGs) based on the hours needed per day/week for nursing and rehabilitation (see chapter on Rehabilitation Settings: Subacute Rehabilitation).
  - Traditional long-term or residential care, where individuals are admitted for custodial care and may additionally get restorative nursing care to maintain function.

Epidemiology
- In the United States, life expectancy at 65 years is 17.6 years (as of 2010).
- It is estimated that the number of NHs in the United States is 16,100, with 1.7 million beds.
- Occupancy is approximately 86% with 1.5 million individuals at both levels for NH care.

The Nursing Home Resident—Facts
- 80% of individuals in NHs are above 65.
- 7% of individuals above 75 and 16% above 85 live in NHs.
- Average age at admission to NH is 79 years.
- 4% have pressure sores at admission
- 40% have heart failure or ischemic heart disease
- 22% have diabetes on admission
- 26% have stroke on admission
- 25% have a diagnosis of dementia; however, 50% to 70% are likely to meet criteria for dementia.
- 20% to 25% have depression
- 75% need assistance in three or more ADLs
- 52% are dependent for eating
- 40% to 60% have bowel and/or bladder incontinence
- 36% have a hearing impairment
- 39% have a visual impairment
- 59% are ambulatory
- 18% walk without assistance or supervision
- 60% have communication problems (comprehension and/or expression)
- Other common medical comorbidities include chronic obstructive pulmonary disease, hypertension, hip fractures, and arthritis
- At age 65, the lifetime risk of NH admission is 46%.

Length of Stay in Nursing Homes
- Less than 90 days: 20%
- ≥90 days: 80%
- Greater than 3 years: 10%

Nursing Homes—Funding/Payors
- Medicaid: A joint federal and state program, which provides health insurance to individuals of all ages with low income and savings, and long-term custodial care in NHs for people who qualify.
- Private pay
- Long-term care insurance
- Medicare and private insurances: pay for skilled or subacute care and hospice care in NHs, not for custodial/traditional long-term care

U.S. Nursing Home Facts
- Average Medicaid NH reimbursement rate: about $150/day
- In all 66.5% of NHs are for profit.
- In all 27.4% of NHs are not for profit.
- In all 6.1% of NHs are government owned.
- On average, NHs operate 107 beds.
- Total NH costs: $120 billion dollars per year
- Ancillary services in NHs: radiology, dialysis, and infusions (42%)

Quality Measures in Nursing Homes
- As the severity of conditions in patients discharged from acute hospitals has increased due to shorter length of stays, NHs have evolved into highly regulated institutions, driven by government and market forces.
- The Omnibus Budget Reconciliation Act (OBRA) of 1987 sets staffing requirements, supports resident's rights by limiting the use of restraints and psychoactive medications, and mandates comprehensive periodic assessments of all residents, with the minimum data set (MDS), which surveys clinical issues directly related to quality of care.
- Additionally, facilities must comply with CMS regulations in the *Code of Federal Regulations*. Each regulation is given a tag number or F-tag. The F-tags indicate that NHs are required to follow stringent regulations.
- Such adherence to regulations is assessed by mandatory site visit surveys every 15 months or if there is a complaint to the state.
- Failure to meet standards leads to penalties for "deficiency" by a corrective action plan, fines, limits on admissions, or facility closure.
- The state identifies residents receiving more than nine drugs. However, since this may be unavoidable, documentation of indication and cost-effective strategies are recommended.

Nursing Home-Specific Medical Issues
- Prevention and screening
- Infections
- Falls
- Malnutrition
- Dehydration
- Incontinence
- Skin breakdown and pressure sores
- Behavioral disturbances
- Polypharmacy

Physiatry in the Nursing Home
- Medical rehabilitative care in NHs is more challenging and rewarding than in any other rehabilitation setting.
- It requires excellent clinical skills, along with a sensitivity to ethical, legal, and interdisciplinary and multidisciplinary issues, along with basic core competencies in geriatrics and an expertise in disability.

Adult Day Care
- This is a community-based option for custodial care, commonly used when caregivers work or need respite.
- It is used for patients who need supervision or assistance with ADLs.
- It can range from nonskilled to skilled, with Medicaid and other insurers covering some services.
- Medicare does not cover custodial care in this setting.
- Offers supervision and recreational activities, as well as clinical assessment and medication management with an on-site registered nurse.
- Adult day care is becoming increasingly popular, due to the flexibility that it provides.

Suggested Readings
Kasper J, O'Malley M. *Changes in Characteristics, Needs, and Payment for Care of Elderly Nursing Home Residents: 1999 to 2004*. Washington, DC: Kaiser Family Foundation; 2007. www.kff.org/medicaid/7663.cfm2

Weiner JM, Freiman MP, Brown D. *Nursing Home Care Quality: Twenty Years after the Omnibus Reconciliation Act of 1987*. Washington, DC: Kaiser Family Foundation; 2007. www.kff.org/medicare/7717.cfm

Zhang NJ, Unruh L, Liu R, et al. Minimum nurse staffing ratios for nursing homes. *Nurs Econ*. 2006;24(2):78–85, 93. © 2006 Jannetti Publications, Inc.

Rehabilitation Settings: Subacute Rehabilitation

Deepthi S. Saxena MD

Description

Subacute rehabilitation is an inpatient medically necessary rehabilitation service for stable patients who do not require acute inpatient hospital or acute rehabilitation, but who still need skilled nursing and advanced therapies greater than what can be met from home.

Need for Subacute Rehabilitation

Subacute rehabilitation is now emerging as the *new paradigm* for rehabilitation with insurers, case managers, primary care physicians, and patients. As criteria for acute inpatient rehabilitation get narrower, more geriatric patients with diagnoses not qualifying for independent rehabilitation facilities (IRFs) are getting admitted for subacute rehabilitation.

Admission and Qualifying Stay Criteria

- Inpatient hospital stay of at least three consecutive days.
- Admission to the subacute unit within a specified time of hospital discharge (generally 30 days).
- Need for services for a condition treated during a qualifying hospital stay; or for one that arose while the patient was in a skilled nursing facility (SNF) for treatment of a condition that was previously treated during a qualifying hospital stay.
- Physician or other qualified practitioner ordered and certified skilled services daily, with the ordering provider's frequent on-site visits.
- The patient must require one or two rehabilitative services daily, with an outcome-focused interdisciplinary approach and a clear discharge plan.
- The patient needs professional, skilled nursing care.
- The patient's mental and physical condition prior to the illness or injury indicates that there is significant potential for improvement.
- The patient is admitted to a Medicare-certified SNF bed.
- Services are reasonable and necessary for the diagnosis or treatment of the condition, that is, are consistent with the nature and severity of the individual's illness or impairment, and with accepted standards of medical practice.
- The patient is medically stable enough to not need acute care.
- The patient must be capable of actively participating in a moderately intensive rehabilitation program, as evidenced by mental status, responsiveness to verbal or visual stimuli, and the ability to follow simple commands.
- The patient is expected to show measurable functional improvement within 7 to 14 days of admission to the program, depending on the underlying diagnosis/medical condition.
- Note: It is adequate to expect reasonable improvement that is of practical value to the individual, measured against their condition at the start of the rehabilitation program.

Goals

Length of stay
- Dependent upon the patient's response to rehabilitation.

Discharge destination
- Usual: home
- Less-preferred alternative: long-term care (LTC).

Types of admission

Short term
- LOS is approximately 2 to 3 weeks.
- Provided by subacute rehabilitation units (SRU) in acute hospitals, free-standing rehabilitation hospitals, and in LTC settings, that is, nursing homes (NHs).

Long term
- The majority of subacute rehabilitation occurs in LTC facilities, that is, NHs, with a LOS of 60 to 100 days.
- The NH does not always allocate a separate unit for subacute rehabilitation patients, but assigns patients to certified beds.

Medicare and Other Insurance
- Medicare and other health insurance programs do not cover custodial care.
- Insurance companies make a distinction between subacute rehabilitation and skilled nursing care, based on the patient's therapy needs.

Covered days
- The Balanced Budget Act (BBA) of 1997 enacted the SNF Prospective Payment System (PPS) reimbursement and Consolidated Billing (CB) requirements.
- Medicare covers 100 days in a single-benefit period under *Part A*. The first 20 of these are fully covered. There are critically important differences in the impact of SNF Consolidated Billing (CB) for Part A.
- *Part B* insurance covers some services rendered during a Part A subacute stay or during a non-Part A stay, including physician services.

Resource utilization groups
- Medicare reimburses subacute rehabilitation under a PPS based on the amount of rehabilitation required, analyzing data from assessments with the minimum data set (MDS) using five resource utilization groups (RUGs):
  - *Ultra High*: 720 minutes/week. At least two disciplines, one discipline at least 5 days/week and one discipline 3 days/week
  - *Very High*: 500 minutes/week. At least one discipline 5 days/week
  - *High*: 325 minutes/week. At least one discipline 5 days/week
  - *Medium*: 150 minutes/week, across three disciplines
  - *Low*: 45 minutes/week, at least 3 days/week.

The Future
- By 2030, the number of adults above the age of 65 in the United States is expected to double to 70 million.
- At least every one in five Americans will fall into this category.
- As more elderly are admitted to subacute rehabilitation, which takes place primarily in the long-term setting, there will be an increasing need for physiatrists to create units with teams in this setting.

Suggested Reading
SNF Consolidated Billing. Program Transmittals: File 5532 CMS web based training modules; 2009. www.cms.gov/zcenter/snf.asp

Rehabilitation Settings: Palliative Care

Kimberly K. Garner MD

Description
Palliative care for the elderly is any form of medical care or treatment that reduces the severity of disease symptoms and stress of illness, rather than striving to cure, delay, or reverse the progression of disease. It can be offered alone or in conjunction with curative care or treatment.

Key Principles
Palliative care may
- Help relieve pain and other distressing symptoms
- Affirm life but regard dying as a normal process
- Intend neither to hasten nor postpone death
- Incorporate psychosocial and spiritual aspects of care
- Encourage patients to live as actively as possible
- Provide a support system to help the family cope
- Use a team approach to address the needs of patients and their families
- Offer treatments that improve the quality of life

Indications
- Palliative care may be appropriate for individuals with serious complex illnesses, whether they are expected to recover, to live with a chronic illness, or progress toward the end of life.
- Because palliative care sees an increasingly wide range of conditions in patients at varying stages of their illness, it follows that palliative care teams offer a range of care. This may range from
  - Managing the physical symptoms in patients receiving treatment for cancer
  - Treating depression in patients with an advanced chronic illness
  - Symptom management for patients in their last days and hours of life

Special Considerations
Palliative care involves multidisciplinary treatments and should be provided by an interdisciplinary team, when possible, consisting of the following:
- Physicians
- Advanced practice nurses
- Registered nurses
- Nursing assistants
- Social workers
- Chaplains
- Pharmacists
- Physiotherapists
- Occupational therapists
- Volunteers
- Families

The team's focus is to optimize the patient's comfort and quality of life.

Finances
In the United States, hospice and palliative care represent two different aspects of care with similar philosophies, but with different payment systems and location of services.
- Palliative care services in the United States are paid by fee-for-service mechanisms, direct hospital support, or philanthropy and are most often provided in acute care hospitals organized around an interdisciplinary consultation service, with or without an acute inpatient palliative care ward.
- Hospice care is provided as a Medicare benefit; similar hospice benefits are offered by Medicaid and most private health insurers.
  - Under the Medicare Hospice Benefit (MHB), a patient signs off their Medicare Part A and enrolls in the MHB with care provided by a Medicare-certified hospice agency.
  - Under terms of the MHB, all costs related to the terminal illness are paid from a per diem rate that the hospice agency receives from Medicare—this includes all services deemed appropriate by the hospice agency including
    - Drugs
    - Equipment
    - Nursing
    - Social service
    - Chaplain visits
    - Other services

Ethics

- Palliative care is based on the principle of autonomy that respects the rights of individuals for self-determination.
- Autonomy can come into conflict with beneficence, when patients, caregivers, or families disagree with the recommendations that health care professionals believe are in the patient's best interest.
- When the patient's or families' interests conflict with the health care providers' recommendation, palliative care physicians may be called in to assist with resolving the conflict because of their advanced knowledge in legal and ethical decision making.

Key Procedural Steps

One of the most important steps in palliative care is to establish the goals of care with patients and their families, using the following principles:

- Ensure a private and comfortable setting for the discussion
- Establish what the patient understands about the current health situation
  - What do you understand about your condition?
- Establish the patient's expectations for treatment
  - What are you hoping for now?
- Discuss options for treatment, including a palliative care approach
- Offer recommendations for treatment
- Respond to emotions
- Establish patient-centered goals
- Restate the patient or caregiver's understanding of the treatment plan (based on the patient's goals)

Anticipated Problems

- Although all these steps may be completed in one discussion, they will frequently need to be readdressed in more than one discussion, depending on the complexity of the issues, the level of understanding of the patient and family, and the emotional responses of the patient and family.

Helpful Hints

- Medications used in the treatment of palliative patients may be used differently than standard medication indications, based on established practices with varying degrees of evidence. Examples include the use of the following:
  - Antipsychotic medications (i.e., haloperidol) to treat nausea
  - Anticonvulsants (i.e., gabapentin) to treat pain
  - Opioids (i.e., morphine) to treat dyspnea
- It is important that clear communication concerning goals of care and nonstandard treatment approaches occurs with patients and their families; this should be documented in the patient's medical chart.
- Alternative routes of medication administration are frequently used, as intravenous access can be difficult to maintain outside a hospital setting. Other routes of administration can include
  - Subcutaneous
  - Sublingual
  - Intramuscular
  - Transdermal
- When establishing goals of care, the health care provider should address code status.
- Cardiopulmonary resuscitation (CPR) for palliative care patients is associated with poor outcomes, as the cause of arrest is usually associated with advanced chronic illness rather than an easily reversible acute cardiopulmonary event.
  - Factors that predict a decreased likelihood to survive for discharge are
    - Sepsis the day prior to CPR
    - Serum creatinine greater than 1.5
    - Metastatic cancer
    - Dementia
    - Dependent status
- When considering discussions about discontinuing medications or treatments, it should be remembered that patients and families may have an emotional reaction to this action.
  - Some will view the medications or the treatments as the final hope for prolonging life or improved function and will resist discontinuation.
  - For others, permission to let go, to accept impending death, and to remove a perceived burden will be welcomed.
  - Health care providers can best help patients and families by focusing discussions around the overall goals of care.
  - When the decision is made with patients and their families to stop a medication, common wisdom supports a gradual dose reduction rather than an abrupt discontinuation of most medicines, if possible.

Suggested Readings

Lynn J, Harrold J. *Handbook for Mortals: Guidance for People Facing Serious Illness.* New York, NY: Oxford University Press; 1999.

Wrede-Seaman L. *Symptom Management Algorithms: A Handbook for Palliative Care.* 2nd ed. Yakima, WA: Intellicard; 1999.

End-of-Life Care

Kimberly A. Curseen MD ■ Sarah E. Harrington MD

Palliative Care
Whole-person care for patients of all ages who are experiencing a debilitating, chronic or life-threatening illness, condition, or injury. The primary goal is to relieve physical and existential suffering associated with the illness. Palliative medicine includes aggressive measures to control pain and other distressing symptoms and can be provided alongside curative care. It can be practiced in a variety of settings, including acute inpatient care, outpatient clinics, home and hospice care, and long-term care.

Comfort Care
Comfort care is palliative care provided to a patient in the terminal phase of an illness. Usually, the patient will elect to forego aggressive interventions and choose care aimed at symptom management at the end-of-life.

Hospice Care
An interdisciplinary program of palliative and supportive services provided both in the home and institutional settings for persons with weeks or months to live, so that they may live as fully and as comfortably as possible.
- Requires two physicians certifying a prognosis of 6 months or less
- Hospice services provide (but are not limited to) physician supervision, nursing services, social work, chaplain support, home aides, respite, durable medical equipment, hospice-related medication coverage, interventions related to comfort, and bereavement support.
- Hospice services can be provided in the location of the home, nursing home, assisted living, inpatient unit, or in a contracted hospital setting.
- Hospice services are covered under Medicare Part A, Medicaid, and most private insurances with little or no out-of-pocket cost to patients. Most hospice programs provide indigent care as well.
- A Do Not Resuscitate (DNR) order is not required to receive hospice care.

Advance Directives
An advance directive is a written document, which provides an instructional framework of patient preferences about what actions should or should not be taken in the event the patient is incapacitated. These documents usually include
- A designated health care proxy or surrogate decision maker
- Wishes concerning life-sustaining treatment, including artificial life support, resuscitation, artificial nutrition and hydration, dialysis, blood product, and so on
- Conditions to guide withdrawal of certain life-sustaining therapies

Resuscitation Preferences
- Cardiopulmonary resuscitation (CPR) is the act of attempting to restore cardiac output and pulmonary ventilation following cardiac arrest and apnea, using artificial respiration and manual chest compression or open-chest cardiac massage. Patients wishing for full resuscitation measures are designated a "Full Code."
- DNR or Do Not Attempt Resuscitation (DNAR) are orders confirmed and written by a medical professional that dictate that in the case of an arrest, patients have identified that they do not wish to receive resuscitative measures.

Rehabilitation in End-of-Life Management
Patients with a terminal illness have many rehabilitation needs, including difficulties with activities of daily living, disruption of usual roles and routines, and anxieties about being a burden to others. Measures of physical function that are traditionally used in rehabilitation medicine such as muscle strength and independence will be difficult benchmarks for this patient population. An alternative framework for measuring rehabilitation outcomes in end-of-life care should be considered. Outcomes such as improving quality of life, fatigue, social participation, and maintaining dignity are all worthwhile goals for patients with a terminal illness. Other practical benefits include decreasing caregiver burden, preserving patient autonomy and independence, and allowing patients more time at home during their final days. Listed below are some of the ways in which

the rehabilitation team can improve the patient's quality of life.
- Occupational therapy can assist patients with improving activities of daily living
- Providing recommendations for appropriate use of durable medical equipment and home modifications
- Providing new techniques for patients and families to cope with their disability and functional decline
- Educating caregivers on safe transfer techniques and other daily patient care issues

Helpful Hints
- Patients with terminal diagnoses may benefit from rehabilitation with focused goals.
- Patients in hospice may have physical, occupational, and speech therapy covered.
- Medicare Part A covers short-term and acute rehabilitation and hospice, but will not pay for concurrent hospice and short-term rehabilitation in a nursing facility.
- If consulted on a patient with limited rehabilitation potential and a terminal diagnosis, consider recommending a palliative care consult.
- Consultative services which may be of benefit to patients at the end of life are: geriatric medicine, geriatric psychiatry, palliative care, pastoral care, behavioral psychology, and social work.

Suggested Readings

Eva G, Wee B. Rehabilitation in end-of-life management. *Curr Opin Support Palliat Care.* 2010;4:158–162.

Hastings Center. *Guidelines on the Terminations of Life-Sustaining Treatment of the Care of the Dying.* Bloomington, IN: Indiana University Press; 1987.

Lynch J, Schuster J, Kabcenell A. *Improving Care for the End of Life: A Sourcebook for Health Care Managers and Clinicians.* New York, NY: Oxford University Press; 2000.

Maxwell T, Martinez J, Knight C. *Unipac 1: The Hospice and Palliative Medicine Approach to Life-Limiting Illness.* Glenview, IL: American Academy of Hospice and Palliative Medicine, 2008.

Index

acetaminophen, 116
AC joint osteoarthritis, 129, 130, 131
activities of daily living (ADLs), 55
acute inpatient rehabilitation, 243, 244
adhesive capsulitis, 129, 130, 131
admission, types of, 253
adnexal structures, age-related changes in, 23
adult day care, 252
advance care directives and health care agents, 231
advance directives, 257
aerobic/cardiovascular exercise, 227
age-related changes
    bone, 4–5
    cardiovascular, 6–7
    central nervous system and cognitive, 8
    gastrointestinal, 10–11
    hearing and vestibular, 12–13
    muscular, 14
    posture and balance, 15–16
    pulmonary, 17–18
    renal, 19–20
    sensory, 21–22
    skin, 23–24
    visual, 25
age-related macular degeneration (ARMD), 201, 202, 203, 206, 207
aging, 2–3
    with developmental disability, 212–214
    with spinal cord injury, 215–217
aka cranial. See giant cell arteritis (GCA)
Alzheimer disease (AD), 30, 135. See also Neurodegenerative diseases
Amitiza, 95
amyotrophic lateral sclerosis (ALS), 40, 138–140
analgesics/nonsteroidal anti-inflammatory drugs, 241
anal ultrasound, 97–98
anemia, 58, 61
ankle, arthritis of, 101–103
anorectal manometry (ARM), 94, 98
anorexia, 11
antagonistic pleiotropic theory, 2
anticholinergics, 242
anticoagulants, 241
anticonvulsants, 241
antidepressants, 241
antiplatelet, 70
    for giant cell arteritis treatment, 186
apoptosis, 2
arthroplasty. See joint replacement

Ativan, 150
autonomy, 224
axial neck pain, 117

B_{12} deficiency, neurologic symptoms of, 61
Babinski sign, 36
balance, normal, 15
balance and mobility, evaluation of, 42
    assessment tools, 42
Balanced Budget Act (BBA) of 1997, 254
balance disorders, 141–142
balance tests, 45
balloon expulsion test, 98
Beck depression inventory (BDI), 53
beneficence, 224
benign paroxysmal positional vertigo (BPPV), 154, 155
benzodiazepines
    and spinal cord injury, 215
Berg balance scale, 43, 47–49
biceps tendinopathy, 129, 130, 131
bleeding, 60
blood disorders, 60–62
blood vessels and age-related changes, 6
bone cell autophagy, 4
bone changes with aging, 4–5
    abnormal bone, 4–5
    normal bone, 4
    physiology, 5
bone mineral density (BMD) testing, 124, 213
bone mineralization, 5
bradykinesia, 36
brain aging, 8
bronchoalveolar lavage (BAL) fluid, 18

canaliculi, 4
cancer, 63
cardiopulmonary resuscitation (CPR), 257
    for palliative care patients, 256
cardiovascular
    amputation, 66–68
    medications, 241
    peripheral arterial disease, 69–71
    syncope and orthostatic hypotension, 72–73
    thromboembolic disease, 74–75
cardiovascular responsiveness and age-related changes, 7
carpal tunnel syndrome (CTS), 143–144
cataracts, 199–200
central auditory processing disorder (CAPD), 196
central auditory testing, 197

central corneal thickness, 202
central nervous system (CNS), aging of, 8
cerebellar examination, 36
cervical myelopathy, 117
cervical radiculopathy, 117
cervical spondylosis, 117
Charcot foot, 145–147
chemo-brain, 64
chemotherapy-induced peripheral neuropathy (CIPN), 63
cholestyramine, 99
chronic kidney disease (CKD)
    epidemiology of, 19
    and frailty, 19–20
chronic lymphocytic leukemia (CLL), 60, 62
chronic myeloid leukemia (CML), 60, 62
cilostazol, 70
claw toe, 34
clock drawing test (CDT), 31
coagulation disorders, 61
cognitive examination, 30–32
COL1a gene, 4
COL1b gene, 4
colchicine, 95
colestipol, 99
colonic motility dysfunction, 93
colon transit studies, 94
comfort care, 257
competence, 224
complementary and alternative medicine (CAM), 218
    awareness, 219–220
    criticism of, 219
    energy/mind–body medicine, 219
    key principles, 218–219
    natural products and supplements, 219
    research and, 219
    topical/specially compounded agents, 219
compound motor action potential (CMAP), 38
conduction system and age-related changes, 6
confidentiality, 224
confusion assessment method (CAM), 31
constipation, 10, 93–95
controversial issues, 225
Cornell scale for depression in dementia, 53
cranial nerve examination, 35
creatinine clearance, estimation of, 236

decision making, 26
deconditioning, 87–88
decubitus ulcers. *See* pressure sores
deep venous thrombosis (DVT), 74
defecography, 94, 98
delirium, 30, 148–150
"demand ischemia," 6
dementia, 30
depression, 76–79
    Beck depression inventory (BDI), 53
    Cornell scale for depression in dementia, 53
    epidemiological studies depression scale, center for, 53–54
    GDS-5 scale, 53
    GDS-short, 52
    Geriatric Depression Scale (GDS), 52
    Zung Self-Rating Depression Scale, 54
dermis, age-related changes in, 23
developmental disability, aging with, 212–214
diabetes mellitus, 80
diabetic foot, 84–86
diabetic retinopathy, 201, 202, 203
DIAPPERS, 208
disequilibrium, treatment for, 155
disposable soma theory, 2
Dix-Hallpike maneuver, 153
dizziness, 151–156
docusate (colace), 95
Do Not Attempt Resuscitation (DNAR), 257
DRIP, 208
driving and medicolegal concerns, 232
driving evaluation, 221–223
    assessment, 221–222
    driver rehabilitation specialist evaluation, 222
    key principles, 221
    physician, ethical and legal responsibilities of, 222
    physician evaluation, 222
    traffic accidents, risk factors for, 221
drop arm test, 34
dry eyes, 25
Dupuytren's contractures, 34, 106
dyskinesia, 36
dysmotility, 93
dysphagia, 157–158
dystonia, 36

elder abuse, 232
electrodiagnosis
    electromyography, 40–41
    nerve conduction studies, 38–39
electromyography (EMG), 40–41
electrotherapy, for pressure sores, 191
endocrine theory, 3
end-of-life care, 225, 257–258
endothelial dysfunction, 6
end stage kidney disease burden in the elderly, 19
enemas, 95
energy/mind–body medicine, 219
epidemiological studies depression scale, center for, 53–54
epidermis, age-related changes in, 23
epigenetic theory, 3
epithelial lining fluid (ELF), 18
esophagus, age-related changes in, 10
ethics, 224–225
    committees, 232
    controversial issues, 225
    definition, 224
    end-of-life care issues, 225
    informed consent, 224

palliative care, 256
principles governing practitioner/patient interactions, 224
euthanasia, 225
evoked potential testing, 197
examination
cognitive, 30–32
musculoskeletal, 33–34
neurologic, 35–37
exercise, 226–227
aerobic/cardiovascular, 227
anticipated problems/complications, 227
balance, 227
benefits of, 227
contraindications to, 227
flexibility, 227
history, 226
physical capability, age-related changes in, 226
physical examination, 226
resistance exercise/muscle strengthening, 227
testing, 226
extrapyramidal system examination, 36

failure to thrive (FTT), 29
falls, 159–161
and gait disorders, 162
injurious, 159
in Parkinson's disease (PD), 171–172
syncopal, 159
fecal incontinence (FI), 96–99
feet testing, 34
ferritin, 62
ferrous sulfate, 62
fibromyalgia, 182–184
50/50 rule, 68
finger arthritis, 104–105
fluorescein angiography, 206
frailty, 29, 89–90
Frailty Index (FI), 89, 90
frailty syndrome, 91
freezing of gait, 171
Fried model, 89–90
frontal release reflexes, 36
frontotemporal dementia (FT), 30
Fullerton advanced balance scale, 43, 50–51
functional decline
deconditioning, 87–88
frailty, 89–90
sarcopenia, 91–92
functional impairment, person with, 55
functional reach test, 44

gait
disorders, 162–164
tests, 45–46
gall bladder, age-related changes in, 11
gastroesophageal junction, age-related changes in, 10

gastroesophageal reflux disease (GERD), 10
gastrointestinal
changes with aging, 10
constipation, 93–95
fecal incontinence, 96–99
medications, 241
GDS-5 scale, 53
GDS-short, 52
genetic damage, target theory of, 3
genitourinary drugs, 242
Geriatric Depression Scale (GDS), 31, 52
geriatric pain management, 233
gestational diabetes (GDM), 80
GH joint osteoarthritis, 129, 130, 131
giant cell arteritis (GCA), 185–186
glabellar reflex, 36
glaucoma, 201, 202, 204–205, 203
normal tension, 204
primary open-angle (POAG), 204
secondary open-angle, 204
glucocorticoids, 5
for giant cell arteritis treatment, 186
gonioscopy, 202
Good Palliative–Geriatric Practice (GP-GP) algorithm, 239
grasp reflex, 36

hair, age-related changes in, 23
Haldol, 150
hallux valgus, 34
haloperidol, 150
hammer toe, 34
hands testing, 34
Hawkins impingement sign, 33w
health insurance programs, 254
hearing
changes in, 21
impairment, 196–198
loss, and age-related changes, 12
technology, 197
Heart, and age-related changes, 6
Helicobacter pylori infection, 10
hind foot, arthritis of, 101–103
hip
fracture, 108
testing, 34
history, 28–29
Hoffmann reflex, 36
home and environment modifications, 228–230
assessment and modification resources, 229
efficacy of, 229
home environment barriers, 228
home hazards, 228
key principles, 228
physician's role in, 228
home health, 243
home health aides (HHAs), 245

home health care rehabilitation, 245–247
    funding criteria for, 246
    missions, 245
    professionals and paraprofessionals, 245
    Program of All-Inclusive Care for the Elderly (PACE), 246–247
homonymous hemianopsia, 165–166
hospice care, 255, 257
hyoscyamine, 99
hyperbaric oxygen, 194
hypercoagulability, 60
hyperthyroidism and bone metabolism, 5
hypnotics, 241–242
hypoglycemia, 82
hypothyroidism and bone metabolism, 5

immune theory and senescence, 2
impingement syndrome, 129, 130, 131
impingement testing, 33
informed consent, 224
inpatient rehabilitation facilities (IRF), 251
instrumental activities of daily living (IADLs), 55
insurance programs, 254
intervertebral disc degenerative cascade, 114

joint replacement, 111
justice, 224

knees testing, 34
kyphoplasty, 125
kyphoscoliosis, 17

labyrinthitis, treatment for, 154
lactulose, 95
large intestine, age-related changes in, 10
laser trabeculoplasty, 205
laxity, ligamentous, 34
leucopenia, 61
Lewy body dementia, 30
life-sustaining treatments (LSTs), cessation of, 225
liver, age-related changes in, 10
Lomotil, 99
long-term acute care hospital (LTAC), 251–252
    and adult day care, 251–252
long-term care hospitals (LTCHs), 243
loperamide, 99
lorazepam, 150
Lou Gehrig's disease. See amyotrophic lateral sclerosis (ALS)
low back pain (LBP), 114
lubiprostone, 95
lumbar stenosis, 40
lung changes with age, 17–18
    exercise capacity in the elderly, 17
    immunologic changes in the elderly, 18
    lung development and growth, 17
    physiologic changes, 17
    structural changes in the elderly, 17
lymphedema, 63, 64

macular degeneration, 206–207. See also age-related macular degeneration (ARMD)
magnesium hydroxide, 95
magnetic resonance imaging (MRI), 197
manual muscle testing, 33
medically nonbeneficial treatment, 232
medical social workers (MSWs), 245
Medicare, 254
    Medicare Hospice Benefit (MHB), 255
medicolegal concerns, 231–232
    advance care directives and health care agents, 231
    autonomy and beneficence, 231
    driving, 232
    elder abuse, 232
    ethics committees, 232
    key principles, 231
    medically nonbeneficial (futile) treatment, 232
    patient decision-making capacity, assessment of, 231
Ménière's disease, 151, 152
    treatment for, 154–155
mental status examination, 35
metastatic cancer, 233
mild cognitive impairment (MCI), 30
mind–body medicine, 219
minicog assessment instruments for dementia, 31
minimental status exam (MMSE), 31
misoprostol, 95
mitochondrial free radical theory and repair, 3
modified stork test, 115
motor examination, 36
multiple myeloma (MM), 61, 62
muscle bulk, 36
muscle tone, 36
musculoskeletal, 101
    ankle and hindfoot, arthritis of, 101–103
    Dupuytren's contracture and trigger finger, 106–107
    examination, 33–34
    hip fracture, 108–110
    joint replacement, 111–113
    low back pain (LBP), 114–116
    neck pain, 117–119
    osteoarthritis (OA), 120–123
    osteoporosis, 124–126
    posterior tibial tendon dysfunction (PTTD), 127–128.
    thumb, fingers, and wrist, arthritis of, 104–105
mutation accumulation theory, 2
myelodysplastic syndrome (MDS), 60, 61, 62
myoclonus, 36

nails, age-related changes in, 23
narcotics, and spinal cord injury, 215
National Center for Complementary and Alternative Medicine (NCCAM), 219, 220
natural products and supplements, 219

neck pain, 117
needle exam. *See* electromyography (EMG)
Neer impingement sign, 33
nerve conduction studies, 38–39
nerve conduction velocity (NCV), 38
neurodegenerative diseases, 135–137
neurologic
   Alzheimer's disease, 135
   amyotrophic lateral sclerosis (ALS), 138–140
   balance disorders, 141–142
   carpal tunnel syndrome, 143–144
   Charcot foot, 145–147
   delirium, 148–150
   dizziness and vertigo, 151–156
   dysphagia, 157–158
   examination, 35–37
   falls, 159–161
   gait disorders, 162–164
   homonymous hemianopsia, 165–166
   neurodegenerative diseases, 135–137
   Parkinson's disease (PD), 167–172
   spinal cord injury (SCI), 173–175
   stroke, 176–178
   traumatic brain injury (TBI), 179–181
nonmaleficence, 224
nonsteroidal anti-inflammatory drugs (NSAIDs), 116
nursing homes (NHs), 251–252
   funding/payors, 252
   length of stay in, 251
   physiatry in, 252
   quality measures in, 252
nursing home/subacute rehabilitation, 243

occupational therapists, 245
occupational therapy, for Parkinson's disease (PD), 169
olanzapine, 149
olfaction and taste, changes in, 21
one-leg stance test, 42
optical coherence topography (OCT), 202, 207
organ-specific changes with aging, 10
   esophagus, 10
   gall bladder, 11
   gastroesophageal junction, 10
   large intestine, 10
   liver, 10
   pancreas, 10
   small intestine, 10
   stomach, 10
   tongue, 10
osteoarthritis (OA), 120–123
osteoclasts, 4
osteocytes, 4
osteopenia, 56
osteoporosis, 63, 124, 213, 216
   evaluation of, 56
otoacoustic emission (OAE) testing, 197
outpatient therapy, 243

oxygen consumption and age-related changes, 6–7

pad testing, 209
painful arc sign, 33
pain management, 233–234
palliative care, 255–256, 257
palmomental reflex, 36
pancreas, age-related changes in, 10
Parkinson's disease (PD), 167–170
   falls in, 171–172
Part B insurance, 254
patellofemoral pain, 34
pathologic reflexes, 36
patient decision-making capacity, assessment of, 231
pelvic floor dysfunction/disorders, 93
pentoxifylline, 70
peripheral arterial disease (PAD), 69
pharmacologic prescriptions, 241
pharmacology, 235
   anticipated problems, 237
   key principles, 235
   pharmacodynamics, 235–236
   pharmacokinetics, 235
   polypharmacy management, 238–240
   prescribing, procedural steps in, 236
physical activity, 226. *See also* Exercise
   benefits of, 227
   recommended types of, 227
physical capability, age-related changes in, 226
physical therapists (PTs), 245
physical therapy, for Parkinson's disease (PD), 169
physician, ethical and legal responsibilities of, 222
physician assessment of driving-related skills (ADRS), 222
physician-assisted suicide (PAS), 225
plasma cells, 60
platelets, 60, 61
Polycythemia Vera (PV), 61, 62
polyethylene glycol, 95
polymyalgia rheumatica (PMR), 187–188
polypharmacy management, 238–240
postacute rehabilitation, evaluation for, 243–244
posterior pelvic pain provocation test, 115
posterior tibial tendon dysfunction (PTTD), 127–128
posture, 15
prediabetes, 80
prednisone, for polymyalgia rheumatica treatment, 188
presbyopia, 25
prescribing
   additional considerations, 242
   pharmacologic prescriptions, 241–242
   procedural steps in, 236
   therapy prescriptions, 242
"prescribing cascade," 239
pressure sores, 189–191, 215
primary open-angle glaucoma (POAG), 204
principles governing practitioner/patient interactions, 224
problem wound, 192–195

Program of All-Inclusive Care for the Elderly (PACE), 246–247
protein error theory, 3
protein matrix, 4
protein modification theory, 3
pudendal nerve terminal motor latency (PNTML), 98
pulmonary changes with age. *See* lung changes with age

quetiapine, 149

rate of living theory, 3
red blood cell, 60
reflexes, 33
rehabilitation settings, 243
    differences in, 251
    home health care, 245–247
    long-term acute care hospital and adult day care, 251–252
    palliative care, 255–256
    postacute rehabilitation, evaluation for, 243–244
    subacute rehabilitation, 253–254
resistance exercise/muscle strengthening, 227
resource utilization groups, 254
rheumatologic
    fibromyalgia, 182–184
    giant cell arteritis (GCA), 186
    polymyalgia rheumatica (PMR), 187–188
Rinne test, 153
risperidone, 149
Risperdal, 149
Romberg test, 42
rotator cuff tendinopathy/tears, 33–34, 129, 130, 131

Saint Louis University mental status exam (SLUMS), 31
sarcopenia, 14, 91–92
Scandinavian total ankle replacement (STAR), 102
senescence, 2
senile cataract. *See* cataracts
"senile emphysema" pattern, 17
sensory examination, 36
sensory system and age-related changes, 21
Seroquel, 149
shoulder pain, 129–131
shoulder testing, 33
    impingement testing, 33
    rotator cuff testing, 33–34
skilled nursing facility (SNF), 251
skin
    pressure sores, 189–191
    problem wound, 192–195
slump sit test, 115
small intestine, age-related changes in, 10
snout reflex, 36
social work/case coordination, 243
somatosensation, changes in, 21
somatosensory system and age-related changes, 21
sorbitol, 95
speech therapy, for Parkinson's disease (PD), 169

spinal cord injury (SCI), 173–175
    aging with, 215–217
spinal stenosis, 132–133
spine testing, 33
stem cell/progenitor cell theory, 3
stomach, age-related changes in, 10
stroke, 176–178
subacute rehabilitation, 253–254
subcutaneous tissue, age-related changes in, 23
suicide, 225
supraspinatus test, 33–34

Tai Chi, 142
tegaserod, 95
temporal arteritis. *See* giant cell arteritis (GCA)
therapy prescriptions, 242
thumb, joint arthritis of, 104
Tinetti's Balance and Gait Index, 43
    mobility assessment and, 45–46
tobacco and problem wound, 195
Toe-Brachial Index (TBI), 193
tongue, age-related changes in, 10
topical/specially compounded agents, 219
traffic accidents, risk factors for, 221
"transitions of care," 251
traumatic brain injury (TBI), 179–181
    related drugs to, 242
tremor, 36
trigger digits, 106–107
trigger finger, 34
type 1 diabetes mellitus (T1DM), 80
type 2 diabetes mellitus (T2DM), 80

ulcer management, 85–86
ultrasound, for pressure sores, 191
urinary incontinence (UI), 208–210
    acute incontinence, 208
    established incontinence, 208
    functional urinary incontinence, 208
    overflow incontinence, 210
    transient incontinence, 208

vascular dementia, 30, 135
venous thromboembolism (VTE), 74
veracity, 224
vertebrobasilar insufficiency, treatment for, 155
vertebroplasty, 125
vertigo, 151–156
vestibular dysfunction and age-related changes, 12–13
vestibular neuronitis, 151, 152–153, 154, 155
vestibular system
    changes in, 21
    testing, 197
virtue, 224
vision
    age-related macular degeneration, 25, 201, 202
    cataracts, 199–200, 201, 202, 203

changes in, 21
diabetic retinopathy, 201, 202, 203
glaucoma, 201, 202, 204–205, 203
macular degeneration, 206–207
Visual Analog Scale (VAS), 233

Weber–Rinne test, 153
white blood cell, 60
wound
assessment, 189
care, 190
dressing, 190–191, 194
management, 190
trauma, treatment of, 194

Zung Self-Rating Depression Scale, 54
zygapophyseal (facet) joint degenerative cascade, 114
zyprexa, 149